Sepsis

Editors

MANU SHANKAR-HARI
MERVYN SINGER

CRITICAL CARE CLINICS

www.criticalcare.theclinics.com

Consulting Editor
JOHN A. KELLUM

January 2018 • Volume 34 • Number 1

ELSEVIER

1600 John F. Kennedy Boulevard • Suite 1800 • Philadelphia, Pennsylvania, 19103-2899

http://www.theclinics.com

CRITICAL CARE CLINICS Volume 34, Number 1
January 2018 ISSN 0749-0704, ISBN-13: 978-0-323-56633-9

Editor: Colleen Dietzler
Developmental Editor: Casey Potter

Critical Care Clinics (ISSN: 0749-0704) is published quarterly by Elsevier Inc., 360 Park Avenue South, New York, NY 10010-1710. Months of issue are January, April, July, and October. Business and Editorial Offices: 1600 John F. Kennedy Blvd., Suite 1800, Philadelphia, PA 19103-2899. Customer Service Office: 6277 Sea Harbor Drive, Orlando, FL 32887-4800. Periodicals postage paid at New York, NY and additional mailing offices. Subscription prices are $234.00 per year for US individuals, $619.00 per year for US institution, $100.00 per year for US students and residents, $279.00 per year for Canadian individuals, $776.00 per year for Canadian institutions, $309.00 per year for international individuals, $776.00 per year for international institutions and $150.00 per year for Canadian and foreign students/residents. To receive student/resident rate, orders must be accompanied by name of affiliated institution, date of term, and the signature of program/residency coordinator on institution letterhead. Orders will be billed at individual rate until proof of status is received. Foreign air speed delivery is included in all *Clinics* subscription prices. All prices are subject to change without notice. POSTMASTER: Send address changes to *Critical Care Clinics*, Elsevier Periodicals Customer Service, 11830 Westline Industrial Drive, St. Louis, MO 63146. **Customer Service: 1-800-654-2452 (US). From outside of the US, call 1-314-447-8871. Fax: 1-314-447-8029. E-mail: journalscustomerservice-usa@ elsevier.com (for print support) or journalsonlinesupport-usa@elsevier.com (for online support).**

Reprints. For copies of 100 or more of articles in this publication, please contact the Commercial Reprints Department, Elsevier Inc., 360 Park Avenue South, New York, NY 10010-1710. Tel.: 212-633-3874; Fax: 212-633-3820; E-mail: reprints@elsevier.com.

Critical Care Clinics is also published in Spanish by Editorial Inter-Medica, Junin 917, 1er A, 1113, Buenos Aires, Argentina.

Critical Care Clinics is covered in *MEDLINE/PubMed (Index Medicus), EMBASE/Excerpta Medica, Current Concepts/ Clinical Medicine, ISI/BIOMED,* and *Chemical Abstracts.*

Contributors

CONSULTING EDITOR

JOHN A. KELLUM, MD, MCCM
Professor of Critical Care Medicine, Medicine, Bioengineering and Clinical & Translational Science, Director, Center for Critical Care Nephrology, Vice Chair for Research, Department of Critical Care Medicine, University of Pittsburgh School of Medicine, Pittsburgh, Pennsylvania, USA

EDITORS

MANU SHANKAR-HARI, MSc, MD, PhD, MB BS, FRCA, FFICM
NIHR Clinician Scientist, Intensive Care Unit, Guy's and St Thomas' NHS Foundation Trust, ICU Support Offices, St Thomas' Hospital, Division of Infection, Inflammation and Immunity, King's College London, Guy's Hospital, London, United Kingdom

MERVYN SINGER, MB BS, MD, FRCP(Lon), FRCP(Edin), FFICM
Professor of Intensive Care Medicine, Division of Medicine, UCL Bloomsbury Institute for Intensive Care Medicine, University College London, London, United Kingdom

AUTHORS

JOHN BOYD, MD
Centre for Heart Lung Innovation, St. Paul's Hospital, Vancouver, British Columbia, Canada

ANDREW CONWAY-MORRIS, MB ChB, PhD, FFICM
NIHR Clinical Lecturer, Division of Anaesthesia, Department of Medicine, John V Farman Intensive Care Unit, Addenbrooke's Hospital, University of Cambridge, Cambridge, United Kingdom

DEENA KELLY COSTA, PhD, RN
Assistant Professor, Department of Systems, Populations and Leadership, School of Nursing University of Michigan, Ann Arbor, Michigan, USA

HERNANDO GOMEZ, MD, MPH
Center for Critical Care Nephrology, The CRISMA (Clinical Research, Investigation, and Systems Modeling of Acute Illness) Center, Department of Critical Care Medicine, University of Pittsburgh, Pittsburgh, Pennsylvania, USA

DAVID GRIMALDI, MD, PhD
Department of Intensive Care, Erasme Hospital, Université libre de Bruxelles, Brussels, Belgium

JAN GUNST, MD, PhD
Clinical Division and Laboratory of Intensive Care Medicine, Department of Cellular and Molecular Medicine, KU Leuven, Leuven, Belgium

NICOLAI HAASE, MD, PhD
Department of Intensive Care, Rigshospitalet, University of Copenhagen, Copenhagen, Denmark

PETER B. HJORTRUP, MD, PhD
Department of Intensive Care, Rigshospitalet, University of Copenhagen, Copenhagen, Denmark

LARS B. HOLST, MD, PhD
Department of Intensive Care, Rigshospitalet, University of Copenhagen, Copenhagen, Denmark

CATHERINE INGELS, MD, PhD
Clinical Division and Laboratory of Intensive Care Medicine, Department of Cellular and Molecular Medicine, KU Leuven, Leuven, Belgium

JOHN A. KELLUM, MD, MCCM
Professor of Critical Care Medicine, Medicine, Bioengineering and Clinical & Translational Science, Director, Center for Critical Care Nephrology, Vice Chair for Research, Department of Critical Care Medicine, University of Pittsburgh School of Medicine, Pittsburgh, Pennsylvania, USA

JOHN C. MARSHALL, MD, FRCSC
Professor of Surgery, University of Toronto, Departments of Surgery and Critical Care Medicine, St. Michael's Hospital, Toronto, Ontario, Canada

MORTEN H. MØLLER, MD, PhD
Department of Intensive Care, Rigshospitalet, University of Copenhagen, Copenhagen, Denmark

GUILLAUME MONNERET, PharmD, PhD
Laboratoire d'Immunologie, Cellular Immunology Laboratory, EA 7426 PI3 "Pathophysiology of Injury-induced Immunosuppression," Université Claude Bernard Lyon I, Hospices Civils de Lyon, bioMérieux, Hôpital Edouard Herriot, Lyon, France; TRIGGERSEP (TRIal Group for Global Evaluation and Research in SEPsis), F-CRIN Network, France

ANDERS PERNER, MD, PhD
Department of Intensive Care, Rigshospitalet, University of Copenhagen, Copenhagen, Denmark

RACHEL POOL, MD
Department of Anesthesiology, University of Pittsburgh Medical Center, Pittsburgh, Pennsylvania, USA

HALLIE C. PRESCOTT, MD, MSc
Assistant Professor, Department of Internal Medicine, University of Michigan, VA Center for Clinical Management Research, Health Services Research and Development Center of Innovation, North Campus Research Center, Ann Arbor, Michigan, USA

THOMAS RIMMELÉ, MD, PhD
EA 7426 PI3 "Pathophysiology of Injury-induced Immunosuppression," Université Claude Bernard Lyon I, bioMérieux, Departement of Anesthesiology, Hospices Civils de Lyon, Hôpital Edouard Herriot, Lyon, France

BARRET RUSH, MD
Division of Critical Care Medicine, St. Paul's Hospital, Vancouver, British Columbia, Canada

JAMES A. RUSSELL, MD
Centre for Heart Lung Innovation, St. Paul's Hospital, Vancouver, British Columbia, Canada

BRENDON P. SCICLUNA, PhD
Division of Laboratory Specialties, Center for Experimental and Molecular Medicine, Department of Clinical Epidemiology, Biostatistics and Bioinformatics, Academic Medical Center, University of Amsterdam, Amsterdam, The Netherlands

MANU SHANKAR-HARI, MSc, MD, PhD, MB BS, FRCA, FFICM
NIHR Clinician Scientist, Intensive Care Unit, Guy's and St Thomas' NHS Foundation Trust, ICU Support Offices, St Thomas' Hospital, Division of Infection, Inflammation and Immunity, King's College London, Guy's Hospital, London, United Kingdom

MERVYN SINGER, MB BS, MD, FRCP(Lon), FRCP(Edin), FFICM
Professor of Intensive Care Medicine, Division of Medicine, UCL Bloomsbury Institute for Intensive Care Medicine, University College London, London, United Kingdom

BOURKE TILLMANN, MD
Clinical Associate, Department of Critical Care Medicine, Sunnybrook Health Sciences Centre, Toronto, Ontario, Canada

GREET VAN DEN BERGHE, MD, PhD
Clinical Division and Laboratory of Intensive Care Medicine, Department of Cellular and Molecular Medicine, KU Leuven, Leuven, Belgium

TOM VAN DER POLL, MD
Professor, Division of Laboratory Specialties, Center for Experimental and Molecular Medicine, Division of Infectious Diseases, Academic Medical Center, University of Amsterdam, Amsterdam, The Netherlands

TJITSKE S.R. VAN ENGELEN, MD
Division of Laboratory Specialties, Center for Experimental and Molecular Medicine, Academic Medical Center, University of Amsterdam, Amsterdam, The Netherlands

FABIENNE VENET, PharmD, PhD
Laboratoire d'Immunologie, Cellular Immunology Laboratory, EA 7426 PI3 "Pathophysiology of Injury-induced Immunosuppression," Université Claude Bernard Lyon I, Hospices Civils de Lyon, bioMérieux, Hôpital Edouard Herriot, Lyon, France

JEAN-LOUIS VINCENT, MD, PhD
Department of Intensive Care, Erasme Hospital, Université libre de Bruxelles, Brussels, Belgium

WILLEM JOOST WIERSINGA, MD
Professor, Division of Laboratory Specialties, Center for Experimental and Molecular Medicine, Division of Infectious Diseases, Academic Medical Center, University of Amsterdam, Amsterdam, The Netherlands

JULIE WILSON, MB ChB
Academic Clinical Fellow, Intensive Care Unit, Guy's and St Thomas' NHS Foundation Trust, ICU Support Offices, St Thomas' Hospital, Division of Infection, Inflammation and Immunity, King's College London, Guy's Hospital, London, United Kingdom

PAUL E. WISCHMEYER, MD, EDIC
Professor of Anesthesiology and Surgery, Department of Anesthesiology, Duke University School of Medicine, Director of Perioperative Research, Duke Clinical Research Institute, Durham, North Carolina, USA

HANNAH WUNSCH, MD, MSc
Staff Physician, Department of Critical Care Medicine, Sunnybrook Health Sciences Centre, Associate Professor, Department of Anesthesia, Interdepartmental Division of Critical Care Medicine, University of Toronto, Toronto, Ontario, Canada

Contents

The word *sepsis* dates back more than 2 millennia but has, over the past 2 centuries, come to be applied first to the clinical state evoked by invasive infection and, more recently, to describe the syndrome resulting from the host response to infection. Further refinements embodied in the recently published Sepsis-3 definition underline the concept of a dysregulated immune response resulting in potentially modifiable life-threatening organ dysfunction. This review summarizes the evolution and limitations of efforts to characterize a common and complex disorder.

Sepsis is a global public health concern. Internationally it contributes to more than 5 million deaths annually. Although rates are variable between countries, over the past 40 years reported incidence has continued to increase. Aside from potential differences in patient populations, the variation in reported rates also reflects differences in identification strategies, access to health care, and awareness of the diagnosis. Factors such as age, sex, socioeconomic status, comorbid disease, and type and site of infection affect the development of and outcomes from sepsis. Although advances have been made in treatment, its impact remains substantial.

Sepsis is caused by a dysregulated host response to infection. Immune responses determine the characteristics of sepsis. The body's protection against infection involves danger signal surveillance and recognition from nonself, effector functions in response to sensing danger signals, homeostatic regulation, and generation of immunologic memory. During sepsis, the immune system is activated by pathogen-associated and host-derived molecular patterns. Detecting these molecular patterns generates multisystem responses. Impaired organ function remote to the site of infection is the unifying feature. The processes by which an appropriate response to a microbial invader change from adaptive to maladaptive and dysregulated remain unclear.

The fundamental features of septic shock are vasodilation, increased permeability, hypovolemia, and ventricular dysfunction. Vasodilation owing to increased nitric oxide and prostaglandins is treated with vasopressors (norepinephrine first). Increased permeability relates to several pathways (Slit/Robo4, vascular endothelial growth factor, angiopoietin 1 and 2/Tie2 pathway, sphingosine-1-phosphate, and heparin-binding protein), some of which are targets for therapies. Hypovolemia is common, and crystalloid is recommended for fluid resuscitation. Cardiomyocyte-inflammatory interactions decrease contractility, and dobutamine is recommended to increase cardiac output. There is benefit in decreasing the heart rate in selected patients with esmolol. Ivabradine is a novel agent for heart rate reduction without decreasing contractility.

Sepsis-associated organ dysfunction involves multiple responses to inflammation, including endothelial and microvascular dysfunction, immune and autonomic dysregulation, and cellular metabolic reprogramming. The effect of targeting these mechanistic pathways on short- and long-term outcomes depends highly on the timing of therapeutic intervention. Furthermore, there is a need to understand the adaptive or maladaptive character of these mechanisms, to discover phase-specific biomarkers to guide therapy, and to conceptualize these mechanisms in terms of resistance and tolerance.

Sepsis induces profound neuroendocrine and metabolic alterations. During the acute phase, the neuroendocrine changes are directed toward restoration of homeostasis and also limit unnecessary energy consumption in the setting of restricted nutrient availability. Such changes are probably adaptive. In patients not recovering quickly, a prolonged critically ill phase may ensue, with different neuroendocrine changes, which may represent a maladaptive response. Whether stress hyperglycemia should be aggressively treated or tolerated remains a matter of debate. Until new evidence from randomized controlled trials becomes available, preventing severe hyperglycemia is recommended. Evidence supports withholding parenteral nutrition in the acute phase of sepsis.

It is now well established that profound immunosuppression develops within a few days after sepsis onset in patients. This should be considered additional organ failure because it is associated with an increased rate of nosocomial infections, mortality, and long-term complications, thus constituting the rationale for immunomodulation in patients. Nevertheless, the efficacy of such therapeutic strategy in improving deleterious outcomes in sepsis remains to be demonstrated. Results from clinical trials based on interleukin 7 and granulocyte macrophage colony-stimulating factor immunoadjuvant therapies in patients with septic shock are expected for 2018.

comorbidity and resulting in varying degrees and combinations of organ dysfunction. Protocolized care with rigid goals may suit populations, assuming the evidence-lite recommendations are beneficial, but not necessarily individual patients. A personalized approach to management is rational and preferable. Other than clinical heterogeneity, a range of biological signatures exist in sepsis, and these fluctuate over the disease course. Subsets of patients with sepsis can display distinct biological signatures that may potentially be used to identify suitability for different treatments and titration to optimal effect.

Despite decades of sepsis research, no specific therapies for sepsis have emerged and current management still relies on source control, antibiotics, and organ support. With improved understanding of sepsis pathophysiology and the development of new techniques to enable better characterization of patients with sepsis, clinical trials are beginning to better target new interventions at those patients most likely to respond. This article discusses advances in sepsis therapeutics designed to improve endothelial cell function, purify the blood to help restore immune homeostasis, and provide immunostimulation for patients with immune exhaustion.

Although acute survival from sepsis has improved in recent years, a large fraction of sepsis survivors experience poor long-term outcomes. In particular, sepsis survivors have high rates of weakness, cognitive impairment, hospital readmission, and late death. To improve long-term outcomes, in-hospital care should focus on early, effective treatment of sepsis; minimization of delirium, distress, and immobility; and preparing patients for hospital discharge. In the posthospital setting, medical care should focus on addressing new disability and preventing medical deterioration, providing a sustained period out of the hospital to allow for recovery.

CRITICAL CARE CLINICS

ISSUE OF RELATED INTEREST

Emergency Medicine Clinics of North America, February 2017 (Vol. 35, Issue 1)
Severe Sepsis Care in the Emergency Department
Jack Perkins and Michael E. Winters, *Editors*

THE CLINICS ARE AVAILABLE ONLINE!
Access your subscription at:
www.theclinics.com

Preface

Caring for Sepsis Patients: An Update

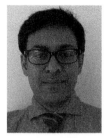 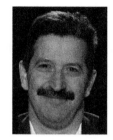

Manu Shankar-Hari, MSc, MD, PhD, MB BS, FRCA, FFICM

Mervyn Singer, MB BS, MD, FRCP(Lon), FRCP(Edin), FFICM

Editors

Sepsis is a common illness and is recognized in the recent World Health Organization resolution as a global health priority.[1] In February 2016, the definitions of sepsis were updated with the emphasis on organ dysfunction being triggered by a dysregulated host response to infection. Septic shock was redefined as a subset of sepsis carrying a worse prognosis. Explicit clinical criteria were published for identifying sepsis, septic shock, and infected patients at risk of bad outcomes.[2–4]

The new sepsis definitions emphasized reliability, feasibility, and validity attributes, and these have been generally confirmed in recently published epidemiology studies. Despite issues surrounding coding, the incidence of sepsis is increasing due to an aging population and increasing medical interventions. Many patients who survive their sepsis-related hospitalization continue to suffer from longer-term morbidity and increased risk of death.[5–10]

Despite the significant advances in our understanding of the pathobiology of sepsis, sepsis management remains largely supportive, with no specific treatments shown to be of benefit. Tailoring treatments based on biological (clinical and laboratory) patient characteristics will likely add further benefit over and above that achieved through improving the general quality of care as recommended by the Surviving Sepsis Campaign guidelines. Furthermore, a number of novel treatments are in the pipeline. To achieve this goal, our focus is now on both identifying septic patients most likely to benefit from specific interventions or who are at greatest risk of bad outcomes and exploring novel trial designs to identify specific treatments in identified subpopulations.[11–14]

Crit Care Clin 34 (2018) xiii–xv
https://doi.org/10.1016/j.ccc.2017.10.001
0749-0704/18/© 2017 Published by Elsevier Inc.

criticalcare.theclinics.com

This issue of *Critical Care Clinics* is dedicated to providing a comprehensive update to practicing physicians on the epidemiology and biology of sepsis, ongoing controversies, clinical care, and novel treatment strategies.

Manu Shankar-Hari, MSc, MD, PhD, MB BS, FRCA, FFICM
Department of Critical Care Medicine
ICU Offices
Guy's and St Thomas' Hospital
NHS Foundation Trust
London SE1 7EH, United Kingdom

Mervyn Singer, MB BS, MD, FRCP(Lon), FRCP(Edin), FFICM
Intensive Care Medicine
University College London
Cruciform Building, Gower Street
London WC1E 6BT, United Kingdom

E-mail addresses:
manu.shankar-hari@kcl.ac.uk (M. Shankar-Hari)
m.singer@ucl.ac.uk (M. Singer)

REFERENCES

1. Reinhart K, Daniels R, Kissoon N, et al. Recognizing sepsis as a global health priority—a WHO resolution. N Engl J Med 2017;377(5):414–7.

2. Singer M, Deutschman CS, Seymour CW, et al. The Third International Consensus Definitions for Sepsis and Septic Shock (Sepsis-3). JAMA 2016;315(8):801–10.

3. Seymour CW, Liu VX, Iwashyna TJ, et al. Assessment of clinical criteria for sepsis: for the Third International Consensus Definitions for Sepsis and Septic Shock (Sepsis-3). JAMA 2016;315(8):762–74.

4. Shankar-Hari M, Phillips GS, Levy ML, et al. Developing a new definition and assessing new clinical criteria for septic shock: for the Third International Consensus Definitions for Sepsis and Septic Shock (Sepsis-3). JAMA 2016; 315(8):775–87.

5. Raith EP, Udy AA, Bailey M, et al. Prognostic accuracy of the SOFA score, SIRS criteria, and qSOFA score for in-hospital mortality among adults with suspected infection admitted to the intensive care unit. JAMA 2017;317(3):290–300.

6. Russell JA, Lee T, Singer J, et al. The Septic Shock 3.0 definition and trials: a vasopressin and septic shock trial experience. Crit Care Med 2017;45(6):940–8.

7. Freund Y, Lemachatti N, Krastinova E, et al. Prognostic accuracy of Sepsis-3 criteria for in-hospital mortality among patients with suspected infection presenting to the emergency department. JAMA 2017;317(3):301–8.

8. Shankar-Hari M, Ambler M, Mahalingasivam V, et al. Evidence for a causal link between sepsis and long-term mortality: a systematic review of epidemiologic studies. Crit Care 2016;20(1):101.

9. Prescott HC, Osterholzer JJ, Langa KM, et al. Late mortality after sepsis: propensity matched cohort study. BMJ 2016;353:i2375.

10. Prescott HC, Langa KM, Iwashyna TJ. Readmission diagnoses after hospitalization for severe sepsis and other acute medical conditions. JAMA 2015;313(10): 1055–7.

11. Rhodes A, Evans LE, Alhazzani W, et al. Surviving Sepsis Campaign: International Guidelines for Management of Sepsis and Septic Shock: 2016. Intensive Care Med 2017;43(3):304–77.
12. Hotchkiss RS, Sherwood ER. Immunology. Getting sepsis therapy right. Science 2015;347(6227):1201–2.
13. Prescott HC, Calfee CS, Thompson BT, et al. Toward smarter lumping and smarter splitting: rethinking strategies for sepsis and acute respiratory distress syndrome clinical trial design. Am J Respir Crit Care Med 2016;194(2):147–55.
14. Shankar-Hari M, Rubenfeld GD. The use of enrichment to reduce statistically indeterminate or negative trials in critical care. Anaesthesia 2017;72(5):560–5.

Sepsis Definitions
A Work in Progress

John C. Marshall, MD, FRCSC

KEYWORDS

- Sepsis • Systemic inflammatory response syndrome • Stratification
- Organ dysfunction • Shock • Epidemiology

KEY POINTS

- The concept of sepsis is ancient and predates by millennia the understanding of the role of infection.
- Inherent in this concept is the notion that the resultant disease is effected through the innate response of the host, and manifested as physiologic organ dysfunction.
- A focus on improved definition serves to support early recognition of the at-risk patient to expedite appropriate anti-infectious and supportive care.
- Improved definitions also facilitate an understanding of epidemiology and of the global burden of disease.
- Existing definitions have not empowered the development of specific biologic therapies, and the process of definition is inherently a work in progress.

The recognition that infection is a transmissible disease caused by the invasion of healthy tissues by pathogenic microorganisms was a product of multiple scientific advances in the nineteenth century. Over evolutionary history, however, the dynamic interactions between microbes and their multicellular hosts have shaped the immune system and become imprinted in the genome. The consequence is an enormously complex process, at once fundamental to survival and one of the leading causes of death on the planet.[1] It follows that the description and understanding of this process has been a continuing challenge, rooted in the history of human sentience and continuing imperfectly to this day.

WHAT IS A DEFINITION, AND WHY IS IT IMPORTANT?

A definition, according to the Merriam-Webster dictionary, is "... an explanation of the meaning of a word ..." (https://www.merriam-webster.com/dictionary/definition).

Disclosure: Dr J.C. Marshall reports receiving reimbursement as a member of Data Safety Monitoring Boards for AKPA Pharma and GlaxoSmithKline and consultancy fees from Bristol Meyers Squibb and Regeneron Therapeutics.
Departments of Surgery and Critical Care Medicine, St. Michael's Hospital, 4th Floor Bond Wing, Room 4-007, 30 Bond Street, Toronto, ON M5B 1W8, Canada
E-mail address: marshallj@smh.ca

A word may have meaning because people create that meaning and agree on the criteria that define it—an inning in baseball is defined as 3 outs by each team, a kilogram is defined as the weight of a bar of platinum, and marriage is defined as the legal union between 2 individuals. Equally, a word may have meaning because data derived from the scientific process establish a plausible constraint: a year is the time required for the earth to revolve around the sun, sandstone is that form of rock resulting from the compression of sand, and cancer is a disease characterized by the abnormal proliferation of transformed cells. A definition delimits what something is and, as importantly, what it is not. A crow is a bird because of an implicit consensus on what makes a living organism a bird; it is not a flying insect for precisely the same reason. Definitions enable ordering the world—to describe it and so to modify it.

By defining sepsis, the parameters of a disease process are established—what it is as well as what it is not—and by implication, a range of interventions that might modify its course is established. A process is characterized from multiple perspectives—pathophysiology, clinical phenotype, prognosis, and potential to respond to therapeutic intervention. A definition may subserve some, but not all, these goals. The definition of cancer as an abnormal proliferation of biologically transformed cells provides a foundation for considering acute myelogenous leukemia and peritoneal liposarcoma as examples of a common pathologic process but provides no insight into common mechanisms of modifying the clinical course of disease.

The ongoing challenge of defining sepsis underlines this complexity. Sepsis is the clinical syndrome resulting from an acute host response to a threat. That response is clinically heterogeneous and not amenable to simple diagnostic criteria; conversely, it is evoked by a highly diverse group of threats. Efforts to define sepsis predate by millennia the contemporary understanding of the role of microbial infection. Conversely, contemporary definitions ignore the fact that the underlying biological process is not unique to infection but rather reflects a conserved response to danger in a variety of forms. The process of definition requires that arbitrary, human-imposed limitations be applied.

Medical definitions describe populations of patients whose clinical trajectory is shaped by a common process and who might, therefore, benefit from interventions that target that process. The validation of a medical definition, however, requires more than consensus: it requires that the definition reliably inform one or more treatment approaches that can be shown to alter clinical outcomes, that it converts a syndrome to a disease.

The evolving construct of sepsis reflects this process, a process that remains unfinished.

ANCIENT PERSPECTIVES

The Egyptians were the first to articulate a medical construct of sepsis. As outlined in the Ebers Papyrus (1500 BCE), they believed that a disease-producing force designated as whdw, pronounced "ukhedu," originated in the intestine and could, under some circumstances, pass into the body and produce disease, whose manifestations included suppuration and fever.[2]

The word, sepsis, is of Greek origin, first appearing in the epics of Homer, and denoting the rotting of flesh.[3] Hippocrates (460–370 BCE) is generally credited with the first definition of sepsis. He postulated that living things die and decay through 1 of 2 processes. Sepsis was the process of death and decay associated with illness, putrefaction, and a foul smell; pepsis, on the other hand, was decay that resulted in well-being, exemplified as the digestion of food or the fermentation of grapes to produce wine.[2]

Aulus Cornelius Celsus (25 BCE—50 CE) proposed the cardinal manifestations of inflammation—*rubor, calor, dolor,* and *tumor* —to which Galen of Pergamon (129–200 CE) added a fifth—*functio laesa.* In describing the characteristic features of a local response to infection, they provided, perhaps better than contemporary authors, a description of the cardinal features of systemic inflammation—vasodilatation, fever, altered mentation, capillary leak, and organ dysfunction (**Table 1**).

INFECTION AND THE GERM THEORY OF DISEASE

Although microscopic life forms had been visualized by van Leeuwenhoek in 1676 after the invention of the microscope, it was not until the nineteenth century with the work of European scientists, such as Pasteur, Semmelweis, and Koch, that the concept of spontaneous generation gave way to the recognition that autonomous minute unicellular organisms were the vectors of infectious diseases. Robert Koch with his eponymous postulates established the criteria for demonstrating infectivity and transmissibility. This revolutionary new insight fundamentally transformed the human world, opening the door to simple but powerful new anti-infectious strategies, such as handwashing, chlorination of the water supply, pasteurization, immunization, and a spectrum of public health measures. The impact at a societal level was profound: over the twentieth century, the mortality of infectious diseases fell more than 10-fold (**Fig. 1**),[4] while the population of the planet increased from a relatively stable level of less than 1 billion individuals in the nineteenth century to upward of 7 billion people today.

The identification of bacteria and fungi created the new scientific discipline of microbiology and led to the identification of substances—often of microbial origin—that could kill bacteria or inhibit their capacity to proliferate. Antibiotics and more efficacious means of controlling local infection through source control measures emerged as the cornerstone of the treatment of infection. Although unquestionably one of the great advances of modern clinical medicine, the development of antibiotics did not so much reduce the prevalence or lethality of infection as alter the microbiology of infection, shifting the commonly isolated species from exogenous organisms to endogenous ones.[5]

As the role of bacteria came to be better understood, the meaning of the word sepsis came to denote systemic, and typically severe, infection. The first recorded use of the word in this context appeared in 1876 (https://www.merriam-webster.com/dictionary/sepsis). *Stedman's Medical Dictionary* from the 1970s (stedmansonline.com) defines sepsis as "... the presence of pus-forming organisms in the bloodstream ...". At the same time, however, it was becoming apparent that the lethality of infection reflected something much more than the uncontrolled proliferation of microorganisms.

Table 1 The cardinal signs of inflammation	
Local	**Systemic**
Rubor (redness)	Vasodilatation
Calor (heat)	Fever
Dolor (pain)	Confusion, discomfort
Tumor (swelling)	Edema; increased capillary permeability
Functio laesa (loss of function)	Organ dysfunction

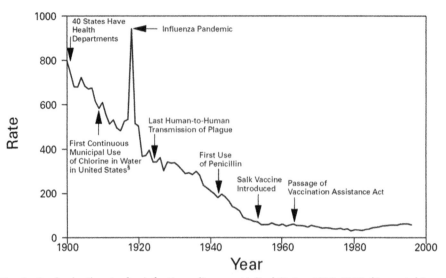

Fig. 1. Crude death rate for infectious diseases, United States 1900–1996. (*From* Achievements in public health, 1900-1999: control of infectious diseases. MMWR Morb Mortal Wkly Rep 1999;48(29):621. Available at: https://www.cdc.gov/mmwr/preview/mmwrhtml/mm4829a1.htm.)

SEPSIS AS THE RESPONSE OF THE HOST

Pfeiffer in the nineteenth century had shown that the illness associated with experimental infection did not require the organism to be viable and capable of proliferation. He deduced that some toxic factor, intrinsic to the organism, was responsible for the clinical syndrome and coined the word, *endotoxin*, to describe this factor.[6] Subsequent work revealed endotoxin to be a complex lipopolysaccharide that makes up much of the cell wall of gram-negative bacteria and that is widely prevalent in the environment. The identification of specific microbial toxins provided a further therapeutic target. It was becoming apparent, however, that intoxication per se was inadequate to explain the pathogenesis of clinical sepsis.

Studies by Coley in the late nineteenth century and by a variety of investigators in the mid-twentieth century, suggested that bacteria could elicit responses in the host. These, rather than the direct toxic effects of the bacterium, were responsible for the clinical phenotype of infection. Coley demonstrated that an extract from tissues infected with *Streptococci* could induce the killing of tumor cells.[7] Carswell and colleagues[8] subsequently showed the responsible factor to be a host-derived protein that they termed, *tumor necrosis factor* (*TNF*). With the demonstration by Tracey and colleagues[9] that TNF was also responsible for the lethality of experimental endotoxin challenge, a new potential therapeutic target was identified. Work in the 1950s suggested that a macrophage-derived factor could induce fever in an experimental animal; this factor was subsequently identified to be a protein, termed *interleukin 1*.[10]

A classical study established the importance of the host response in the lethality of endotoxin challenge.[11] A random gene mutation in an inbred mouse strain—the C3h HeN mouse—had resulted in a separate strain, the C3h HeJ strain, that was resistant to endotoxin. Michalek and coworkers[11] irradiated mice of both strains to eliminate their native bone marrow, then transplanted these irradiated mice with bone marrow from the opposite strain. When they challenged these chimeric animals with endotoxin, lethality was seen only in the animals with C3h HeN marrow-derived cells. It was not the intrinsic toxicity of endotoxin that killed them: they were dying because their own marrow cells were recognizing and responding to endotoxin. It was subsequently shown that the genetic defect in the C3h HeJ mouse was a single point mutation in a cell surface receptor, called *toll-like receptor* (*TLR*) *4*, that enables innate immune cells to recognize and respond to endotoxin.[12]

The list of endogenous molecules that contribute to the adverse consequences of experimental infection is long: more than 130 separate species have been shown to modulate survival in experimental murine endotoxemia.[13] These are potential therapeutic targets, but their number and diversity underline the complexity of the clinical challenge. The effort to treat infection by targeting the detrimental host response—so far largely unsuccessful—has fueled the latest efforts to define sepsis and to refine these definitions.

SEPSIS SYNDROME AND THE CONTEMPORARY CHALLENGE OF DEFINITION

A small randomized clinical trial conducted in the 1970s provided the first suggestion that the host response could be a therapeutic target. Schumer[14] treated a cohort of patients with sepsis with large doses of methylprednisolone or placebo and reported that steroids reduced mortality from 39% to 11%. Several years later, Ziegler and colleagues[15] reported that an antiserum directed against the lipid A moiety of endotoxin could improve the survival of patients with gram-negative infections, particularly in the face of shock. The stage was set for the current generation of sepsis trials, however it was unclear how potential candidates should be identified.

The late Roger Bone and colleagues[16] led the first such trial, evaluating the effects of high dose methylprednisolone (30 mg/kg) or placebo in patients with severe sepsis and septic shock. These investigators recognized that they need to recruit septic patients early in the course of their illness and usually before cultures were available. They thus proposed diagnostic criteria that they termed, *sepsis syndrome*,[17] using these as entry criteria for the trial. In the absence of epidemiologic data or robust prior consensus, the criteria comprised documented or suspected infection, in conjunction with systemic signs of inflammation and evidence of organ dysfunction (**Box 1**). On the one hand, these criteria were pragmatic and had reasonable face validity. On the other hand, however, it was evident that there was no common biochemical mediator response underlying them but rather a very heterogeneous group of disorders with respect to the site and bacteriology of infection, and the nature of the response

---

Box 1
Sepsis syndrome

Documented or suspected infection, in association with
- Fever (>38.3°C) or hypothermia (<35.6°C)
- Tachycardia (>90 beats per minute)
- Tachypnea (≥20 breaths per minute or mechanically ventilated)
- At least 1 manifestation of organ dysfunction
  - Altered mentation
  - Hypoxemia
  - Elevated lactate
  - Oliguria (<30 mL or 0.5 mL/kg urine output per hour)

Data from Bone RC, Fisher CJ, Clemmer TP, et al. A controlled clinical trial of high-dose methylprdenisolone in the treatment of severe sepsis and septic shock. N Engl J Med 1987;317:653–8.

evoked in the host.[18] When the trial failed to show benefit from corticosteroids, the intervention, rather than the trial design and diagnostic criteria, was blamed for the lack of efficacy, a pattern since repeated in more than 100 phase II and phase III clinical trials of putative therapies.[13]

THE AMERICAN COLLEGE OF CHEST PHYSICIANS/SOCIETY OF CRITICAL CARE MEDICINE SEPSIS DEFINITIONS CONFERENCE, 1991

Dissatisfaction with the sepsis syndrome criteria and an emerging need articulated by several pharmaceutical companies planning trials of novel mediator-targeted therapy prompted the American College of Chest Physicians and the Society of Critical Care Medicine to host a consensus conference outside Chicago in August 1991.[19] The charges for the conference were to develop new definitions for sepsis and organ failure and criteria for the use of novel therapies.

The conference differentiated infection as a microbial phenomenon from the response that infection evoked in the host; the latter was considered to be sepsis. *Infection* was defined as the invasion of normally sterile host tissues by viable microorganisms and *sepsis* as the systemic host response to that tissue invasion. This distinction, however, raised additional questions and considerations. A systemic response to invasive infection was more often an appropriate and adaptive process that enabled the host to more effectively clear the infection: sepsis, as defined, could be either beneficial or detrimental. To address this, the conference proposed the term, *severe sepsis*, defined as sepsis in association with organ dysfunction to differentiate those cases of harm outweighing the benefits of a response. Finally, the term, *septic shock*, was proposed to describe cases of sepsis in which hypotension was present, and tissue oxygenation impaired. A consequence of these new definitions was the recommendation that the word, *septicemia*, be abandoned as imprecise.

A second consequence of these definitions arose through the recognition that the clinical syndrome of sepsis could also be seen in association with noninfectious diseases, such as trauma, burns, or pancreatitis. Thus a new concept was proposed— *systemic inflammatory response syndrome (SIRS)*—defined as a clinical syndrome of systemic inflammation independent of its triggering cause. Sepsis represented infection associated with a systemic host response, recognizing that the response could exist in the absence of infection, and that infection could exist in the absence of a systemic host response: the familiar Venn diagram of sepsis and SIRS emerged (**Fig. 2**).

Importantly, the 1991 conference did not propose specific criteria for SIRS: these appeared only after the conference, to meet the needs of companies seeking consensus criteria to facilitate the design of clinical trials. The SIRS criteria, variants of the sepsis syndrome criteria, were promulgated without a priori data; it was not surprising when they were subsequently shown to be predictive of a higher risk of death[20] because the criteria include 4 of the 12 variables of the APACHE (Acute Physiology and Chronic Health Evaluation) II score.

The conference also proposed the terminology, *multiple organ dysfunction syndrome (MODS)*, in preference to such earlier formulations of the concept as multiple organ failure. The refined terminology emphasized 2 core features of the process— that it represented a continuum of severity, rather than a categorical state that either was or was not present and that the process was potentially reversible.

THE SECOND SEPSIS DEFINITIONS CONFERENCE, 2001

As concepts from the 1991 conference came to be disseminated and adopted, an undercurrent of dissatisfaction about the formulation of SIRS began to evolve—not so

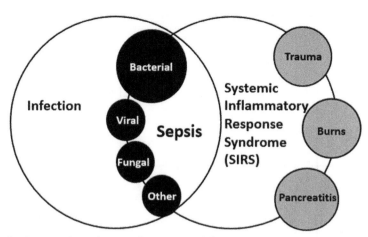

Fig. 2. Infection, sepsis, and SIRS. Infection was defined as the presence of microorganisms in normally sterile tissues; the resulting host systemic response was called the SIRS. Sepsis was said to be present when infection resulted in SIRS, recognizing that SIRS can also be a consequence of a sterile inflammatory process such as is seen in multiple trauma, burns, or pancreatitis. (*Adapted from* Bone RC, Balk RA, Cerra FB, et al. ACCP/SCCM Consensus Conference. Definitions for sepsis and organ failure and guidelines for the use of innovative therapies in sepsis. Chest 1992;101:1644–55.)

much with the concept as with the nonspecific nature of the criteria that defined it and with the fact that the definitions had been promulgated by an exclusively North American group.[21] Moreover, the articulation of a novel set of definitions had largely failed to resolve the inherent heterogeneity of sepsis, while clinical trials of biologic therapies conducted using these new definitions had yielded disappointing results. Thus, a second consensus conference was held in 2001, this time bringing together representatives from 5 professional societies.[22]

The 2001 definitions conference reaffirmed the concepts and terms from the 1991 conference but proposed an expanded set of criteria to define SIRS and presented a template for a novel stratification system for sepsis—the predisposition, insult, response, organ dysfunction (PIRO) model (**Table 2**).[22]

The PIRO concept is an effort to develop a stratification system for critical illness patterned on the tumor, node, metastasis (TNM) model widely used in staging cancer.[23] The underlying concept is that a multidimensional approach is needed to stratify patients to guide the multimodal management of sepsis. Just as therapies targeting the primary tumor—surgery and radiotherapy—are most efficacious in the absence of regional or distant spread, so interventions targeting the inciting infection are more effective in the absence of advanced organ dysfunction. Conversely, just as spread to regional lymph nodes identifies a patient with cancer who is more likely to benefit from adjuvant systemic therapy, so evidence of an activated systemic response may identify patients more likely to benefit from treatments that target the host response. The PIRO model proceeds from the hypothesis that the optimal treatment of the individual patient with sepsis requires independent consideration of baseline predisposing factors (both genetics and acquired comorbidities), the nature and site of the infection, the nature and magnitude of the resulting host response, and the presence, type, and degree of organ dysfunction. Two considerations bear emphasis. First, PIRO is not primarily a prognostic model: its objective is not to predict survival but rather to predict potential response to specific therapies. Second, at this

Table 2
The predisposition, insult, response, organ dysfunction model

Domain	Present	Future	Rationale
Predisposition	Premorbid illness with reduced probability of short-term survival. Cultural or religious beliefs, age, gender.	Genetic polymorphisms in components of inflammatory response (eg, TIR, TNF, IL-1, CD14); enhanced understanding of specific interactions between pathogens and host diseases.	In the present, premorbid factors impact on the potential attributable morbidity and mortality of an acute insult; deleterious consequences of insult heavily dependent on genetic predisposition (future).
Insult infection	Culture and sensitivity of infecting pathogens; detection of disease amenable to source control.	Assay of microbial products (LPS, mannan, bacterial DNA); gene transcript profiles.	Specific therapies directed against inciting insult require demonstration and characterization of that insult.
Response	SIRS, other signs of sepsis, shock, CRP.	Nonspecific markers of activated inflammation (eg, PCT or IL-6) or impaired host responsiveness (eg, HLA-DR); specific detection of target of therapy (eg, protein C, TNF, PAF).	Both mortality risk and potential to respond to therapy vary with nonspecific measures of disease severity (eg, shock); specific mediator-targeted therapy is predicated on presence and activity of mediator.
Organ dysfunction	Organ dysfunction as number of failing organs or composite score (eg, MODS, SOFA, LOD system, PEMOD, PELOD).	Dynamic measures of cellular response to insult—apoptosis, cytopathic hypoxia, cell stress.	Response to pre-emptive therapy (eg, targeting microorganism or early mediator) not possible if damage already present; therapies targeting the injurious cellular process require that it be present.

Abbreviations: CRP, C-reactive protein; HLA-DR, human leukocyte antigen-DR; IL, interleukin; LPS, lipopolysaccharide; PAF, platelet-activating factor; PCT, procalcitonin; PELOD, pediatric logistic organ dysfunction; PEMOD, pediatric multiple organ dysfunction.

stage of its evolution, it is a hypothesis that still lacks the large scale empiric testing that could convert it into a useful tool for research and clinical management.

SEPSIS-3

The third international effort to refine sepsis definitions was a collaboration between the North American Society of Critical Care Medicine and the European Society of Intensive Care Medicine. It evolved through a series of face-to-face and online meetings over the course of several years; the resultant articles were published in 2016.[24–26]

The Third International Consensus Definitions for Sepsis and Septic Shock (Sepsis-3) initiative introduced a new definition for sepsis, defining it as "life-threatening organ dysfunction caused by a dysregulated host response to infection."[24] Several nuances of this revised definition merit comment. By identifying the clinical phenotype of sepsis as organ dysfunction, the definition eliminated the need for the terminology, severe sepsis, and shifted the focus from the concept to its clinical consequence—organ dysfunction. In addition, in describing the host response as dysregulated, the definition acknowledged the apparent paradox that manifestations of over-activation and suppression of the immune response could coexist and that the resulting syndrome was neither hyperinflammation nor immunosuppression but rather something more complex.

The conference opted to not propose a definition for infection but rather focused on identifying clinical criteria that, among patients presenting with suspected or proved infection, identified a subset at increased risk of adverse outcome. In contrast to earlier iterations, this was accomplished not by expert opinion but by querying large electronic databases that included a spectrum of patients from the emergency department, hospital ward, and ICU. Three variables were identified that independently predicted a risk of in-hospital death or an ICU stay of 3 days or longer—a respiratory rate greater than 22 breaths per minute, a systolic blood pressure less than 100 mm Hg, and a Glasgow Coma Scale score of 13 or less. For pragmatic reasons, a Glasgow Coma Scale score of less than 15, that is, any abnormal mentation, was adopted because the model including this slight modification was essentially similar. The model was termed, *quick sequential (sepsis-related) organ failure assessment (SOFA)*; the presence of any 2 of these criteria proved to have superior ability to predict imminent deterioration than greater than or equal to 2 SIRS criteria, particularly for patients outside the critical care unit.

The conference also defined septic shock as " … a subset of sepsis in which profound circulatory, cellular and metabolic abnormalities are associated with a greater risk of mortality than with sepsis alone."[26] Changes in definition reflected an evolving realization that the biological abnormalities of the septic shock state extended beyond simple circulatory insufficiency and included fundamental changes in cellular metabolism and function.

Sepsis-3 advances the description of sepsis in several important ways. In emphasizing organ dysfunction as the defining feature of the aberrant host response, it both defines a phenotype and opens the door to considering noninfectious causes of organ dysfunction within the sepsis framework, reflecting recent understanding that the host response to infection is not specific to infection but can be activated by a spectrum of stimuli that represent acute threats to normal host homeostasis. It shifts the process of definition revision from one grounded in expert opinion to one informed by clinical data. And, in describing the result as Sepsis-3, it acknowledges that the process of definition is an unfinished one that will be further changed and refined as understanding of clinical biology evolves.

Sepsis-3, however, has limitations. It is not a tool to facilitate the early diagnosis of infection but rather a framework to identify, among patients with suspected or documented infection, those at greatest risk of imminent deterioration. Nor are the quick-SOFA criteria valid criteria for identifying patients who might be enrolled in trials of novel therapies. Although they identify risk of deterioration and adverse outcome, they do not resolve the inherent heterogeneity in that risk and have not been validated on the basis of their potential to predict response to therapy. They are likely to prove no better than sepsis syndrome or SIRS criteria in delineating a homogeneous population for treatment. Finally, the process through which the definitions were developed has been criticized for the lack of diversity of the panel, in particular, the absence of women and clinicians working in low-income and middle-income countries.

ORGAN DYSFUNCTION AS THE SEPSIS PHENOTYPE

There is an intriguing symmetry in the evolution of ancient perspectives on inflammation and contemporary perspectives on sepsis. It was more than a century after Galen articulated his 4 cardinal signs of local inflammation that Celsus added a fifth—loss of function. It was 25 years after contemporary definitions that organ dysfunction became a defining feature of systemic inflammation in the Sepsis-3 definition. The incorporation of functional deficit in both definitions reflects the fact that inflammation is an adaptive and protective process and only becomes a pathologic one when homeostasis is impacted to the point that biological function is impaired.

Organ dysfunction in sepsis, or more generally in critical illness, is a complex concept and has proved challenging to operationalize in practice. Although there several similar scores that have been developed as tools to quantify the extent of organ dysfunction—the SOFA score,[27] the multiple organ dysfunction (MOD) score,[28] the logistic organ dysfunction (LOD) score,[29] and the Brussels score[30]—they share common shortcomings and are based on concepts from more than 2 decades ago.

First, each makes the assumption that global physiologic dysfunction is reliably reflected in the dysfunction of 6 organ systems—respiratory, renal, cardiovascular, gastrointestinal, neurologic, and hematologic. Not included, for example, are the immune, musculoskeletal, and endocrine systems, despite that abnormal function in each of these is common in patients with sepsis. With advancing knowledge of the critical role played by the microbiome and by its derangements in critical illness, the normal host flora might reasonably be considered a further system whose function is deranged in critical illness. Parsing a systemic process into discrete derangements in 6 arbitrarily defined systems may well be arbitrary, although it is acknowledged that most of these systems can be independently supported using critical care technology.

Second, dysfunction within each system is reduced to a simple abnormality in 1 or more variables that may or may not reflect the function of the entire system—platelet numbers for the hematologic system or bilirubin for the liver. For a system, such as the gastrointestinal tract, a simple descriptor has yet to be identified.

Third, septic and other critically ill patients frequently have preexisting comorbidities that impair organ function; the differentiation of baseline preexisting deficits from acute and potentially reversible ones may be difficult.

Finally, the interaction between organ dysfunction and ICU support is complex and one that varies with approaches to patient management. The SOFA score, for example, quantifies cardiovascular dysfunction as the dose of vasoactive agent used to support blood pressure. This is a reflection of a clinical decision, however, not an objective clinical state; thresholds for the use of vasoactive agents are variable, and blood pressure itself can be impacted by the use of sedation. Similarly, the use of mechanical ventilation is not an intrinsic state of a patient but a decision by the clinician. Equally, the use of hemodialysis can lower the creatinine level without altering kidney function and, when used in isolation, may create an artifact. Many measures of organ dysfunction are not so much a reflection of abnormal patient physiology as of prevailing ICU practice. This is all the more important as it is becoming apparent that ICU support—while instituted as a life-sustaining intervention—can itself cause further harm in the form of exacerbated organ dysfunction.[31]

These limitations notwithstanding, the construct of acute and potentially reversible organ dysfunction does embody the clinically important consequences of sepsis and raises key questions for future work. Should defining organ dysfunction on the basis of the ICU interventions used to support individual systems be continued, or can organ dysfunction be better defined by common cellular abnormalities, such as alterations in metabolism or in the kinetics of regulated cell death? If organ dysfunction is the phenotype and a dysregulated host response the cause, should acute organ dysfunction secondary to noninfectious causes be considered sepsis? If not, what terminology should be adopted? Do different predisposing genetic and premorbid factors or differential biochemical response profiles underlie differing patterns of acute organ dysfunction? If not, why does organ dysfunction take the form of severe acute respiratory distress syndrome (ARDS) in some patients and hematologic or renal dysfunction in others?

SUMMARY: SEPSIS DEFINITIONS ARE A WORK IN EVOLUTION

The articulation of the latest version of sepsis definitions as Sepsis-3 reflects an explicit understanding that these are simply the latest iteration of an ongoing effort to characterize a complex and highly heterogeneous process: they will be supplanted and improved, and these improvements will reflect a better integration of the rapidly evolving understanding of host-microbial interactions and the biology of the acute host response. Yogi Berra once opined,"It's tough to make predictions, especially about the future," so at the risk of misrepresenting the questions that future workers will ask, what follows are some subjective thoughts on residual uncertainties that must be addressed.

Current concepts of sepsis are based on a model of host-microbial interactions that views these as fundamentally adversarial. Although this is a reasonable conclusion when confronted with a life-threatening infection, the bigger picture is that the evolutionary relationship of humans and microbes is better framed as symbiotic. All healthy individuals carry a complex microbial flora that is essential to such processes as the maturation of the immune system and the absorption of foodstuffs from the gastrointestinal tract. Moreover, although there may be in excess of 1 billion different species of microorganisms on the planet, fewer than 2 dozen of these are commonly responsible for infection in critically ill patients. Future definitions of sepsis will need to embrace the concept that normal host-microbial homeostasis is fundamental to health and that sepsis represents a disruption of this advantageous state.

The focus of contemporary formulations of sepsis is bacterial infection. Viruses are also able, however, to evoke a septic response, as are bacterial products, such as endotoxin. Endotoxemia is common in critical illness and in a variety of noninfectious disorders, such as congestive heart failure, chronic renal failure, and cirrhosis. Thus it is appropriate that the concept of sepsis be expanded to include the presence of microbial products in the host. Moreover, the pattern recognition receptors whose engagement initiates a septic response can also be activated by noninfectious stimuli, such as oxidized phospholipids, heat shock proteins, uric acid, and mitochondria—the latter remnants of the ancient invasion of primitive cells by endosymbiotic bacteria.[32] A consideration of what comprises infection is revealing increasing orders of complexity. There is evidence of a blood microbiome that is present in healthy individuals.[33] A strong argument can be made that microbial products such as endotoxin also subserve an important role as a component of normal host defenses against infection, priming the innate immune system for a more effective response.[34]

Contemporary descriptions of sepsis focus on a cause—infection—and a physiologic response—tachycardia, fever, and hypotension. Yet the underlying mechanism is a complex series of biochemical alterations, effected through a profoundly altered pattern of gene expression. These changes are genetically determined, clinically and biochemically heterogeneous, and poorly correlated with simple physiologic perturbations. Moreover, the treatment of sepsis is multimodal, with interventions that target the infection, the deranged physiologic state, and, although not yet a clinical reality, the central biochemical alterations that produce the syndrome. The combination of a complex and biologically heterogeneous disease and a multimodal approach to therapy call out for descriptive systems that can better stratify patients with respect not to their risk of adverse outcome but to their potential to respond to specific treatments. This is the aspiration of the PIRO model, although to date, it remains unrealized.

The challenge is made even greater by virtue of the fact that sepsis as a disease is not shaped solely by the infection and the response of the host but also by the supportive care provided to the patient. In the absence of that care, the outcome is either a brief self-limiting illness or death. Most cases of sepsis on the planet, particularly in low-income and middle-income countries, are treated without access to ICU care and with only rudimentary techniques of anti-infective therapy and supportive care. For this reason, globally important infectious diseases responsible for preventable deaths—malaria, dengue, Ebola, and gastroenteritis, to name a few—are not recognized as sepsis, although they clearly reflect life-threatening organ dysfunction as a result of a dysregulated response to infection. But once support is provided, it becomes another factor contributing to the dysregulated host response. Positive pressure mechanical ventilation exacerbates inflammatory lung injury, enhancing the release of inflammatory mediators,[35] and independently increasing the risk of death.[36] Intravenous fluids pass through the more permeable walls of the microvasculature, resulting in tissue edema, evident in the lung as the early phases of ARDS. Invasive devices disrupt normal physical barriers to infection, whereas antibiotics alter the indigenous flora, factors that contribute to an increased risk of nosocomial infection and further activation of a host response.

Sepsis is immediately recognizable and unusually challenging to define. It is common but also grounded in a remarkably complex and effective homeostatic process that has enabled multicellular organisms to survive in a not infrequently hostile environment. The obsession with definition that has been so prominent over the past quarter century is both trivial and profound. It is trivial in the sense that it has not advanced the development of new therapies or facilitated fundamental new insights into biology. Yet it is of profound importance in that it shapes how a common human illness is conceptualized and how its global impact on the human species is measured. It is an exercise that is destined to continue.

REFERENCES

1. Fleischmann C, Scherag A, Adhikari NK, et al. Assessment of global incidence and mortality of hospital-treated sepsis. current estimates and limitations. Am J Respir Crit Care Med 2016;193:259–72.

2. Majno G. The ancient riddle of (sepsis). J Infect Dis 1991;163:937–45.
3. Geroulanos S, Douka ET. Historical perspective of the word "sepsis". Intensive Care Med 2006;32:2077.
4. Achievements in public health, 1900-1999: control of infectious diseases. MMWR Morb Mortal Wkly Rep 1999;48(29):621–9.
5. Rogers DE. The changing pattern of life-threatening microbial disease. N Engl J Med 1959;261:677–83.
6. Rietschel ET, Cavaillon JM. Endotoxin and anti-endotoxin. The contribution of the schools of Koch and Pasteur: life, milestone-experiments and concepts of Richard Pfeiffer (Berlin) and Alexandre Besredka (Paris). J Endotoxin Res 2002;8: 71–82.
7. Wiemann B, Starnes CO. Coley's toxins, tumor necrosis factor and cancer research: a historical perspective. Pharmacol Ther 1994;64:529–64.
8. Carswell EA, Old LJ, Kassel RL, et al. An endotoxin-induced serum factor that causes necrosis of tumors. Proc Natl Acad Sci U S A 1975;72:3666–70.
9. Tracey KJ, Beutler B, Lowry SF, et al. Shock and tissue injury induced by recombinant human cachectin. Science 1986;234(4775):470–4.
10. Atkins E, Wood WB Jr. Studies on the pathogenesis of fever. II. Identification of an endogenous pyrogen in the blood stream following the injection of typhoid vaccine. J Exp Med 1955;102:499–516.
11. Michalek SM, Moore RN, McGhee JR, et al. The primary role of lymphoreticular cells in the mediation of host responses to bacterial endotoxin. J Infect Dis 1980;141:55–63.
12. Poltorak A, He X, Smirnova I, et al. Defective LPS signaling in C3H/HeJ and C57BL/10ScCr mice: mutations in Tlr4 gene. Science 1998;282:2085–8.
13. Marshall JC. Why have clinical trials in sepsis failed? Trends Mol Med 2014;20: 195–203.
14. Schumer W. Steroids in the treatment of septic shock. Ann Surg 1976;184: 333–41.
15. Ziegler EJ, McCutchan JA, Fierer J, et al. Treatment of gram-negative bacteremia and shock with human antiserum to a mutant Escherichia coli. N Engl J Med 1982;307:1225–30.
16. Bone RC, Fisher CJ, Clemmer TP, et al. A controlled clinical trial of high dose methylprednisolone in the treatment of severe sepsis and septic shock. N Engl J Med 1987;317:654–8.
17. Bone RC, Fisher CJ, Clemmer TP, et al. Sepsis syndrome: a valid clinical entity. Crit Care Med 1989;17:389–93.
18. Casey LC, Balk RA, Bone RC. Plasma cytokines and endotoxin levels correlate with survival in patients with the sepsis syndrome. Ann Intern Med 1993;119: 771–8.
19. Bone RC, Balk RA, Cerra FB, et al. ACCP/SCCM Consensus Conference. Definitions for sepsis and organ failure and guidelines for the use of innovative therapies in sepsis. Chest 1992;101:1644–55.
20. Rangel-Frausto MS, Pittet D, Costigan M, et al. The natural history of the systemic inflammatory response syndrome (SIRS): a prospective study. JAMA 1995;273: 117–23.
21. Vincent JL. Dear SIRS, I'm sorry to say that I don't like you. Crit Care Med 1997; 25:372–4.
22. Levy MM, Fink M, Marshall JC, et al. 2001 SCCM/ESICM/ACCP/ATS/SIS international sepsis definitions conference. Crit Care Med 2003;34:1250–6.

23. Marshall JC. The PIRO (predisposition, insult, response, organ dysfunction) model: towards a staging system for acute illness. Virulence 2014;5:27–35.
24. Singer M, Deutschman CS, Seymour CW, et al. The third international consensus definitions for sepsis and septic shock (sepsis-3). JAMA 2016;315:801–10.
25. Seymour CW, Liu VX, Iwashyna TJ, et al. Assessment of clinical criteria for sepsis: for the third international consensus definitions for sepsis and septic shock (sepsis-3). JAMA 2016;315:762–74.
26. Shankar-Hari M, Phillips GS, Levy ML, et al. Developing a new definition and assessing new clinical criteria for septic shock: for the third international consensus definitions for sepsis and septic shock (sepsis-3). JAMA 2016;315:775–87.
27. Vincent JL, Moreno R, Takala J, et al. The sepsis-related organ failure assessment (SOFA) score to describe organ dysfunction/failure. Intensive Care Med 1996;22: 707–10.
28. Marshall JC, Cook DJ, Christou NV, et al. Multiple organ dysfunction score: a reliable descriptor of a complex clinical outcome. Crit Care Med 1995;23:1638–52.
29. Le Gall JR, Klar J, Lemeshow S, et al. The logistic organ dysfunction system - a new way to assess organ dysfunction in the intensive care unit. JAMA 1996;276: 802–10.
30. Bernard G. The Brussels score. Sepsis 1997;1:43–4.
31. Marshall JC. Critical illness is an iatrogenic disorder. Crit Care Med 2010; 38(Suppl):S582–9.
32. Zhang Q, Raoof M, Chen Y, et al. Circulating mitochondrial DAMPs cause inflammatory responses to injury. Nature 2010;464:104–7.
33. Paisse S, Valle C, Servant F, et al. Comprehensive description of blood microbiome from healthy donors assessed by 16S targeted metagenomic sequencing. Transfusion 2016;56:1138–47.
34. Marshall JC. Lipopolysaccharide: an endotoxin or an exogenous hormone? Clin Infect Dis 2005;41(Suppl 7):S470–80.
35. Ranieri VM, Suter PM, Tortorella C, et al. Effect of mechanical ventilation on inflammatory mediators in patients with acute respiratory distress syndrome. A randomized controlled trial. JAMA 1999;282:54–61.
36. Brower RG, Matthay MA, Morris A, et al. Ventilation with lower tidal volumes as compared with traditional tidal volumes for acute lung injury and the acute respiratory distress syndrome. N Engl J Med 2000;342:1301–8.

Epidemiology and Outcomes

Bourke Tillmann, MD[a], Hannah Wunsch, MD, MSc[a,b,*]

KEYWORDS

- Sepsis • Epidemiology • Incidence • Outcomes • Mortality • Risk factors

KEY POINTS

- Reported sepsis incidence is increasing worldwide.
- Variability in case definition plays a significant role in the differences in reported incidence.
- Reported case fatality rates for sepsis are decreasing, but due to the prevalence of sepsis, the absolute number of patients with sepsis who die has increased.
- Specific risk factors for the development of sepsis include increased age, male gender, the presence of comorbid disease, and lower social economic status.
- The annual hospital cost for severe sepsis in the United States alone is estimated to be more than $24 billion.

INTRODUCTION

Sepsis is a global public health concern. International data demonstrate that sepsis contributes to more than 5 million deaths annually[1] and represents a significant financial burden to patients and society.[2–4] To appropriately evaluate current therapies and guide new treatment, a thorough understanding of the epidemiology of sepsis is essential. This article describes the epidemiology of, and short-term mortality from sepsis, focusing on global variation, risk factors, and special populations. The article also highlights the causes of variation in reported data, and the implications of this variation.

INCIDENCE AND TEMPORAL TRENDS OF SEPSIS

Over the past 40 years (1975–2015), the aggregate global incidence of hospital-treated sepsis is estimated to be 288 sepsis cases per 100,000 person-years.[1]

Disclosure Statement: No conflicts of interest.
[a] Department of Critical Care Medicine, Sunnybrook Health Sciences Centre, 2075 Bayview Avenue, Room D1.08, Toronto, Ontario M4N 3M5, Canada; [b] Department of Anesthesia and Interdepartmental Division of Critical Care Medicine, University of Toronto, 123 Edward Street, Toronto, ON M5G 1E2, Canada
* Corresponding author. Department of Critical Care Medicine, Sunnybrook Health Sciences Centre, 2075 Bayview Avenue, Room D1.08, Toronto, Ontario M4N 3M5, Canada.
E-mail address: hannah.wunsch@sunnybrook.ca

Crit Care Clin 34 (2018) 15–27
http://dx.doi.org/10.1016/j.ccc.2017.08.001
0749-0704/18/© 2017 Elsevier Inc. All rights reserved.
criticalcare.theclinics.com

However, for the latter 10 years (2005–2015), this estimate has increased to 437 sepsis cases per 100,000 person-years, with a similar increase in severe sepsis from 148 cases per 100,000 persons to 270 per 100,000 person-years.[1] These data equate to an estimate of 31.5 million sepsis and 19.4 million severe sepsis cases treated in hospitals around the globe each year.[1] Furthermore, a significant proportion of these patients are treated in intensive care units (ICUs), with estimates ranging from 10% to 20% of all ICU admissions being specifically for severe sepsis or septic shock.[5–11]

However, the incidence of sepsis and severe sepsis is highly variable globally,[12] with data lacking from large parts of the world.[1] Most available data come from high-income countries. More recent data on severe sepsis (**Fig. 1**) demonstrate 2 key findings: (1) the reported incidence of severe sepsis has consistently increased across individual countries with available published data,[1,2,5,13–16] and (2) the reported incidence of severe sepsis is higher in North American than other countries.

Very limited data are available on the epidemiology of sepsis in middle and low-income countries; these economic labels also identify a highly heterogeneous group of countries, ranging from upper middle income, such as Turkey and Brazil,[11,17,18] to low-income countries, such as the Gambia and Uganda.[19,20] However, patients diagnosed with sepsis likely account for a larger proportion of hospital admissions in these countries. For example, in a Brazilian study by Silva and colleagues,[11] over a 1-year time span, 46.9% of all patients admitted to an ICU for more than 24 hours met their definition for sepsis. Additionally, in low-income countries, sepsis may represent an even greater burden on the health care system as a whole.[20]

REASONS FOR VARIABILITY IN REPORTED INCIDENCE OF SEPSIS

Variability in rates of sepsis may be due to differences in underlying populations across countries, but also may be due to detection bias. This includes variability in

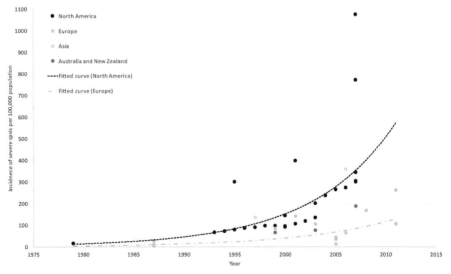

Fig. 1. Incidence of severe sepsis over time per 100,000 population, categorized by region of the world. (*Data from* Fleischmann C, Scherag A, Adhikari NK, et al. Assessment of global incidence and mortality of hospital-treated sepsis. Current estimates and limitations. Am J Respir Crit Care Med 2016;193(3):259–72.)

the strategies used to identify patients with sepsis, policies related to the identification of septic patients, and factors related to hospital presentation.

Case Definitions

Studies that rely on large databases usually use diagnostic codes, whereas cohort studies often use clinical definitions, or a combination of both diagnostic codes and clinical variables. Even within each detection method, differences exist. For example, 4 commonly cited articles use different International Classification of Diseases (ICD), Ninth Revision, Clinical Modification codes to identify patients who have severe sepsis in large databases.[21-24] Gaieski and colleagues[25] used all 4 definitions to examine US hospitalizations between 2004 and 2009, and assessed the incidence of severe sepsis. The estimated incidences ranged from 300 cases per 100,000 persons, with the Dombrovskiy[22] definition up to 1031 cases per 100,000 persons with the Wang definition. Additionally, these patients were of different disease severity. Most patients identified by the methods of Angus[21] and Wang[24] had single-organ system dysfunction (72.4% and 71.9% respectively) whereas only 47.8% and 47.3% of patients identified by Martin[23] and Dombrovskiy were limited to single-organ dysfunction.[25] Further variation in patient identification has occurred over time, as diagnostic codes have been revised and ICD-10 codes introduced. Stiermaier and colleagues[26] found that when using a definition of severe sepsis based on specific ICD-10 codes, their ICD-10–based method identified only one-fifth of the patients classified as having severe sepsis using clinical criteria through chart review.

However, reliance on clinical criteria does not remove variability in estimates due to the reliance on the need for a clinical suspicion (and documentation) of infection as well as differing frequency in the measurement of variables, such as those required for the systemic inflammatory response syndrome criteria in older definitions or quick Sequential Organ Failure Assessment (SOFA) variables (Sepsis-3 definition).[27,28]

Impact of Sepsis-3 Definition on Estimates of Sepsis Epidemiology

Currently few published studies have used the new Sepsis-3 definition, which notably does not include the specific concept of "severe sepsis." One study comparing the incidence of sepsis based on the new Sepsis-3 definition with the incidence of severe sepsis based on the prior 2001 sepsis definition found a similar incidence, identifying 780 cases per 100,000 population with the Sepsis-3 definition and 687 cases with the older definition.[28] However, the actual agreement of cases was approximately 50%, raising the concern of identification of different groups of patients.

It is also important to note that the new Sepsis-3 definition requires some form of organ dysfunction for a patient to be diagnosed as having sepsis. Therefore, the group most likely to be reclassified as nonseptic are those who previously met criteria for sepsis but not severe sepsis. It is quite possible that as more studies use the Sepsis-3 definition, the reported incidence of sepsis may decrease and associated mortality increase.

Policies

As well as the variability in methods for patient identification, specific policies also may impact the detection of sepsis. This phenomenon was examined in a study based in California.[29] Over a 10-year period, 2 different policies were enacted. The first (October 2003), was the issuing of guidance on appropriate sepsis coding by the Centers for Medicare and Medicaid Services, and the second (October 2007), was the revision of the previous diagnosis-related group (DRG) reimbursement system into the medical severity DRG, an attempt to connect reimbursement to medical severity.[29] To examine the impact of these 2 policies, Gohil and colleagues[29] used baseline trends to estimate changes in sepsis rates over time. Based on coding, they found actual rates that were 5 to 10 cases per 1000 patients higher than projected. It is possible that these policy changes led to both an increase in vigilance around cases of possible sepsis and created a more aggressive culture of identifying cases. Additionally, as these policy changes were specific to the United States, they may also play a role in the increased incidence of sepsis seen in the North American literature as compared with both European and international literature.

Access to Care

For a diagnosis of sepsis, individuals must present for care and be evaluated by a clinician who then suspects the diagnosis. Therefore, most studies describe the epidemiology of treated sepsis. This is an important point because (1) the availability of access to care may vary greatly based on both geography and time frame, (2) the time in disease progression at which individuals present for care may vary, and (3) economic factors can play a role in what interventions patients receive. For example, as shown in a study of care in 8 countries, the percentage of patients in the ICU identified as having severe sepsis or septic shock is directly correlated with the overall provision of ICU beds for the population.[30] As such a high percentage of such patients within an ICU may more accurately reflect the scarcity of ICU beds within the country as opposed to a high incidence of sepsis.

SHORT-TERM MORTALITY

Mortality estimates for sepsis vary markedly across studies, depending on the definition, population, resources, and the inclusion or exclusion of different groups representing those with sepsis, severe sepsis, or septic shock. Including the less severely ill (those with sepsis, but without organ dysfunction), estimates of mortality range from 11% to 26% in one review.[1] When limiting studies to severe sepsis, 2 international studies estimated higher mortality rates. A systematic review of studies from 1991 to 2009 found a 28-day mortality rate of 33.2% for the 2 decades, whereas a 3-year international study reported a hospital mortality of 49.6%.[31,32] Similarly, another international study limited to septic shock in the ICU found an in-hospital mortality rate of 52%.[33]

Variability in reported mortality is present across countries as well, with sepsis mortality estimate ranging from 17% in one US study,[34] up to 30% in other high-income European countries,[3,16,26] and 30.9% to 87.3% in middle-income countries.[7,11,17,18,35] For cohorts of patients diagnosed with severe sepsis or septic shock, mortality is similarly variable.[3–11,14,15,25,26,28,36–40] However, studies have consistently found decreasing hospital mortality associated with sepsis over time. For example, in the United States, mortality for patients with severe sepsis was reported to have decreased from 40.0% in 1998 to 17.3% in 2012.[2,29,36] In studies from Europe, mortality has been reported to have decreased from 54.0% (2003) to 43.6% (2013),[3,37] and in Australia and New Zealand from 35.0% in 2000 to 18.4% in 2012.[5] Studies focused solely on septic shock report the same trend.[14,40] It is notable that another consistent finding is reporting of lower mortality in the United States compared with European and other countries (**Fig. 2**). One hypothesis is that specific US policies are leading to a more liberal classification of patients with sepsis and the inclusion of very low-risk individuals. Due to the increasing prevalence of sepsis, even with a decreasing case fatality rate, the absolute number of severe sepsis cases ending in

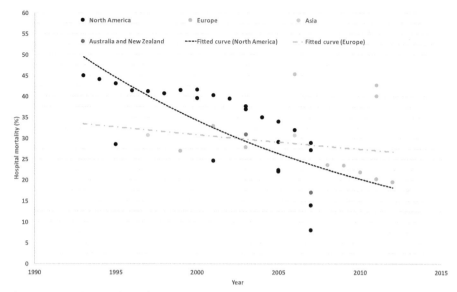

Fig. 2. Hospital mortality of severe sepsis cases over time, categorized by region of the world. (*Data from* Fleischmann C, Scherag A, Adhikari NK, et al. Assessment of global incidence and mortality of hospital-treated sepsis. Current estimates and limitations. Am J Respir Crit Care Med 2016;193(3):259–72.)

death has increased significantly,[13,15,29,41] with up to 1.8 times as many severe sepsis hospitalizations leading to death in 2007 compared with 2000.[13]

ETIOLOGY AND SITE OF INFECTION
Etiology

Based on available epidemiologic data, gram-negative, gram-positive, and culture-negative sepsis are all common causes of sepsis (**Fig. 3**). In cases in which gram-negative organisms were cultured, *Escherichia coli* and *Pseudomonas* were the 2 most frequently reported organisms across multiple countries,[32,38] with *Klebsiella* rates increasing in middle-income countries.[17,35] For cases with gram-positive organisms, *Staphylococcus aureus* was the most common organism cultured followed by *Streptococcus pneumoniae*.[32,38] Of note, methicillin-resistant *S aureus* has been identified in up to 10% of gram-positive infections.[42] In the United States, 47.1% of all severe sepsis admissions identified by Gupta and colleagues[43] were for culture-negative sepsis, and the age-adjusted proportion of culture-negative sepsis hospitalizations increased from 33.9% in 2000 to 43.5% in 2010.

The exact impact of the type of infection on mortality is unclear. Previously, gram-negative bacteremia was associated with a higher mortality compared with gram-positive bacteremia,[44] a finding supported by more recent data from the United Kingdom.[45] However, in nosocomial infections, gram-positive organisms have been associated with higher mortality.[45] Among the more common organisms, *S aureus* and *Pseudomonas* were associated with the highest mortality, whereas *E coli* and *Enterococcus* with the lowest.[32] Additionally, anaerobic and fungal organisms were associated with increased mortality.[32,36,46] However, these data are confounded by the question of appropriate early antibiotic therapy, with further adjustment made

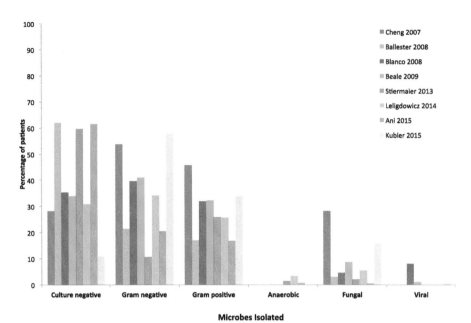

Fig. 3. Selected studies showing the distribution of different categories of microbes isolated in patients with sepsis. Total percentage isolated in any given study is greater than 100%, as in some cases multiple organisms were isolated.

for this factor, one study found that the type of organism was no longer associated with mortality.[47]

Site of Infection

Although hospital-acquired infections are associated with an increased risk of mortality,[10] 53% to 65% of cases are still acquired in the community.[9,33,37,38] For both hospital-acquired and community-acquired infections, the lungs and the abdomen are the 2 most common sites of infection. Pulmonary infections were reported to occur in 28% to 53% of cases,[4,8,9,17,32,33,37,38] and intra-abdominal infections in 19% to 49% of cases[8,9,32,33,37,38] (**Fig. 4**); studies from surgical ICUs reported the higher intra-abdominal infection rates.

The site of infection is thought to play a major role in outcome. Pulmonary and intra-abdominal infections, as well as disseminated infections, are associated with an increased risk of mortality compared with other sites (such as the urinary tract).[9,33,48] Again there is some evidence that the importance of infection site may be attenuated by other factors. Zahar and colleagues[47] demonstrated that when adjusting for all comorbidities, disease severity, and the implementation of appropriate early antibiotics, the site of infection no longer had a major impact on outcome. As described by Cohen and colleagues[44] in their meta-analysis of 510 articles examining the role of the characteristics of an infection in the outcome of sepsis, they found distinct patterns. For example, they found that urosepsis and central venous catheter–associated infections were less likely to cause lethal infections than sepsis associated with pulmonary, intra-abdominal, or soft tissue sources. They also found that specific organisms in each group were associated with very different outcomes, and the relationship between site of infection and organism represents a complex system, not easily captured or summarized in large epidemiologic studies.

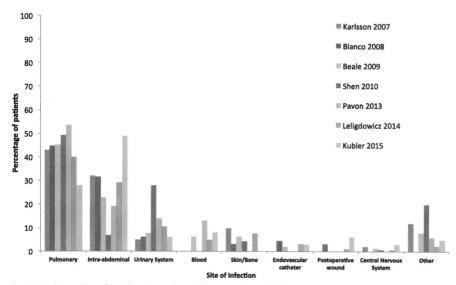

Fig. 4. Selected studies showing the different sites of infection in patients with sepsis.

RISK FACTORS FOR SEPSIS AND MORTALITY
Demographics

Commonly accepted demographic risk factors for acquiring sepsis include male sex and increased comorbid illness.[3,34,49] There is also a strong association with age; after the age of 30, the rate of emergency department visits for sepsis appears to double for each 10-year increase in age.[34] As well as an association with an increased risk of acquiring sepsis, specific risk factors are associated with an increased risk of death. Commonly cited risk factors for mortality include increased age, comorbid disease, number of organs failed, and, as described previously, lack of an identified pathogen.[6,10,15,39] Each additional 10 years of age carries a hazard ratio for mortality of 1.31,[10] with those age 65 and older having an odds ratio for mortality of 3.2 compared with patients younger than 18.[15] As for organ dysfunction, the hazard ratio for each additional point on the SOFA score has been found to be 1.21,[10] and after 3 or more organ system failures, the odds ratio for mortality is as high as 3.89.[15] In a recent review of nearly 250,000 sepsis admissions to ICUs in England, unadjusted mortality was found to vary significantly with organ dysfunction from 18.5% for those with single-organ dysfunction up to 69.9% for those with 5 organ dysfunctions.[48]

Socioeconomic Status and Race

Increasingly evidence demonstrates that low socioeconomic status is associated with a higher likelihood of acquisition of sepsis and higher mortality. In one study looking at the odds of having a positive blood culture on time of admission, it was found that the adjusted odds ratio increased as the patient's neighborhood poverty rate increased, with an odds ratio of 1.5 for those in a neighborhood with a poverty rate ≥40% compared with a neighborhood less than 5%.[50] Additionally, after adjusting for known risk factors, including the year of admission, a lack of health care insurance was associated with an odds ratio for death of 1.4 compared with patients with private insurance.[51] Despite the decreasing mortality rates demonstrated for severe sepsis over time, the mortality difference between privately insured and uninsured patients has remained unchanged.[51]

Race also appears to have an impact on sepsis development and outcome. In the United States, rates of sepsis are significantly higher in black patients compared with the rest of the population (1.98 cases per 1000 US citizens among blacks vs 1.13 cases per 1000 in the rest of the population).[34] Similarly, as measured by hospitalizations for severe sepsis, black patients have a 67% higher severe sepsis rate compared with white patients, despite a lower likelihood of being admitted from the emergency department with an infection (odds ratio for hospital admission 0.7 compared with white patients).[52] Overall, infection and severe sepsis mortality rates are 1.5 and 1.8 times higher in black patients compared with whites,[52] and the rate of death from severe sepsis in black patients exceeds that of white patients by approximately 30 deaths per 100,000 US population per year.[41] The exact underlying social and physiologic mechanisms for these differences are not fully understood, although they are likely multifactorial.

SPECIAL POPULATIONS
Maintenance Dialysis

The incidence for severe sepsis among patients receiving dialysis in very high, with a rate of 145.4 cases per 1000 versus 3.5 per 1000 in the general population.[53] These patients also are younger (64.1 years vs 68.2 years) and are disproportionately black (28.1% vs 11.7%). Additionally, the etiology of severe sepsis in patients receiving dialysis is different, as bloodstream infections with no other source occur far more commonly in these patients than in the general population. Although the same decline in overall mortality rates was seen in patients on maintenance dialysis as in the general population, the risk of mortality for patients on maintenance dialysis with severe sepsis remains significantly higher than that of the general population, with an adjusted odds ratio of 1.26.[53]

Immunodeficiency

Immunodeficiency is common in patients with sepsis. One French study demonstrated that 30.6% of all patients admitted to the ICU with severe sepsis or septic shock were immunocompromised.[9] Although different profiles of immunodeficiency are associated with different risks of death, overall immunodeficiency itself is an independent risk factor for death. The type of organism causing sepsis in these patients is also different, with more Pseudomonas, gram-positive cocci other than pneumococci, mycobacteria, viruses, parasites, and fungi compared with patients who are not immunocompromised. Additionally in immunocompromised patients, these infections more frequently involve multiple sites.[9]

Maternal Sepsis

In the most recent review of maternal deaths in the United Kingdom, sepsis has now been identified as the most common cause of direct maternal death.[54] Similarly, in the United States, the rate of sepsis complicating delivery has been increasing; sepsis now complicates 1 in every 3300 deliveries and severe sepsis 1 in 10,800. Additionally, the risk of sepsis-related death has increased by 10% each year, and currently occurs in 1 in every 105,400 deliveries.[55]

Postoperative Patients

The rates of postoperative sepsis and severe sepsis also have been increasing. Sepsis is now estimated to occur in 1.3% of patients postoperatively, and severe sepsis in 0.9%.[56] Although the mortality rate for postoperative sepsis has decreased, in line with sepsis overall,[56,57] it still represents a significant postoperative risk. Furthermore, the excess hospital charges associated with postoperative severe sepsis have increased from an estimate of $US 119,337 per hospitalization to $US 157,882. Of note, pneumonia remains the most common cause of severe sepsis in postoperative patients (35.2%), with unspecified postoperative infections, including intra-abdominal abscesses, and other wound infections accounting for only 18% of cases.[56]

Trauma Patients

Given their younger age and lack of comorbid illness, trauma patients represent a distinct group of patients at risk for sepsis.[58] The rate of the development of sepsis after traumatic injury varies greatly in the literature from 2% to 10.2%,[58,59] and is linked to the severity of injury. Patients with an Injury Severity Score (ISS) $\geq$15 have a 6-fold increased rate, and those with an ISS $\geq$30 are at a 16-fold increased risk compared with patients with mild injuries.[59] In trauma patients, sepsis is related to multiple adverse outcomes, including increased mortality, increased risk of single and multi-system organ failure, and increased length of ICU and hospital stay.[58,59]

COST OF SEPSIS

Sepsis represents a significant cost to the health care system and the individual affected.

Length of Intensive Care Unit and Hospital Stay

Internationally, the length of ICU stay associated with severe sepsis has been estimated at 14.6 days, and the length of hospital stay at 28.2 days,[32] with variability in ICU length of stay across individual countries. For example, the median ICU length of stay was reported to be 10 days in Canada,[6] 8 to 13 days in Poland,[37] and 10 days in Spain.[38] In the United States, the hospital length of stay for severe sepsis has decreased from 16 days in 1999 to 7 days in 2012.[2,36,41] However, the United States appears to be an outlier with this very short hospital (and therefore ICU) length of stay.

Financial Cost

Regardless of the country of origin, sepsis represents a significant financial cost to both the patient and the health care system. In Germany, it is estimated that the mean expenditure per case of sepsis is €27,468, equaling a total cost of €7.7 billion in 2013 after all the inpatient and subsequent outpatient costs are considered.[3] When examining Asian countries, the costs vary, but remain significant; in Taiwan the median hospital charge increased from $US 1718 in 1997 to $US 2911 in 2006,[4] and in China the median total cost of sepsis care per patient is reported at $US 11,390.[39] Similarly, the median cost of care per patient with sepsis in Brazil is now $US 9632.[18] In the United States, the median charge per hospital stay is $US 55,749 (2012 data) and total hospital cost for severe sepsis patients has been estimated at $US 24.3 billion (2007 data).[2,41]

SUMMARY

Globally, sepsis remains a common and significant cause of mortality, morbidity, and costs of care. Although the increase in incidence can be partially related to changes in detection and differing definitions, international data demonstrate that reported rates of sepsis are increasing. Furthermore, despite the ongoing decrease in associated case mortality, sepsis continues to represent a large cause of death worldwide. As the population continues to age, and patient complexity and burden of multiple comorbid illnesses increases, the impact of sepsis on individuals and the health system will remain substantial.

REFERENCES

1. Fleischmann C, Scherag A, Adhikari NK, et al. Assessment of global incidence and mortality of hospital-treated sepsis. Current estimates and limitations. Am J Respir Crit Care Med 2016;193(3):259–72.
2. Stoller J, Halpin L, Weis M, et al. Epidemiology of severe sepsis: 2008-2012. J Crit Care 2016;31(1):58–62.
3. Fleischmann C, Thomas-Rueddel DO, Hartmann M, et al. Hospital incidence and mortality rates of sepsis: an analysis of hospital episode (DRG) statistics in Germany from 2007 to 2013. Dtsch Arztebl Int 2016;113(10):159–66.
4. Shen HN, Lu CL, Yang HH. Epidemiologic trend of severe sepsis in Taiwan from 1997 through 2006. Chest 2010;138(2):298–304.
5. Kaukonen KM, Bailey M, Suzuki S, et al. Mortality related to severe sepsis and septic shock among critically ill patients in Australia and New Zealand, 2000-2012. JAMA 2014;311(13):1308–16.
6. Martin CM, Priestap F, Fisher H, et al. A prospective, observational registry of patients with severe sepsis: the Canadian Sepsis Treatment and Response Registry. Crit Care Med 2009;37(1):81–8.
7. Phua J, Koh Y, Du B, et al. Management of severe sepsis in patients admitted to Asian intensive care units: prospective cohort study. BMJ 2011;342:d3245.
8. Karlsson S, Varpula M, Ruokonen E, et al. Incidence, treatment, and outcome of severe sepsis in ICU-treated adults in Finland: the Finnsepsis study. Intensive Care Med 2007;33(3):435–43.
9. Tolsma V, Schwebel C, Azoulay E, et al. Sepsis severe or septic shock: outcome according to immune status and immunodeficiency profile. Chest 2014;146(5):1205–13.
10. Pavon A, Binquet C, Kara F, et al. Profile of the risk of death after septic shock in the present era: an epidemiologic study. Crit Care Med 2013;41(11):2600–9.
11. Silva E, Pedro Mde A, Sogayar AC, et al. Brazilian Sepsis Epidemiological Study (BASES study). Crit Care 2004;8(4):60.
12. Jawad I, Lukšić I, Rafnsson SB. Assessing available information on the burden of sepsis: global estimates of incidence, prevalence and mortality. J Glob Health 2012;2(1):010404.
13. Kumar G, Kumar N, Taneja A, et al. Nationwide trends of severe sepsis in the 21st century (2000-2007). Chest 2011;140(5):1223–31.
14. Walkey AJ, Wiener RS, Lindenauer PK. Utilization patterns and outcomes associated with central venous catheter in septic shock: a population-based study. Crit Care Med 2013;41(6):1450–7.
15. Bouza C, López-Cuadrado T, Saz-Parkinson Z, et al. Epidemiology and recent trends of severe sepsis in Spain: a nationwide population-based analysis (2006-2011). BMC Infect Dis 2014;14:3863.
16. Andreu Ballester JC, Ballester F, González Sánchez A, et al. Epidemiology of sepsis in the Valencian community (Spain), 1995-2004. Infect Control Hosp Epidemiol 2008;29(7):630–4.
17. Tanriover MD, Guven GS, Sen D, et al. Epidemiology and outcome of sepsis in a tertiary-care hospital in a developing country. Epidemiol Infect 2006;134(2):315–22.

18. Sogayar AM, Machado FR, Rea-Neto A, et al. A multicentre, prospective study to evaluate costs of septic patients in Brazilian intensive care units. Pharmacoeconomics 2008;26(5):425–34.

19. Hill PC, Onyeama CO, Ikumapayi UN, et al. Bacteraemia in patients admitted to an urban hospital in West Africa. BMC Infect Dis 2007;7:2.

20. Jacob ST, Moore CC, Banura P, et al. Severe sepsis in two Ugandan hospitals: a prospective observational study of management and outcomes in a predominantly HIV-1 infected population. PLoS One 2009;4(11):e7782.

21. Angus DC, Linde-Zwirble WT, Lidicker J, et al. Epidemiology of severe sepsis in the United States: analysis of incidence, outcome, and associated costs of care. Crit Care Med 2001;29(7):1303–10.

22. Dombrovskiy VY, Martin AA, Sunderram J, et al. Rapid increase in hospitalization and mortality rates for severe sepsis in the United States: a trend analysis from 1993 to 2003. Crit Care Med 2007;35(5):1244–50.

23. Martin GS, Mannino DM, Eaton S, et al. The epidemiology of sepsis in the United States from 1979 through 2000. N Engl J Med 2003;348(16):1546–54.

24. Wang HE, Shapiro NI, Angus DC, et al. National estimates of severe sepsis in United States emergency departments. Crit Care Med 2007;35(8):1928–36.

25. Gaieski DF, Edwards JM, Kallan MJ, et al. Benchmarking the incidence and mortality of severe sepsis in the United States. Crit Care Med 2013;41(5):1167–74.

26. Stiermaier T, Herkner H, Tobudic S, et al. Incidence and long-term outcome of sepsis on general wards and in an ICU at the General Hospital of Vienna: an observational cohort study. Wien klin Wochenschr 2013;125(11–12):302–8.

27. Henriksen DP, Laursen CB, Jensen TGG, et al. Incidence rate of community-acquired sepsis among hospitalized acute medical patients—a population-based survey. Crit Care Med 2015;43(1):13–21.

28. Mellhammar L, Wullt S, Lindberg Å, et al. Sepsis incidence: a population-based study. Open Forum Infect Dis 2016;3(4):ofw207.

29. Gohil SK, Cao C, Phelan M, et al. Impact of policies on the rise in sepsis incidence, 2000-2010. Clin Infect Dis 2016;62(6):695–703.

30. Wunsch H, Angus DC, Harrison DA, et al. Variation in critical care services across North America and Western Europe. Crit Care Med 2008;36(10):2787–93, e1–9.

31. Stevenson EK, Rubenstein AR, Radin GT, et al. Two decades of mortality trends among patients with severe sepsis: a comparative meta-analysis*. Crit Care Med 2014;42(3):625–31.

32. Beale R, Reinhart K, Brunkhorst FM, et al. Promoting global research excellence in severe sepsis (PROGRESS): lessons from an international sepsis registry. Infection 2009;37(3):222–32.

33. Leligdowicz A, Dodek PM, Norena M, et al, Co-operative Antimicrobial Therapy of Septic Shock Database Research Group. Association between source of infection and hospital mortality in patients who have septic shock. Am J Respir Crit Care Med 2014;189(10):1204–13.

34. Filbin MR, Arias SA, Camargo CA, et al. Sepsis visits and antibiotic utilization in U.S. emergency departments*. Crit Care Med 2014;42(3):528–35.

35. Chehade AEIH, Chebl RB, Majzoub I, et al. Assessment of sepsis in a developing country: where do we stand? Health Care Curr Rev 2015;3:141.

36. Ani C, Farshidpanah S, Bellinghausen Stewart A, et al. Variations in organism-specific severe sepsis mortality in the United States: 1999-2008. Crit Care Med 2015;43(1):65–77.

37. Kübler A, Adamik B, Durek G, et al. Results of the severe sepsis registry in intensive care units in Poland from 2003-2009. Anaesthesiol Intensive Ther 2015;47(1):7–13.

38. Blanco J, Muriel-Bombín A, Sagredo V, et al. Incidence, organ dysfunction and mortality in severe sepsis: a Spanish multicentre study. Crit Care 2008;12(6):R158.

39. Cheng B, Xie G, Yao S, et al. Epidemiology of severe sepsis in critically ill surgical patients in ten university hospitals in China. Crit Care Med 2007;35(11):2538–46.

40. Kadri SS, Rhee C, Strich JR, et al. Estimating ten-year trends in septic shock incidence and mortality in United States Academic Medical Centers using clinical data. Chest 2017;151(2):278–85.

41. Lagu T, Rothberg MB, Shieh MSS, et al. Hospitalizations, costs, and outcomes of severe sepsis in the United States 2003 to 2007. Crit Care Med 2012;40(3):754–61.

42. Vincent JL, Rello J, Marshall J, et al. International study of the prevalence and outcomes of infection in intensive care units. JAMA 2009;302(21):2323–9.

43. Gupta S, Sakhuja A, Kumar G, et al. Culture-negative severe sepsis: nationwide trends and outcomes. Chest 2016;150(6):1251–9.

44. Cohen J, Cristofaro P, Carlet J, et al. New method of classifying infections in critically ill patients. Crit Care Med 2004;32(7):1510–26.

45. Morgan MP, Szakmany T, Power SG, et al. Sepsis patients with first and second-hit infections show different outcomes depending on the causative organism. Front Microbiol 2016;7:207.

46. Ng K, Schorr C, Reboli AC, et al. Incidence and mortality of sepsis, severe sepsis, and septic shock in intensive care unit patients with candidemia. Infect Dis (Lond) 2015;47(8):584–7.

47. Zahar JR, Timsit JF, Garrouste-Orgeas M, et al. Outcomes in severe sepsis and patients with septic shock: pathogen species and infection sites are not associated with mortality. Crit Care Med 2011;39(8):1886–95.

48. Shankar-Hari M, Harrison DA, Rowan KM. Differences in impact of definitional elements on mortality precludes international comparisons of sepsis epidemiology-a cohort study illustrating the need for standardized reporting. Crit Care Med 2016;44(12):2223–30.

49. Sakr Y, Elia C, Mascia L, et al. The influence of gender on the epidemiology of and outcome from severe sepsis. Crit Care 2013;17(2):R50.

50. Mendu ML, Zager S, Gibbons FK, et al. Relationship between neighborhood poverty rate and bloodstream infections in the critically ill. Crit Care Med 2012;40(5):1427–36.

51. Kumar G, Taneja A, Majumdar T, et al. The association of lacking insurance with outcomes of severe sepsis: retrospective analysis of an administrative database*. Crit Care Med 2014;42(3):583–91.

52. Mayr FB, Yende S, Linde-Zwirble WT, et al. Infection rate and acute organ dysfunction risk as explanations for racial differences in severe sepsis. JAMA 2010;303(24):2495–503.

53. Sakhuja A, Nanchal RS, Gupta S, et al. Trends and outcomes of severe sepsis in patients on maintenance dialysis. Am J Nephrol 2016;43(2):97–103.

54. Cantwell R, Clutton-Brock T, Cooper G, et al. Saving mothers' lives: reviewing maternal deaths to make motherhood safer: 2006-2008. The eighth report of the confidential enquiries into maternal deaths in the United Kingdom. BJOG 2011;118(Suppl 1):1–203.

55. Bauer ME, Bateman BT, Bauer ST, et al. Maternal sepsis mortality and morbidity during hospitalization for delivery: temporal trends and independent associations for severe sepsis. Anesth Analg 2013;117(4):944–50.
56. Bateman BT, Schmidt U, Berman MF, et al. Temporal trends in the epidemiology of severe postoperative sepsis after elective surgery: a large, nationwide sample. Anesthesiology 2010;112(4):917–25.
57. Vogel TR, Dombrovskiy VY, Lowry SF. Trends in postoperative sepsis: are we improving outcomes? Surg Infect (Larchmt) 2009;10(1):71–8.
58. Wafaisade A, Lefering R, Bouillon B, et al. Epidemiology and risk factors of sepsis after multiple trauma: an analysis of 29,829 patients from the trauma registry of the German Society for Trauma Surgery. Crit Care Med 2011;39(4):621–8.
59. Osborn TM, Tracy JK, Dunne JR, et al. Epidemiology of sepsis in patients with traumatic injury. Crit Care Med 2004;32(11):2234–40.

Immune Activation in Sepsis

Andrew Conway-Morris, MB ChB, PhD, FFICM[a,b,*], Julie Wilson, MB ChB[c,d], Manu Shankar-Hari, MSc, MD, PhD, MB BS, FRCA, FFICM[c,d]

KEYWORDS

- Sepsis • Inflammation • Immunosuppression

KEY POINTS

- Sepsis is a dysregulated multisystem response to infection.
- The immune responses begin as compartmentalized, progressive processes of microbial recognition, followed by triggering and amplification of inflammation and homeostatic regulation.
- How these immune responses become dysregulated and maladaptive remains a key conundrum.

INTRODUCTION

Sepsis is defined as life-threatening organ dysfunction caused by a dysregulated host response to infection.[1] These dysregulated host responses underpin the clinical phenotypes that range from a mild, self-limiting illness to a severe progressive illness resulting in multiorgan failure and death. A complex, interlinked system of cells, receptors, secreted proteins, enzymes, and structural and chemical defense elements such as epithelium and associated antimicrobial proteins, together referred to as the immune system, protect the human body from infection. This protection involves four interlinked tasks: danger signal surveillance and recognition from nonself, effector functions in response to sensing danger signals, homeostatic regulation, and generation of immunologic memory in certain situations. Functionally distinct innate and adaptive immune systems work in synergy to perform these tasks. In this article, a simple conceptual overview is provided of the current understanding of these dysregulated immune responses in sepsis.

All authors declare that they have no conflicts of interest.
[a] Division of Anaesthesia, Department of Medicine, Addenbrooke's Hospital, University of Cambridge, Hills Road, Box 93, Cambridge CB2 0QQ, UK; [b] John V Farman Intensive Care Unit, Addenbrooke's Hospital, Hills Road, Cambridge, CB2 0QQ, UK; [c] Intensive Care Unit, Guy's and St Thomas' NHS Foundation Trust, ICU Support Offices, St Thomas' Hospital, 1st Floor, East Wing, London SE1 7EH, UK; [d] Division of Infection, Inflammation and Immunity, King's College London, Guy's Hospital, 3rd Floor, Borough Wing, Great Maze Pond, London SE1 9RT, UK
* Corresponding author.
E-mail address: mozza@doctors.org.uk

Overview of Innate and Adaptive Immune System Response to Pathogens

Pathogens access a normally sterile area following breach of either epithelial or mucosal barriers (infection). The innate immune system is the first line of defense against infections (surveillance and recognition of nonself). The innate immune system consists of cells of myeloid lineage with the ability to clear and kill pathogens by phagocytosis (such as granulocytes, monocytes/macrophages, and dendritic cells) and the complement system of proteins, aside from epithelial- and mucosa-associated structural and chemical defense mechanisms.

Innate immunity to infection can be broadly categorized into two categories:

An immediate response (0–4 hours), where the infection is recognized by preformed, nonspecific, and broadly specific effectors such as the complement system

An early induced immune response (beyond 4 hours) with recruitment and activation of effector cells that rely on evolutionarily conserved pattern recognition receptors (PRRs) of danger signals for infection clearance

Innate immune cells with the ability to process and present antigens (antigen-presenting cells; APCs), in particular dendritic cells, form a link to the adaptive immune system. These inform the adaptive immune cells of danger, on the need to generate a specific immune response against the inciting pathogen, and also provide essential initiating signals for these responses. This occurs in secondary lymphoid organs such as spleen, lymph nodes, and mucosal-associated lymphoid tissues (MALT). The adaptive immune system consists of 2 major cell types: B and T lymphocytes. These cells express specific antigen-detecting receptors on the cell surface: B cell receptors (BCRs) and T cell receptors (TCRs). In contrast to the innate immune cell PRRs, the adaptive immune cell receptors have antigen specificity, (ie, the ability to individually identify different antigens as opposed to common patterns on antigens). This specificity is a product of creation of a diverse repertoire of receptors, plus selection and clonal expansion of the adaptive immune cells.

Complement and Coagulation Cascades in Sepsis

On breaching the epithelial surface barrier, the pathogen encounters complement system proteins (C), a group of soluble proteins produced by the liver that circulate normally in an inactive form. The complement system can be activated by antibody-coated pathogens (classical pathway), by the pathogen alone (alternative pathway), and by carbohydrate-binding proteins (eg, mannose-binding lectin, ficolins) that coat the pathogens (lectin pathway). All three pathways converge on generating a C3 convertase enzyme that cleaves the complement protein C3 into C3a and C3b. C3b remains on the pathogen surface as a potent opsonin that is recognized by phagocytes. C3a is released into the circulation, acting as a potent proinflammatory molecule that recruits more phagocytes to the site of infection. In sepsis, the complement system undergoes massive activation with deleterious effects. This is predominantly mediated by the activated complement molecules C3a and C5a, the anaphylatoxins.[2] The systemic activation of the coagulation and fibrinolytic systems results in deposition of fibrin and formation of microthrombi in the microcirculation; this may contribute to the impaired microcirculation seen in sepsis.[3] Activated complement products, C5a in particular, activate the coagulation system via tissue factor,[4] while thrombin from the activated coagulation cascade cleaves C5 into C5a and C5b independent of its upstream pathways.[5] This illustrates the positive feedback loop seen in sepsis between the dysregulated, systemic activation of the complement, coagulation, and fibrinolytic cascades, exacerbating tissue damage and organ dysfunction.[6,7]

Danger Signals and Sepsis

The first step in the pathobiology of sepsis is detection of the presence of pathogens within a normally sterile tissue or body cavity. This is achieved by leukocyte recognition of pathogen-associated molecular patterns (PAMPs). Microorganisms express a range of molecules that are structurally or metabolically critical, such as lipopolysaccharide (LPS), peptidoglycan, flagellin, and double-stranded RNA. The tissue damage that occurs with established infection also generates danger signals. These danger-associated molecular patterns (DAMPs) or alarmins include, among others, heat shock proteins (HSPs),[8] cathelicidins,[9] uric acid,[10] fibrinogen, free cellular and mitochondrial DNA, and high-mobility group box-1 (HMGB-1). DAMPs activate a variety of receptors including RAGE, Toll-like receptors (TLRs) and specific receptors such as IL (interleukin)-1R.[11] As these DAMPs are related to illness severity, it is likely that the dysregulated host response in sepsis is influenced by these DAMPs.[12,13]

Danger Signal Sensors

Unifying characteristics of these danger signals (DAMPs and PAMPs) are conserved molecular patterns that can be easily sensed by pattern recognition receptors (PRRs) on leukocytes. These PRRs are germline-encoded receptors present on both the cell surface and intracellularly. Five subclasses of PRRs have been described thus far: TLRs, nucleotide oligomerization domain-like receptors (NODs or NLRs), retinoic acid-inducible gene (RIG-1)-like receptors, C-type lectin receptors, and absence-in-melanoma 2 (AIM-2)-like receptors.[14] The sensing of PAMPs or DAMPs by PRRs upregulates the transcription of genes involved in inflammation. PRRs can recognize a wide range of microbial membrane components from gram-positive bacteria, gram-negative bacteria, atypical organisms, parasites, viral nucleic acids, and yeasts.

Transduction of Danger Signals by Pattern Recognition Receptors

Ligation of PRRs triggers intracellular signaling pathways that depend on MyD88 or TRIF.[15] These pathways transduce PRR signals into an inflammatory response via activation of inflammasome protein complexes[16] and by induction of inflammatory gene transcription via nuclear factor kappa-B (NF-KappaB).[17] The inflammasome is a multimeric protein complex that assembles in the cytosol following PRR signaling, cleaving precursor proteins (eg, pro- IL-1beta) into active cytokines (eg, IL-1beta).[18] These usually assist in eliminating the pathogen, resulting in resolution of the infection. However, excessive systemic activation of inflammatory pathways outside the normal homeostatic regulations may drive the host toward organ dysfunction (ie, sepsis).[19]

Amplification

The process whereby signals from pattern recognition receptors are transduced into inflammatory cytokine release results in an exponential amplification of multiple immune responses through feedback loops. A key molecule that provides exponential amplification is nuclear factor kappa B (NF-kappaB). This increases transcription of precursor proteins (eg, pro-IL-1beta), so providing further substrate for the inflammasome. The products of inflammasome activation can in turn induce further NF-kappaB activation in neighboring cells,[20] leading to a self-sustaining and amplifying inflammatory response. Conversely, a recently identified negative feedback loop involving NF-KappaB-mediated elimination of damaged mitochondria will constrain inflammasome activation.[21] A greater understanding of how these positive and negative feedback loops interact will bring crucial new insights into the processes by which inflammation spreads from the site of primary infection to the systemic manifestations that characterize sepsis.

Host Response Patterns in Sepsis

The plethora of immune responses in sepsis, mostly characterized using whole blood leukocyte transcriptome profiles, will generate two distinct immune response patterns. In pattern 1, both pro- and anti-inflammatory responses generated by innate and adaptive immune cells are present at the onset of the sepsis illness. Early deaths are thought to occur from excessive innate immune system-driven inflammation. Recovery is characterized by restoration of homeostasis in both adaptive and innate immune systems, with resolution of inflammation and recovery of immune cell paresis. In this pattern, late deaths are caused by a progressive and adaptive immune system impairment resulting in immunosuppression. This pattern of immune response in sepsis is conventional wisdom and is supported by identification of immunosuppression phenotypes in immune cells observed from the spleen and lung in patients who die from protracted sepsis. Indirect evidence supporting this hypothesis is the lack of response to anti-inflammatory therapies in all sepsis trials to date. Pattern-2 is similar to pattern-1, where both pro- and anti-inflammatory responses are activated at the onset of sepsis illness, and early deaths are also caused by an excessive, innate immune system-driven inflammation. Likewise, recovery of illness is characterized by restoration of homeostasis in both adaptive and innate immune systems, with resolution of inflammation and recovery of immune cell paresis. However, in this pattern, the late deaths are caused by intractable inflammation-induced organ injury, although immunosuppression does occur during the late phase. This pattern of immune responses is supported by observations from young patients suffering from trauma and in endotoxin-related effects in volunteers. Indirect evidence to support this pattern of response comes from pneumonia cohorts who have subclinical inflammation well beyond the acute phase assessed using IL-6 and IL-10 profiling, associated with worse survival characteristics.[22]

Cytokines and Other Mediators in Sepsis

Following detection of PAMPs from infecting pathogens and DAMPs generated secondary to tissue injury associated with the infection, the innate immune cells and the adaptive immune cells generate a plethora of pro- and anti-inflammatory cytokines that mediate the systemic responses seen in sepsis. Cytokines are small proteins (<25 kDa) released by immune cells that act in an autocrine, paracrine, and endocrine manner. Proinflammatory cytokines that are well characterized in sepsis include interleukin (IL)-1, -6, -8, and -12; tumor necrosis factor (TNF); macrophage inhibitory factor (MIF); and the interferons. Cytokines with anti-inflammatory effects include IL-4, -6 and -10, and TGF-β. Chemoattractant cytokines (chemokines) promote leukocyte migration. These have a prefix CC or CXC depending on whether there are 2 cysteine residues adjacent to each other (CC) or separated by another amino acid (CXC); they act via the receptors CCR1-9 or CXCR1-6, respectively. A summary of the likely sources and roles of cytokines and other mediators in sepsis is shown in **Table 1**.

Compartmentalization of Host Responses

The presence of systemic inflammation is pathognomonic of sepsis, yet the presence and manifestations of immune activation are not uniform across the body spaces and organs. In human sepsis, the ready accessibility to blood makes this the best understood compartment. It is also the likely conduit by which a focus of infection at one site can produce organ damage at a distant site.[70] However, the apparently

Table 1
Summary of the sources, usual function and identified roles in sepsis pathophysiology of cytokines and soluble immune mediators

Cytokine	Main Source	Normal Physiologic Role	Evidence in Sepsis
Proinflammatory			
IL-1β	Monocytes, macrophages	Immune cell proliferation and differentiation	↓Serum levels[23] and ↓monocyte mRNA Levels in septic shock[24] ↑serum levels in non-survivors[25] Levels frequently raised at tissue site of infection[26]
IL-6	T cells, macrophages	Stimulates B and T lymphocytes; has both pro- and anti-inflammatory actions	↑Serum levels vs controls[25,27] Serum levels correlate with septic shock[28] and disease severity[29] Persistently ↑serum levels associated with increased risk of death[30] Decreasing trend in serum levels associated with better prognosis[31]
IL-8	Macrophages, Endothelial cells	Promotes Granulocyte chemotaxis, induces phagocytosis, stimulates angiogenesis	↑Serum[27] and tissue[26] Levels vs controls ↑serum levels associated with increased risk of sepsis in burns[32] Persistently higher serum levels seen in patients with sepsis compared with uncomplicated infection[33] Predictor of 28-d mortality[34]
IL-12	Dendritic cells, macrophages, lymphoblastoid cells	Induces differentiation of Th1 cells from naïve T cells	↑serum levels vs controls[25] Serial increase in serum levels noted in survivors vs non-survivors[35] Impaired monocyte IL-12 production associated with increased risk of sepsis post-operatively[36]

(continued on next page)

Table 1
(continued)

Cytokine	Main Source	Normal Physiologic Role	Evidence in Sepsis
IL-17	Th17 cells	Induces synthesis of a wide variety of cytokines and chemokines	↑percentage of IL-17-producing T cells vs controls[37] May have a role in development of renal failure in septic shock[38] Animal models suggest that neutralisation of IL-17 may improves outcomes[39]
IL-18	Macrophages, monocytes	Induces production of a wide variety of cytokines and chemokines	↑serum levels vs controls[27,29] Increased plasma levels associated with poor outcome[40] May be able to distinguish between Gram-positive and -negative infections[41]
IL-33	Macrophages, mast cells, dendritic cells, endothelial cells, fibroblasts	Induces production of cytokines by eosinophils, mast cells and Th2 cells	↑serum levels vs controls[42] May contribute to sepsis-induced immunosuppression through promoting expansion of regulatory T cells[43]
TNF-α	Activated macrophages, CD4+ T cells, NK cells, neutrophils, eosinophils and mast cells	Activates inflammatory cascade	↑serum levels vs controls[27] Associated with development of renal failure[44] Potential as therapeutic target[45]
IFN-β	Monocytes, fibroblasts	Stimulates chemokine and cytokine production, activates adaptive immunity; also has some anti-inflammatory effects	Evidence of contribution to both hyperinflammatory and immunosuppressed states[46] Inhibits secretion of pro-inflammatory cytokines[47]

IFN-γ	CD4 and CD8 T cells, NK cells	Activator of macrophages Important in anti-viral immunity	↑serum levels but ↓ in septic shock[48] ↓production by NK cells[49]
GM-CSF	T cells, macrophages, mast cells	Stimulates neutrophil, monocyte and macrophage development from stem cells	↑serum levels in non-survivors[50] Potential therapeutic agent[51]
Macrophage migration inhibitory factor (MIF)	Monocytes, macrophages; endothelial/epithelial cells	Recruitment of leukocytes to sites of inflammation Inhibits immune cell apoptosis Counter-acts glucocorticoid-induced suppression of inflammatory response	↑serum levels vs controls[52] Levels correlate with mortality[53]
Monocyte chemotactic protein (MCP)-1	Macrophages, monocytes, dendritic cells	Recruits CD4 T cells, monocytes, and dendritic cells to site of inflammation	↑serum levels in non-survivors[27] May play a role in the development of liver and lung injury in sepsis[54]
Leukotrienes	Leukocytes, mast cells, neutrophils	Regulation of inflammatory mediators, neutrophil chemotaxis	↑serum levels vs controls, but ↓ production in non-survivors[55] Potential role for leukotriene inhibitors suggested by animal studies[56]

(continued on next page)

Table 1
(continued)

Cytokine	Main Source	Normal Physiologic Role	Evidence in Sepsis
Anaphylotoxins (C3a, C5a)	Plasmalytic cascade, multiple mechanisms of activation	Recruits and activates neutrophils, monocytes and macrophages	Direct role in vasodilatation and capillary leak, and recruitment of immune cells to sites of organ damage[2] Excessive levels can impair neutrophil antimicrobial responses[57]
Anti-inflammatory			
IL-1ra	Monocytes, macrophages, neutrophils, fibroblasts	Anti-inflammatory; binds IL-1 receptor and so prevents IL-1 binding	↑serum levels vs controls[58] ↑serum levels in septic shock compared with uncomplicated sepsis[59]
IL-4	Activated T cells, mast cells, basophils, eosinophils	Promotes proliferation of B and T cells. Promotes differentiation of CD4 T cells into Th2 cells. Induces release of IL-13 from macrophages.	IL-4 mRNA expression higher in sepsis survivors[60] In mouse studies blockade of IL-4 prevents shift toward Th-2 profile, and improves survival[61]
IL-10	B cells, CD4+ Th2 cells, monocytes	Inhibits synthesis of pro-inflammatory cytokines by macrophages and helper T cells	↑serum levels in sepsis vs controls,[27] and in septic shock compared with uncomplicated sepsis[27] Sustained upregulation associated with worse prognosis[62] Mediator of monocyte endotoxin tolerance[63]
IL-11	Epithelial cells, fibroblasts	Induces expression of IL-4; inhibits production of IFN-γ and IL-2	Uncertain role in human sepsis, animal studies suggest increased mRNA levels[64]

IL-13	Th2 cells	Inhibits pro-inflammatory cytokine production Associated with prolonged monocyte survival	↑serum levels in non-survivors[65] ↑serum levels in septic shock.[62] Mouse studies suggest a protective role in a model of fecal peritonitis through suppression of inflammatory cytokines in tissues[66]
IL-35	Regulatory T cells	Converts naïve T cells into regulatory T cells Stimulates proliferation of regulatory T cells	↑serum levels vs controls, with levels correlating with severity[67]
TGF-β	Macrophages, smooth muscle cells	Inhibits B cell proliferation Promotes development of CD4 T cells into Th17 cells Inhibits activated macrophages	Negative effects on T cell and NK cell function suggested by animal models[68]
Prostaglandin E₂	Macrophages, antigen-presenting cells	Inhibition of B and T cell proliferation Promotion of T cell apoptosis	Some evidence from animal studies of a role in sepsis-induced immunosuppression[69]

hyperinflammatory cytokine levels and recruitment of immune cells at the site of infection may not be reflected in the blood compartment,[71] and septic plasma may have a net immunosuppressive effect.[63] In conditions such as pneumonia[26] and abscess formation,[72] immune cell function is frequently as (if not more) impaired in cells taken from the site of infection as in cells taken from the blood compartment.

Gene transcription responses to an infective insult also vary markedly from organ to organ.[73] This is particularly the case in the lung, which is among the most common sites of secondary organ damage. In contrast to other phagocytes resident in other tissues, alveolar macrophages do not demonstrate tolerance to lipopolysaccharide.[74] Indeed, they may demonstrate enhanced TNF-alpha release following a prior insult such as trauma-haemorrhage.[75] These differential and compartmentalized responses may explain the typical patterns of infection focus and organ damage commonly seen in patients with sepsis.

How Immune Responses Become Dysregulated Remains Unclear

Identifying the mediators involved in sepsis, the sequence of events, and the points at which adaptive inflammatory responses descend into maladaptive processes is extremely challenging. Patients usually present after the septic insult is apparent. The lag time between onset and presentation is often not objectively quantifiable. As noted, blood is the most commonly studied body fluid but seldom reflects the compartmentalization and differences in regional immune responses.[26,72] Investigators are therefore obliged to rely in part on data acquired from animal models, which are imperfect guides to human disease.[76,77] It seems likely that differential regulation of the host response, by a combination of genetic, physiologic, and microbiological factors, interacts with the initial insult to trigger the systemic activation of inflammation that characterizes the early phases of sepsis. Animal models and human studies suggest an early rise in proinflammatory molecules such as IL-1 and TNF-alpha, which, in blood at least, tend to peak early (within minutes) before declining.[18] Slightly later responses involve molecules such as IL-6,[78] monocyte chemotactic proteins 1 and 2 (MCP-1 and 2),[79] and IL-8,[80] as well as anti-inflammatory molecules such as IL-10 and the soluble TNF and IL-1 receptors.[18] Later mediators include HMGB-1.[81] Interestingly, as predictors of outcome in sepsis, the magnitude of the anti-inflammatory response (as gauged by IL-10 concentrations) performs better than the proinflammatory response (as gauged by TNF-alpha, IL-1, IL-6, and IL-8).[82]

In summary, sepsis remains a clinical and biological challenge. The immune system has provided therapeutic targets and will continue to do so. Understanding how these immune response modulators will alter the amplified feedback host response loops in sepsis is necessary to inform future therapy.

REFERENCES

1. Singer M, Deutschman CS, Seymour CW, et al. The third international consensus definitions for sepsis and septic shock (Sepsis-3). JAMA 2016;315:801–23.

2. Ward PA. The dark side of C5a in sepsis. Nat Rev Immunol 2004;4:133–42.

3. Zhou JS, Friend DS, Feldweg AM, et al. Prevention of lipopolysaccharide-induced microangiopathy by gp49B1: evidence for an important role for gp49B1 expression on neutrophils. J Exp Med 2003;198:1243–51.

4. Kambas K, Markiewski MM, Pneumatikos IA, et al. C5a and TNF-alpha up-regulate the expression of tissue factor in intra-alveolar neutrophils of patients with the acute respiratory distress syndrome. J Immunol 2008;180:7368–75.

5. Wetsel RA, Kolb WP. Expression of C5a-like biological activities by the fifth component of human complement (C5) upon limited digestion with noncomplement enzymes without release of polypeptide fragments. J Exp Med 1983;157: 2029–48.

6. Rittirsch D, Flierl MA, Ward PA. Harmful molecular mechanisms in sepsis. Nat Rev Immunol 2008;8:776–87.

7. Amara U, Flierl MA, Rittirsch D, et al. Molecular intercommunication between the complement and coagulation systems. J Immunol 2010;185:5628–36.

8. Wheeler DS, Chase MA, Senft AP, et al. Extracellular Hsp72, an endogenous DAMP, is released by virally infected airway epithelial cells and activates neutrophils via Toll-like receptor (TLR)-4. Respir Res 2009;10:31.

9. Yu J, Mookherjee N, Wee K, et al. Host defense peptide LL-37, in synergy with inflammatory mediator IL-1beta, augments immune responses by multiple pathways. J Immunol 2007;179:7684–91.

10. Liu-Bryan R, Scott P, Sydlaske A, et al. Innate immunity conferred by Toll-like receptors 2 and 4 and myeloid differentiation factor 88 expression is pivotal to monosodium urate monohydrate crystal-induced inflammation. Arthritis Rheum 2005;52:2936–46.

11. Bianchi ME. DAMPs, PAMPs and alarmins: all we need to know about danger. J Leukoc Biol 2007;81:1–5.

12. Dorward DA, Lucas CD, Doherty MK, et al. Novel role for endogenous mitochondrial formylated peptide-driven formyl peptide receptor 1 signaling in acute respiratory distress syndrome. Thorax 2017 [pii:thoraxjnl-2017–210030] [Epub ahead of print].

13. Nakahira K, Kyung S-Y, Rogers AJ, et al. Circulating mitochondrial DNA in patients in the ICU as a marker of mortality: derivation and validation. PLoS Med 2013;10:e1001577. Vincent J-L, editor.

14. Kawasaki T, Kawai T. Toll-like receptor signaling pathways. Front Immunol 2014;5: 461.

15. Mogensen TH. Pathogen recognition and inflammatory signaling in innate immune defenses. Clin Microbiol Rev 2009;22:240–73.

16. Guo H, Callaway JB, Ting JP-Y. Inflammasomes: mechanism of action, role in disease, and therapeutics. Nat Med 2015;21:677–87.

17. Beutler BA. TLRs and innate immunity. Blood 2009;113:1399–407.

18. Thijs LG, Hack CE. Time course of cytokine levels in sepsis. Intensive Care Med 1995;21:S258–63.

19. Matsuda N, Hattori Y. Systemic inflammatory response syndrome (SIRS): molecular pathophysiology and gene therapy. J Pharmacol Sci 2006;101:189–98.

20. Kasza A. IL-1 and EGF regulate expression of genes important in inflammation and cancer. Cytokine 2013;62:22–33.

21. Zhong Z, Umemura A, Sanchez-Lopez E, et al. NF-κB restricts inflammasome activation via elimination of damaged mitochondria. Cell 2016;164:896–910.

22. Kellum JA, Kong L, Fink MP, et al. Understanding the inflammatory cytokine response in pneumonia and sepsis: results of the genetic and inflammatory markers of sepsis. Arch Intern Med 2007;167:1655–63.

23. Giamarellos-Bourboulis EJ, van de Veerdonk FL, Mouktaroudi M, et al. Inhibition of caspase-1 activation in Gram-negative sepsis and experimental endotoxemia. Crit Care 2011;15:R27.

24. Fahy RJ, Exline MC, Gavrilin MA, et al. Inflammasome mRNA expression in human monocytes during early septic shock. Am J Respir Crit Care Med 2008; 177:983–8.

25. Mera S, Tatulescu D, Cismaru C, et al. Multiplex cytokine profiling in patients with sepsis. APMIS 2011;119:155–63.
26. Conway Morris A, Kefala K, Wilkinson TS, et al. Diagnostic importance of pulmonary interleukin-1{beta} and interleukin-8 in ventilator-associated pneumonia. Thorax 2010;65:201–7.
27. Chaudhry H, Zhou J, Zhong Y, et al. Role of cytokines as a double-edged sword in sepsis. In Vivo 2013;27:669–84.
28. Wu H-P, Chen C-K, Chung K, et al. Serial cytokine levels in patients with severe sepsis. Inflamm Res 2009;58:385–93.
29. Feng M, Sun T, Zhao Y, et al. Detection of serum interleukin-6/10/18 levels in sepsis and its clinical significance. J Clin Lab Anal 2016;30:1037–43.
30. Gomez HG, Gonzalez SM, Londo o JM, et al. Immunological characterization of compensatory anti-inflammatory response syndrome in patients with severe sepsis. Crit Care Med 2014;42:771–80.
31. Punith K, Kumar R, Ravi Kumar VN, et al. Cytokine profile in elderly patients with sepsis. Indian J Crit Care Med 2009;13:74–8.
32. Kraft R, Herndon DN, Finnerty CC, et al. Predictive value of IL-8 for sepsis and severe infections after burn injury. Shock 2015;43:222–7.
33. Macdonald SPJ, Stone SF, Neil CL, et al. Sustained elevation of resistin, NGAL and IL-8 are associated with severe sepsis/septic shock in the emergency department. PLoS One 2014;9:e110678–9. Stover CM, ed.
34. Livaditi O, Kotanidou A, Psarra A, et al. Neutrophil CD64 expression and serum IL-8: sensitive early markers of severity and outcome in sepsis. Cytokine 2006;36: 283–90.
35. Wu H-P, Shih C-C, Lin C-Y, et al. Serial increase of IL-12 response and human leukocyte antigen-DR expression in severe sepsis survivors. Crit Care 2011;15: R224.
36. Hensler T, Heidecke CD, Hecker H, et al. Increased susceptibility to postoperative sepsis in patients with impaired monocyte IL-12 production. J Immunol 1998; 161:2655–9.
37. Colo Brunialti MK, Santos MC, Rigato O, et al. Increased percentages of T helper cells producing IL-17 and monocytes expressing markers of alternative activation in patients with sepsis. PLoS One 2012;7:e37393. Cunha-Neto E, editor.
38. Maravitsa P, Adamopoulou M, Pistiki A, et al. Systemic over-release of interleukin-17 in acute kidney injury after septic shock: clinical and experimental evidence. Immunol Lett 2016;178:68–76.
39. Flierl MA, Rittirsch D, Gao H, et al. Adverse functions of IL-17A in experimental sepsis. FASEB J 2008;22:2198–205.
40. Emmanuilidis K, Weighardt H, Matevossian E, et al. Differential regulation of systemic IL-18 and IL-12 release during postoperative sepsis: high serum IL-18 as an early predictive indicator of lethal outcome. Shock 2002;18:301–5.
41. Oberholzer A, Steckholzer U, Kurimoto M, et al. Interleukin-18 plasma levels are increased in patients with sepsis compared to severely injured patients. Shock 2001;16:411–4.
42. Xu H, Turnquist HR, Hoffman R, et al. Role of the IL-33-ST2 axis in sepsis. Mil Med Res 2017;4:3.
43. Nascimento DC, Melo PH, Pi eros AR, et al. IL-33 contributes to sepsis-induced long-term immunosuppression by expanding the regulatory T cell population. Nat Commun 2017;8:14919.

44. Xu C, Chang A, Hack BK, et al. TNF-mediated damage to glomerular endothelium is an important determinant of acute kidney injury in sepsis. Kidney Int 2014;85: 72–81.
45. Lv S, Han M, Yi R, et al. Anti-TNF-α therapy for patients with sepsis: a systematic meta-analysis. Int J Clin Pract 2014;68:520–8.
46. Rackov G, Shokri R, De Mon MÁ, et al. The role of IFN-β during the course of sepsis progression and its therapeutic potential. Front Immunol 2017;8:762–8.
47. Yoo C-H, Yeom J-H, Heo J-J, et al. Interferon gamma protects against lethal endotoxic and septic shock through SIRT1 upregulation. Sci Rep 2014;4:262–8.
48. Li J, Li M, Su L, et al. Alterations of T helper lymphocyte subpopulations in sepsis, severe sepsis, and septic shock: a prospective observational study. Inflammation 2014;38:995–1002.
49. Souza-Fonseca-Guimaraes F, Parlato M, Philippart F, et al. Toll-like receptors expression and interferon-γ production by NK cells in human sepsis. Crit Care 2012;16:R206.
50. Perry SE, Mostafa SM, Wenstone R, et al. Low plasma granulocyte-macrophage colony stimulating factor is an indicator of poor prognosis in sepsis. Intensive Care Med 2002;28:981–4.
51. Meisel C, Schefold JC, Pschowski R, et al. Granulocyte-macrophage colony-stimulating factor to reverse sepsis-associated immunosuppression: a double-blind, randomized, placebo-controlled multicenter trial. Am J Respir Crit Care Med 2009;180(7):640–8.
52. Grieb G, Merk M, Bernhagen J, et al. Macrophage migration inhibitory factor (MIF): a promising biomarker. Drug News Perspect 2010;23:257–64.
53. Bozza FA, Gomes RN, Japiassú AM, et al. Macrophage migration inhibitory factor levels correlate with fatal outcome in sepsis. Shock 2004;22:309–13.
54. Ramnath RD, Ng SW, Guglielmotti A, et al. Role of MCP-1 in endotoxemia and sepsis. Int Immunopharmacol 2008;8:810–8.
55. Baenkler M, Leykauf M, John S. Functional analysis of eicosanoids from white blood cells in sepsis and SIRS. J Physiol Pharmacol 2006;57(Suppl 12):25–33.
56. Benjamim CF, Canetti C, Cunha FQ, et al. Opposing and hierarchical roles of leu-kotrienes in local innate immune versus vascular responses in a model of sepsis. J Immunol 2005;174(3):1616–20.
57. Morris AC, Brittan M, Wilkinson TS, et al. C5a-mediated neutrophil dysfunction is RhoA-dependent and predicts infection in critically ill patients. Blood 2011;117: 5178–88.
58. Kasai T, Inada K, Takakuwa T, et al. Anti-inflammatory cytokine levels in patients with septic shock. Res Commun Mol Pathol Pharmacol 1997;98:34–42.
59. Carlyn CJ, Andersen NJ, Baltch AL, et al. Analysis of septic biomarker patterns: prognostic value in predicting septic state. Diagn Microbiol Infect Dis 2015;83: 312–8.
60. Wu H, Wu C, Chen C, et al. The interleukin-4 expression in patients with severe sepsis. J Crit Care 2008;23:519–24.
61. Song GY, Chung CS, Chaudry IH, et al. IL-4-induced activation of the Stat6 pathway contributes to the suppression of cell-mediated immunity and death in sepsis. Surgery 2000;128:133–8.
62. Bozza FA, Salluh JI, Japiassú AM, et al. Cytokine profiles as markers of disease severity in sepsis: a multiplex analysis. Crit Care 2007;11:R49.
63. Fumeaux T, Pugin JRM. Role of interleukin-10 in the intracellular sequestration of human leukocyte antigen-DR in monocytes during septic shock. Am J Respir Crit Care Med 2002;166:1475–82.

64. Chang M. Endogenous interleukin-11 expression is increased and prophylactic use of exogenous IL-11 enhances platelet recovery and improves survival during thrombocytopenia associated with experimental group B streptococcal sepsis in neonatal rats. Blood Cells Mol Dis 1996;22:57–67.

65. Collighan N, Giannoudis PV, Kourgeraki O, et al. Interleukin 13 and inflammatory markers in human sepsis. Br J Surg 2004;91:762–8.

66. Matsukawa A, Hogaboam CM, Lukacs NW, et al. Expression and contribution of endogenous IL-13 in an experimental model of sepsis. J Immunol 2000;164: 2738–44.

67. Cao J, Xu F, Lin S, et al. IL-35 is elevated in clinical and experimental sepsis and mediates inflammation. Clin Immunol 2015;161:89–95.

68. Souza-Fonseca-Guimaraes F, Parlato M, Fitting C, et al. NK cell tolerance to TLR agonists mediated by regulatory T cells after polymicrobial sepsis. J Immunol 2012;188:5850–8.

69. Brogliato AR, Antunes CA, Carvalho RS, et al. Ketoprofen impairs immunosuppression induced by severe sepsis and reveals an important role for prostaglandin E2. Shock 2012;38:620–9.

70. Cavaillon J-M, Annane D. Compartmentalization of the inflammatory response in sepsis and SIRS. J Endotoxin Res 2006;12:151–70.

71. Dehoux MS, Boutten A, Ostinelli J, et al. Compartmentalized cytokine production within the human lung in unilateral pneumonia. Am J Respir Crit Care Med 1994; 150:710–6.

72. Hart PH, Spencer LK, Nulsen MF, et al. Neutrophil activity in abscess-bearing mice: comparative studies with neutrophils isolated from peripheral blood, elicited peritoneal exudates, and abscesses. Infect Immun 1986;51:936–41.

73. Chinnaiyan AM, Huber-Lang M, Kumar-Sinha C, et al. Molecular signatures of sepsis: multiorgan gene expression profiles of systemic inflammation. Am J Pathol 2001;159:1199–209.

74. Fitting C, Dhawan S, Cavaillon J-M. Compartmentalization of tolerance to endotoxin. J Infect Dis 2004;189:1295–303.

75. Molina PE, Bagby GJ, Stahls P. Hemorrhage alters neuroendocrine, hemodynamic, and compartment-specific TNF responses to LPS. Shock 2001;16:459–65.

76. Mestas J, Hughes CCW. Of mice and not men: differences between mouse and human immunology. J Immunol 2004;172:2731–8.

77. Dyson A, Singer M. Animal models of sepsis: why does preclinical efficacy fail to translate to the clinical setting? Crit Care Med 2009;37:S30–7.

78. Damas P, Ledoux D, Nys M, et al. Cytokine serum level during severe sepsis in human IL-6 as a marker of severity. Ann Surg 1992;215:356–62.

79. Bossink AW, Paemen L, Jansen PM, et al. Plasma levels of the chemokines monocyte chemotactic proteins-1 and -2 are elevated in human sepsis. Blood 1995;86: 3841–7.

80. Hack CE, Hart M, van Schijndel RJ, et al. Interleukin-8 in sepsis: relation to shock and inflammatory mediators. Infect Immun 1992;60:2835–42.

81. Gibot S, Massin F, Cravoisy A, et al. High-mobility group box 1 protein plasma concentrations during septic shock. Intensive Care Med 2007;33:1347–53.

82. Gogos C, Kotsaki A, Pelekanou A, et al. Early alterations of the innate and adaptive immune statuses in sepsis according to the type of underlying infection. Crit Care 2010;14:R96.

Pathophysiology of Septic Shock

James A. Russell, MD[a],*, Barret Rush, MD[b], John Boyd, MD[a]

KEYWORDS

- Septic shock • Sepsis • Vasodilation • Permeability • Cardiac dysfunction
- Contractility • Nitric oxide • Cytokines

KEY POINTS

- Fundamental features of septic shock reviewed herein are vasodilation, increased permeability, hypovolemia, and ventricular dysfunction.
- Appreciation of the pathophysiology provides a basis for developing novel therapies.
- Increased permeability relates to several pathways (Slit/Robo4, vascular endothelial growth factor, angiopoietin 1 and 2/Tie2 pathway, sphingosine-1-phosphate, and heparin-binding protein), some of which are targets for therapies.

INTRODUCTION

Fundamental features of septic shock reviewed herein are vasodilation, increased permeability, hypovolemia, and ventricular dysfunction. Appreciation of the pathophysiology provides a basis for developing novel therapies.

PERIPHERAL VASODILATION

An integral feature of septic shock is hypotension.[1] Although cardiac dysfunction and hypovolemia contribute to the hypotension, loss of vascular smooth muscle reactivity causing peripheral vasodilation is the major mechanism.[1] Peripheral vasodilation occurs after the failure of normal mechanisms to vasoconstrict vascular smooth muscle. Peripheral levels of catecholamines are dramatically increased in patients with septic shock, with values correlating with sepsis severity, yet there is peripheral vasodilation indicating decreased responsiveness to natural vasoconstrictors.[2,3] There is also

Disclosure: See last page of article.
[a] Department of Medicine, Centre for Heart Lung Innovation, St. Paul's Hospital, 1081 Burrard Street, Vancouver, British Columbia V6Z 1Y6, Canada; [b] Division of Critical Care Medicine, St. Paul's Hospital, 1081 Burrard Street, Vancouver, British Columbia V6Z 1Y6, Canada
* Corresponding author. Centre for Heart Lung Innovation, Division of Critical Care Medicine, St. Paul's Hospital, 1081 Burrard Street, Vancouver, British Columbia V6Z 1Y6, Canada.
E-mail address: Jim.Russell@hli.ubc.ca

evidence of activation of the renin–angiotensin system, as well as a deficiency of vasopressin.[4] Once these regulatory mechanisms are overwhelmed, peripheral vasodilation and hypotension develop rapidly.

Vasodilation in sepsis is mediated mainly by two mechanisms: increased nitric oxide (NO) and prostacyclin synthesis. A calcium-independent NO synthase is induced by endotoxin interaction with vascular endothelial cells, leading to increased levels of NO.[5] Prostacyclin is released by endothelial cells in response to both endotoxin and inflammatory cytokines.[6,7] However, the relative role of prostaglandins in the pathophysiology of human sepsis is diminished by the lack of effect on clinical outcomes seen with ibuprofen (a prostaglandin synthesis inhibitor) in a large multicenter randomized controlled trial.[8]

Adrenomedullin is a pleiotropic vasodilating hormone and a cardiac depressant, levels of which are increased in septic shock[9] and associated with increased mortality.[9,10] Adrenomedullin blockade is a putative strategy to improve hemodynamics and outcomes of septic shock. An antiadrenomedullin antibody decreased mortality,[11] increased responsiveness to norepinephrine,[12] and improved renal function in murine cecal ligation and perforation sepsis models.[11,12]

Other mechanisms of vasodilation in sepsis have been identified recently that may be targets for future therapies. Activation of the transient receptor potential vanilloid type 4 (TRPV4) channel has been demonstrated to induce vascular leak and may be involved in the inflammatory cascade, leading to peripheral vasodilation.[13] Pharmacologic inhibition of TRPV4 signaling improved outcomes in both murine endotoxin and cecal ligation and perforation sepsis models.[14]

Norepinephrine, Epinephrine, and Phenylephrine

The cornerstone of current management of patients with vasodilatory septic shock involves the infusion of catecholamines. Norepinephrine as well as epinephrine act on both α-1 and α-2 adrenergic receptors causing vasoconstriction, as well as β-1 and β-2 receptors, increasing cardiac output. Norepinephrine is the suggested first-line agent for hypotension in septic shock, a strong recommendation based on moderate evidence.[15] Norepinephrine, and indeed virtually all vasopressors,[16] can cause excessive vasoconstriction and decrease vital organ perfusion leading to peripheral, myocardial, cerebral, and gut ischemia. Furthermore, norepinephrine has potentially adverse immune effects[17] that limit its safety in septic shock.

Although some trials show that epinephrine is comparable with norepinephrine[18] or norepinephrine plus dobutamine,[19] epinephrine use as a first-line agent is discouraged owing to concerns regarding splanchnic vasoconstriction, tachyarrhythmias, and generation of lactate that may interfere with lactate-guided resuscitation management.[15]

Phenylephrine is a pure α-agonist catecholamine vasopressor that is commonly used as a short-term vasopressor by anesthesiologists in an operative setting. There are concerns regarding splanchnic vasoconstriction leading to gut ischemia with long-term use of phenylephrine and it is not recommended for routine prolonged resuscitation of hypotension in sepsis.[15] A national US shortage of norepinephrine recently led to a natural experiment to compare outcomes of septic shock before, during, and after the shortage.[20] Phenylephrine was the most commonly used vasopressor in this shortage period, during which time a higher mortality was seen compared with the periods with an adequate norepinephrine supply.[20] This information also suggests the primacy of norepinephrine over phenylephrine as vasopressor of first choice in septic shock.

Dopamine

Dopamine acts on both α- and β-adrenergic receptors, and has additional activity on dopaminergic (DA1 and DA2) receptors that vasodilate splanchnic and renal vasculature at low doses, thereby increasing splanchnic and renal perfusion. Initially, the potentially beneficial increased renal perfusion properties of low-dose dopamine were thought to improve renal function in sepsis; however, a large randomized controlled trial found no difference in renal replacement rates, urine output, time to renal recovery, or survival in patients who received dopamine versus placebo.[21] Although dopamine has historically been used as a first-line vasopressor for septic shock, concerns about proarrhythmic properties and other adverse events have removed it from the Surviving Sepsis Guidelines.[15] De Backer and colleagues[22] reported that dopamine increased the risk of tachyarrhythmias and needed to be discontinued more often than norepinephrine. Dopamine can still be considered for select patients who are bradycardic, but routine use is not recommended.[15]

Vasopressin

Vasopressin is a nonapeptide potent vasopressor hormone released by the posterior pituitary gland in response to hypotension.[23] Vasopressin stimulates a family of receptors—V1a for vasoconstriction, V1b for stimulation of adrenocorticotrophic hormone release, V2 for antidiuretic effects, oxytocin (a vasodilator), and purinergic receptors (of limited relevance to septic shock). Vasopressin paradoxically induces synthesis of NO,[24] limiting vasopressin's vasoconstrictor actions, but preserving renal perfusion in animal models[25] and potentially contributing to vasopressin/NO-induced cardiac depression.

Activation of V1a receptors on vascular smooth muscle induces vasoconstriction via a catecholamine-independent pathway. There is a deficiency of vasopressin in septic shock and low-dose vasopressin infusion has been shown to decrease norepinephrine requirements, maintain blood pressure, and increase urine output in small cohorts of patients with septic shock.[26–28] However, a large randomized, controlled trial of vasopressin versus norepinephrine (VASST [Vasopressin and Septic Shock Trial]) found no overall difference in mortality, but a trend toward benefit with vasopressin in patients with less severe septic shock.[29] The use of vasopressin was associated with lower plasma cytokine levels,[30] especially in those patients with less severe shock. There was also a potentially beneficial interaction of vasopressin and corticosteroids in septic shock—lower mortality with the combination—perhaps because of synergistic effects on vascular responsiveness, immunity, or other actions.[31] Despite findings from VASST that vasopressin improved renal function more than norepinephrine,[32] a recent randomized, controlled trial found no difference in renal function (the primary endpoint), albeit a significantly decreased use of renal replacement therapy[33] with vasopressin. Furthermore, no outcome effect was seen on interaction with corticosteroids. Vasopressin is recommended by the Surviving Sepsis Guidelines[15] to reduce catecholamine dose or to achieve target mean arterial pressure in patients not responding to norepinephrine. Highly selective V1a receptor agonists (selepressin[34–38]) have been investigated in patients with refractory septic shock (discussed elsewhere in this article). Large pivotal, randomized, controlled trial(s) are needed to define the safety and efficacy of selepressin.

Methylene Blue

This pharmaceutical dye was traditionally used to treat methemoglobinemia or as a dye marker. Methylene blue inhibits guanylate cyclase, which prevents smooth muscle relaxation by nitrogen-based vasodilators such as NO.[39,40] Exploitation of this catecholamine-independent pathway has been used as a rescue therapy for refractory vasoplegia after cardiopulmonary bypass. There have also been observational studies in patients with refractory septic shock. Administration of methylene blue was associated with increased mean arterial pressure and decreased catecholamine requirements. Prior attempts to directly target NO synthase have been shown to be associated with higher rates of mortality in septic shock.[41] Thus, the interaction between augmentation of NO and outcomes in septic shock are likely multifactorial. Unfortunately, no large multicenter randomized trial has addressed clinical outcomes in septic shock patients receiving methylene blue, thus limiting recommendations for its use.[42]

Angiotensin II

Recent attention has focused on the potential role angiotensin II may play in refractory septic shock.[43,44] Angiotensin II is the crucial effector molecule of the renin–angiotensin hormone system and plays a major role in regulating vascular tone during hypotension. Polymorphisms of the angiotensin II receptor associated protein (AGTRAP) gene were associated with worse outcomes in patients with septic shock.[45] The recent ATHOS-3 trial (Angiotensin II for the Treatment of High-Output Shock 3) added angiotensin II or placebo to patients with refractory shock on maximum doses of conventional vasopressors.[46] Angiotensin II increased mean arterial pressure, decreased norepinephrine requirements, and improved cardiovascular organ dysfunction; mortality was not significantly lower with angiotensin II than placebo (46% vs 54%; $P = .12$).

Inotropic Agents to Complement Vasopressors in Septic Shock

The depressed cardiac contractility of septic shock is discussed elsewhere in this article. Vasopressors increase afterload and this could further decrease cardiac output in patients with septic shock, especially if they have concomitant sepsis-induced or underlying decreased cardiac contractility. Thus, inotropic agents such as dobutamine are commonly added to norepinephrine[19] and vasopressin[29,47] to increase cardiac output, but with side effects such as increased heart rate, myocardial oxygen consumption, and tachyarrhythmias.

ENDOTHELIAL INJURY, VASCULAR LEAK, AND PERMEABILITY

Endothelial injury is a near universal feature of the pathophysiology of septic shock and is mediated by cellular—mainly leukocyte mediated—and humoral mediators. Endothelial dysfunction is important in sepsis, often leading to hypotension, inadequate organ perfusion, shock, and death, in part because of acute vascular dysfunction and leakage. Sepsis activates circulating neutrophils and increases their rolling, adhesion, and diapedesis between endothelial cells to combat the infecting microorganisms in tissue. Neutrophils adherent to endothelial cells release into the tight space between the neutrophil and the endothelial cell a range of mediators including prostaglandins, reactive oxygen species, and proteases, as well as coagulation activation and coagulation-derived proteases.[1] These substances mediate endothelial dysfunction, a major phenotype of which is increased endothelial permeability.

Increased fluid balance is associated with increased mortality in septic shock. This can occur owing to either overresuscitation causing hypervolemia and increased hydrostatic pressure—an iatrogenic cause—or to increased vascular permeability such that there is increased vascular leak at normal or even decreased hydrostatic pressure. The Frank-Starling principle states that increased capillary transmural hydrostatic pressure (eg, owing to fluid overload) increases transmural fluid leak into the tissue interstitium, causing organ edema and, ultimately, organ dysfunction. Tissue edema causes pulmonary, cerebral, cardiac, and renal dysfunction in animal models of sepsis.[48–51] Furthermore, edema impairs oxygen and metabolite diffusion, changes tissue architecture, blocks capillary blood flow and lymphatic drainage, and modifies intercellular interaction.[52]

The association between tissue edema and organ dysfunction may explain why patients with sepsis and high fluid balance have worse outcomes. Increased edema impairs oxygenation and increases work of breathing (owing to pulmonary edema), intraabdominal hypertension contributes to organ (especially renal) hypoperfusion and dysfunction,[53] and cerebral edema decreases level of consciousness increasing the risk of aspiration and nosocomial pneumonia,[54] all of which increase mortality.[55]

Sepsis also causes endothelial dysfunction leading to increased vascular permeability,[56] thereby exacerbating transmural vascular leak at any given transmural hydrostatic pressure, and creating a vicious cycle: (i) sicker patients have greater increases in endothelial permeability, (ii) sicker patients have greater third space fluid losses, so they need more fluid input, and (iii) if fluid input increases transmural hydrostatic pressure even modestly, then sicker patients will have greater fluid leakage into tissues, increasing organ edema, organ dysfunction and mortality. Emerging well-defined mediators of increased permeability in sepsis include heparin-binding protein (HBP), soluble thrombomodulin, angiopoietin-2 (ANG2), and natriuretic peptides.[57–60]

The ALBIOS (Albumin Italian Outcome Sepsis) multicenter open-label randomized, controlled trial assessed supplementation of 20% albumin in 1810 adult patients with severe sepsis or septic shock.[61,62] Although no overall difference was seen between groups in the primary outcome (28-day mortality), in patients with septic shock there was a significant decrease in 90-day mortality in those receiving albumin (relative risk, 0.88). This is possibly explained by the oncotic, antiinflammatory, and NO-scavenging properties of albumin. Another hypothesis is that albumin may blunt the early fluid losses caused by increased endothelial permeability. We consider ALBIOS supportive for the concept of limiting fluid balance through limiting permeability, tissue edema, and organ dysfunction.

Therapies That Limit Increased Endothelial Permeability Could Limit Fluid Requirements and the Risk of Fluid Overload

Several pathways modulate endothelial permeability including HBP, the Slit/Robo4, vascular endothelial growth factor, the ANG1 and ANG2/Tie2 pathway, and sphingosine-1-phosphate (S1P). These pathways have been or could be targeted as potential therapies to minimize increased permeability in septic shock.

HBP increases vascular leakage in septic shock by inducing loss of endothelial barrier integrity, thereby increasing vascular permeability (**Fig. 1**). Administration of HBP in a murine model rapidly induced acute lung injury, similar to that observed after lipopolysaccharide administration.[63] The presence of heparan sulfate and chondroitin sulfate moieties on the endothelial cell surface is required for HBP-induced increased permeability.[63] HBP increases permeability through an interaction with luminal cell surface glucosaminoglycans, which then activates the protein kinase C and Rho-kinase pathways.[63] Heparins are potential inhibitors of excessive HBP-induced increased permeability.[63] HBP also increases renal tubular cell inflammation (increased IL-6) and is a marker of increased risk of acute kidney injury.[64] Thus, plasma HBP may be a marker of endothelial dysfunction and is associated with a worse prognosis in sepsis.[65,66]

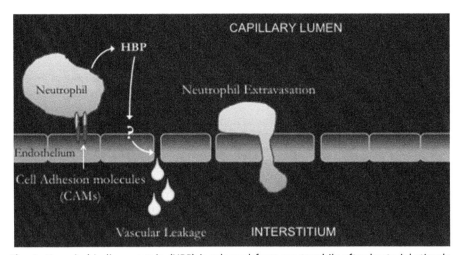

Fig. 1. Heparin-binding protein (HBP) is released from neutrophils after bacterial stimulation, binds to receptors (still unidentified), and increases endothelial cell permeability causing vascular leakage of fluid from the capillary lumen to the interstitium.

The central role of the Slit/Robo4 interaction and vascular endothelial growth factor was best shown by the observation that intervention with recombinant Slit in an endotoxin model of septic shock decreased endotoxin-induced increased permeability, mediated in part by vascular endothelial cadherin and acute mortality.[67] Vascular endothelial cadherin and p120-catenin are components of the endothelial cell junction complex that binds endothelial cells together throughout the vasculature and thus prevents increased permeability and neutrophil migration between endothelial cells into tissues. However, when the vascular endothelial cadherin/p120-catenin complex is disrupted, such as by increased vascular endothelial growth factor, the endothelial junctions are disrupted, neutrophils can migrate between endothelial cells, and vascular permeability is increased. Slit protein is protective because it acts to minimize vascular endothelial cadherin/p120-catenin disruption. Interestingly, the benefits of Slit on permeability do not depend on decreasing cytokine levels. ANG-2 blocks the Ang-1/Tie-2 interaction that stabilizes these junctions.

The balance between ANG1 and ANG2 also mediates vascular permeability, with ANG1 playing a protective role and ANG2 an injurious role. ANG1 (produced primarily by pericytes) protects against vascular leakage by constitutively maintaining interendothelial junctions and has antiinflammatory properties.[68] In contrast, ANG2 increases vascular leakage by competing with ANG1 for binding to Tie-2.[69] We showed that increased plasma ANG2 and an increase in the ANG2/ANG1 ratio are associated with increased fluid balance, organ dysfunction, and mortality in septic shock.[70] In a murine model of sepsis, the administration of ANG2 antibody attenuated lipopolysaccharide-induced hemodynamic changes and reduced mortality.[60] ANG2 inhibitors are in development in cancer; ANG2 is an angiogenesis factor important in metastatic cancer[71,72]; such ANG2 inhibitors, if safe enough, could be useful for preventing increased permeability and so decreasing organ dysfunction and mortality in septic shock.

S1P, a signaling lipid, and the S1P receptor S1PR3 also modulate and control endothelial barrier function as a protective factor and so prevent increased endothelial permeability. S1P is also an angiogenic factor maintaining endothelial cell function.[73]

S1P levels are increased in both animal models and human sepsis, and are associated with increased organ dysfunction and mortality.[74] Levels of apolipoprotein M, a carrier of S1P in plasma, are decreased in sepsis.[75] Human genetic studies also emphasize the role of S1P in sepsis: single nucleotide polymorphisms of the promoter of the S1PR3 gene (alleles −1899G and −1785C) were associated with lower plasma S1PR3 protein levels and decreased sepsis-associated acute respiratory distress syndrome risk in cohort studies.[76] S1P therapeutic targeting[77,78] has had some success in renal injury[79] and lung[73,80] injury models of sepsis showing potential benefits in septic shock. Activated protein C also had beneficial actions on the S1P pathway[81,82] but, despite early signs of efficacy[83] and clinical approval, activated protein C proved ineffective in improving outcomes in a second pivotal trial in septic shock.[84]

The vasopressin pathway may also modulate and be a target to prevent increased permeability in septic shock. The V1a receptor seems to be promising as a more specific target based on exciting preliminary preclinical studies of selective V1a agonism[85] such as by selepressin.[86,87] Selepressin decreased lung wet/dry weight, lung edema, and cumulative fluid balance to a greater extent than vasopressin in an ovine fecal peritonitis sepsis model.[35] Selepressin also lowered IL-6 and nitrite/nitrate levels with indirect beneficial effects on vascular permeability through decreasing the inflammatory response.[35] A phase IIA blinded, placebo-controlled randomized, controlled trial of selepressin versus placebo in septic shock demonstrated that selepressin lowered positive fluid balance, and led to more rapid weaning of norepinephrine.[38] A phase IIB/III randomized, controlled trial of selepressin versus placebo in human septic shock is ongoing currently and will evaluate the efficacy, safety and, specifically, potential fluid balance benefits of selepressin (NCT02508649).

Accordingly, we suggest an important and novel pathway for therapies of septic shock such as recombinant Slit protein, HBP inhibitors, and selepressin that target mediators of increased endothelial permeability and vascular leak in septic shock. These agents could mitigate limit fluid requirements and the risk of volume overload, and thereby decrease acute organ dysfunction and mortality.

HYPOVOLEMIA AND VOLUME RESUSCITATION

Patients with septic shock are almost always hypovolemic to varying extents because of obvious fluid losses (diarrhea, vomiting) or increased insensitive losses (fever, tachypnea). In addition, as described, there may be ongoing fluid losses because of redistribution of fluid from the vascular to the extravascular space owing to increased vascular permeability. Direct measurement of the degree of fluid losses is not possible; a decline in plasma radiolabeled albumin can be used to measure protein loss and implied vascular permeability,[88,89] but this is not feasible as a routine clinical tool. Hemoconcentration may be an indirect marker of such fluid redistribution, but does not address how much fluid has been redistributed.

The first step of resuscitation in septic shock is volume resuscitation to restore adequate perfusion.[15] Two ongoing controversies regarding fluids in septic shock are: (i) How much fluid is needed and how does one monitor the adequacy of fluid resuscitation? and (ii) What type of fluid?

How Much Fluid? How Does One Monitor Adequacy of Fluid Resuscitation?

The latest Surviving Sepsis Guidelines[15] recommend at least 30 mL/kg over the first 3 hours and frequent reassessment of hemodynamic status that includes clinical and noninvasive as well as invasive technology to complement clinical assessments. Dynamic assessments are recommended over static assessments.[15] The original

Rivers trial of early goal-directed therapy showed that measuring and targeting a central venous oxygen saturation of greater than 70% decreased overall fluid resuscitation volumes and decreased mortality. This study led to widespread uptake of early goal-directed therapy in clinical practice with suggestions of benefit.[90] However, 3 recent multicenter trials of early goal-directed therapy[90–92] did not validate Rivers' findings with no difference in mortality or hospital stay compared with usual care. Interestingly, these trials wanted to recruit patients early in the emergency department and so had 1000 mL fluid as one of the inclusion criteria. We[93] and others[94] have shown that increased positive fluid balance is associated with increased mortality in septic shock, and recommend caution regarding fluid resuscitation in septic shock,[95,96] targeting adequate perfusion.

What Type of Fluid?

The Surviving Sepsis Guidelines[15] recommend crystalloids should be used for initial fluid resuscitation. A weak recommendation was given for balanced solutions or normal saline (although some studies show superiority of balanced solutions) supplemented by albumin[61] if "substantial crystalloid volumes are required." Starch solutions are specifically not recommended for use because of adverse renal and mortality effects.[97,98]

MYOCARDIAL DYSFUNCTION DURING SEPTIC SHOCK: PATHOGENESIS AND THERAPY
Pathogenesis of Sepsis-Induced Cardiac Dysfunction

Cardiomyocytes are terminally differentiated cells dedicated to highly coordinated contraction, generating cardiac output and arterial pressure. This contractile function of cardiomyocytes is impacted by how they recognize and respond to danger signals (primarily bacterial cell wall components) with a complex inflammatory and functional response.[50,99–109] Within minutes of "recognizing" bacterial infection via cell membrane innate immune Toll-like receptors, cardiomyocytes secrete proinflammatory cytokines and chemokines that initiate a local inflammatory response and recruit inflammatory cells.[110–113] Cardiomyocytes concurrently express high levels of the cell surface adhesion molecule ICAM-1, which interacts first externally with newly recruited inflammatory cells and the extracellular matrix and, second, within the cell with actin filaments to reduce contractile efficiency.[106,109,114–117] Cardiomyocytes also produce 2 small calcium regulated molecules (S100A8 and S100A9) that reduce calcium flux in septic cardiac dysfunction.[118] This cardiomyocyte inflammatory program rapidly leads to decreased cardiomyocyte contractility (**Fig. 2**) through reduced calcium transients and interference with excitation–contraction coupling.

RATIONAL DIAGNOSIS OF ACUTE SEPTIC HEART FAILURE

It has been recognized since the early 1980s that sepsis can stun the heart and cause acute circulatory failure.[119] At initial presentation and before fluid resuscitation, it is not evident who will progress to acute heart failure, because patients naïve to fluids and vasopressor therapy generally present with hypotension (mean arterial pressure $\leq$65 mm Hg) and tachycardia (HR >100 bpm).[91] Once the mean arterial pressure is restored with intravenous fluids and norepinephrine, patients with heart failure, either alone or in conjunction with vasodilatory shock, might benefit from additional intervention(s).

How can the treating team reliably identify depressed cardiac contractility in patients resuscitated by fluids and vasopressors? Placement of a pulmonary arterial catheter allows invasive measurement of cardiac output and stroke volume; central

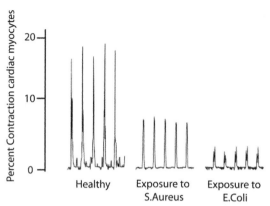

Fig. 2. Mouse cardiomyocytes normally demonstrate 18% to 20% fractional shortening upon contraction. After exposure to saturating doses of heat-killed *Staphylococcus aureus* and *Escherichia coli*, the cardiomyocytes rapidly produce ICAM-1 which disrupts the cellular cytoskeleton, and S100A8 and S100A9, which reduce calcium flux. The net result is an extreme reduction in cardiac contractility by 4 hours. (*Adapted from* Boyd JH, Mathur S, Wang Y, et al. Toll-like receptor stimulation in cardiomyocytes decreases contractility and initiates an NF-kappaB dependent inflammatory response. Cardiovasc Res 2006;72(3):384–93.)

or mixed venous oxygen saturation provides an estimate of oxygen delivery versus oxygen consumption. A low central or mixed venous oxygen saturation (<70%) reflects increased oxygen extraction, a state furthering that metabolic demand exceeds oxygen delivery[120] owing to increased demand, reduced oxygen delivery (most commonly low cardiac output; less commonly low oxygen content), or both. Logically, one would attempt to increase oxygen delivery but a strategy titrating inotropes to thermodilution-derived cardiac output or oxygen saturation did not improve either organ function or survival in a multicenter randomized, controlled trial of 762 patients with shock.[121] So-called flow-directed therapy titrating inotropic agents according to mixed venous oxygen saturation, obtained from central venous or pulmonary artery catheters, is no longer recommended because several randomized, controlled trials demonstrated either no benefit or harm.[90–92,121,122] The time, risks (related to insertion of the catheter), variability of operator-dependent thermodilution measurements over time and the lack of sensitivity and precision[123] has rendered pulmonary arterial catheter and, possibly, central venous oximetry rarely indicated.

Direct visualization of the heart by transthoracic ultrasound imaging to estimate left ventricular ejection fraction provides an immediate, noninvasive measure of ventricular performance. Importantly, if ultrasound imaging is used too early in the resuscitation process when the patient is still hypotensive, it can overestimate cardiac function owing to low afterload (low systemic vascular resistance and systemic blood pressure). Conversely, if left ventricular ejection fraction is measured before norepinephrine is begun the beneficial effect of norepinephrine-augmented preload on cardiac performance will be missed.

The effects of norepinephrine plus fluid on left ventricular performance was evaluated by ultrasound imaging in 105 patients with septic shock.[124] Thirty-four patients (32%) had a decreased left ventricular ejection fraction (≤45%). After the administration of norepinephrine, 50% of these patients increased stroke volume and improved other measures of cardiac performance in a preload-dependent fashion. This small study begins to clarify the optimal timing of ultrasound imaging, likely best done after fluid resuscitation and the initiation of vasopressors. In our own observational cohort study (n = 220) of resuscitation guided by ultrasound imaging, 25% of patients had reduced left ventricular contractility after administration of fluids and norepinephrine.[125]

Therapy for Acute Sepsis-Induced Heart Failure: Should We Reject Inotropic and Chronotropic Agents and Focus on Increasing Diastolic Filling Time?

Clinicians have generally focused on strategies that acutely increase cardiac output in patients with acute sepsis-induced cardiac dysfunction by infusing potent β-adrenergic agonists such as dobutamine, norepinephrine, dopamine, and/or epinephrine. Several large, well-conducted, randomized, controlled trials in septic shock show no differences in mortality between norepinephrine versus epinephrine,[18] norepinephrine plus dobutamine versus epinephrine,[19] vasopressin versus norepinephrine,[29,33] and dopamine versus norepinephrine,[126] but fewer tachyarrhythmias with norepinephrine versus dopamine.[127] However, we suggest that these clinical trials were all underpowered to detect feasible mortality differences.

β-Agonists have variable chronotropic and inotropic potencies so it is of great interest to compare mortality and adverse event rates. After 30 to 50 mL/kg intravenous fluid resuscitation, heart rate often decreases from about 110 to 120 bpm on presentation to about 95 to 100 bpm. Which β-agonist the clinician selects determines in part the subsequent hemodynamic changes. Dopamine and epinephrine have the greatest chronotropy, both increasing heart rate by 15% when compared with norepinephrine.[18,126,127] Despite this increased heart rate, at equipotent doses (as judged by maintenance of mean arterial pressure) and there were no differences in cardiac output. Vasopressin is recommended for norepinephrine-refractory shock[15] and facilitates so-called decatecholaminization.[34] Vasopressin, when added to norepinephrine, reduces heart rate by about 10%, an effect induced in part by a reduction of nearly 50% in norepinephrine dose as well as direct bradycardic effects of vasopressin via baroreceptors.[125] However, in VASST, the vasopressin and norepinephrine groups had similar cardiac outputs because more patients in the vasopressin group had dobutamine added to their care.[47]

What other drugs can decrease heart rate in septic shock and could be of benefit? A more impressive reduction in heart rate was seen during infusion of the ultrashort-acting β-blocker esmolol in human septic shock, with up to a 20% reduction in heart rate and suggestions of improved survival.[128] Levosimendan, a calcium-sensitizing agent, exerts its main hemodynamic effect via increased heart rate (>10% compared with norepinephrine), with either no change or a decline in stroke volume[129]; however, it did not affect outcomes compared with norepinephrine in human septic shock.

There is growing evidence that therapies that decrease heart rate may be better than therapies that increase heart rate in septic shock. Our metaanalysis of large, randomized, controlled trials of hemodynamic support during septic shock (**Fig. 3**) revealed that strategies associated with lower heart rate (vasopressin, esmolol) were either significantly associated with or trended toward improved survival and less severe adverse events (generally tachyarrhythmias). Therapies that increased heart rate (levosimendan, epinephrine, dopamine), however, trended toward decreased survival.

How could drugs that increase heart rate worsen outcomes of septic shock? In the seminal description of stress-induced cardiomyopathy owing to sudden emotional distress, the most significant abnormality was catecholamine levels (norepinephrine and epinephrine) that were, remarkably, 2- to 5-fold higher than catecholamine levels taken from patients with acute myocardial infarction.[130,131] Catecholamine levels

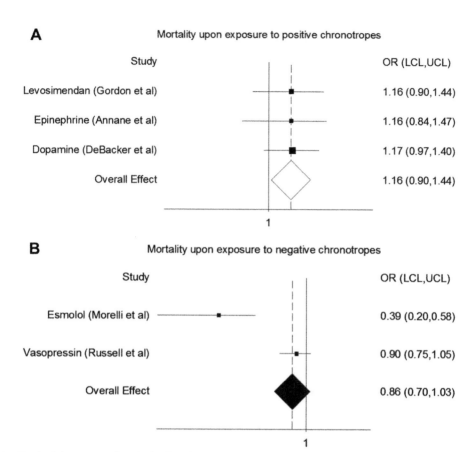

Fig. 3. (A) Compared with the first-line agent norepinephrine, dopamine, epinephrine, and levosimendan all increase heart rate during the first 24 hours by 15%. In each case, there is a trend toward higher mortality with the higher heart rate. Both dopamine and levosimendan use resulted in a large increase in tachyarrhythmias compared with norepinephrine. (B) Vasopressin resulted in a 10% reduction in heart rate during the first 24 hours, whereas esmolol resulted in a 20% decrease. LCL, lower confidence limit; UCL, upper confidence limit.

peaked on the first day at a norepinephrine equivalent dose of 3.5 ng/mL. Plasma catecholamine levels during norepinephrine infusion for septic shock ranged from 3 to 170 ng/mL.[131] Thus, it is possible, indeed likely, that an inflamed (septic) heart is injured because of the increased catecholamine-induced chronotropy and catecholamine-induced heart damage.

Therapies to Reduce Heart Rate Beyond Esmolol

An agent that decreases heart rate but does not affect cardiac contractility might have benefits in septic shock. Ivabradine is a novel agent recommended by the 2016 American Heart Association heart failure guidelines for heart rate reduction without danger of impairing contractility.[132] Ivabradine selectively acts on the I_f (funny) sodium–potassium ion current, which is most important in the sinoatrial node, is regulated by the autonomic nervous system[132] and, importantly, inhibits the sinoatrial node without altering cardiac contractility. Decreased heart rate without decreased contractility may offer a significant advantage over β-blockers during septic shock. Indeed, authors have demonstrated that ivabradine retains its potency during endotoxemia[133] and improves microcirculatory function in preclinical models of abdominal sepsis.[134] We look forward to human data as this drug becomes more widely available.

DISCLOSURE

Dr J.A. Russell reports patents owned by the University of British Columbia (UBC) that are related to PCSK9 inhibitor (s) and sepsis and related to the use of vasopressin in septic shock. Dr J.A. Russell is an inventor on these patents. Dr J.A. Russell is a founder, director, and shareholder in Cyon Therapeutics Inc (developing a sepsis therapy). Dr J.A. Russell has share options in Leading Biosciences Inc. Dr J.A. Russell is a shareholder in Molecular You Corp. Dr J.A. Russell reports receiving consulting fees from Cubist Pharmaceuticals (now owned by Merck; formerly was Trius Pharmaceuticals; developing antibiotics), Leading Biosciences (developing a sepsis therapeutic), Ferring Pharmaceuticals (manufactures vasopressin and is developing selepressin), Grifols (sells albumin), La Jolla Pharmaceuticals (developing angiotensin II; Dr J.A. Russell chairs the DSMB of a trial of angiotensin II in septic shock), CytoVale Inc (developing a sepsis diagnostic), Asahi Kesai Pharmaceuticals of America (AKPA) (developing recombinant thrombomodulin). Dr J.A. Russell reports having received an investigator-initiated grant from Grifols that is provided to and administered by UBC.

REFERENCES

1. Angus DC, van der Poll T. Severe sepsis and septic shock. N Engl J Med 2013; 369:840–51.
2. Benedict CR, Rose JA. Arterial norepinephrine changes in patients with septic shock. Circ Shock 1992;38:165–72.
3. Sylvester JT, Scharf SM, Gilbert RD, et al. Hypoxic and co hypoxia in dogs: hemodynamics, carotid reflexes, and catecholamines. Am J Physiol 1979;236: H22–8.
4. Cumming AD, Driedger AA, McDonald JW, et al. Vasoactive hormones in the renal response to systemic sepsis. Am J Kidney Dis 1988;11:23–32.
5. Cobb JP, Danner RL. Nitric oxide and septic shock. JAMA 1996;275:1192–6.
6. Zardi EM, Zardi DM, Dobrina A, et al. Prostacyclin in sepsis: a systematic review. Prostaglandins Other Lipid Mediat 2007;83:1–24.
7. Araujo AV, Ferezin CZ, Rodrigues GJ, et al. Prostacyclin, not only nitric oxide, is a mediator of the vasorelaxation induced by acetylcholine in aortas from rats submitted to cecal ligation and perforation (CLP). Vasc Pharmacol 2011;54: 44–51.
8. Bernard GR, Wheeler AP, Russell JA, et al. The effects of ibuprofen on the physiology and survival of patients with sepsis. The ibuprofen in sepsis study group. N Engl J Med 1997;336:912–8.
9. Caironi P, Latini R, Struck J, et al. Circulating biologically active adrenomedullin (bio-ADM) predicts hemodynamic support requirement and mortality during sepsis. Chest 2017. http://dx.doi.org/10.1016/j.chest.2017.03.035.
10. Lundberg OH, Bergenzaun L, Ryden J, et al. Adrenomedullin and endothelin-1 are associated with myocardial injury and death in septic shock patients. Crit Care 2016;20:178.

11. Struck J, Hein F, Karasch S, et al. Epitope specificity of anti-adrenomedullin antibodies determines efficacy of mortality reduction in a cecal ligation and puncture mouse model. Intensive Care Med Exp 2013;1:22.

12. Wagner K, Wachter U, Vogt JA, et al. Adrenomedullin binding improves catecholamine responsiveness and kidney function in resuscitated murine septic shock. Intensive Care Med Exp 2013;1:21.

13. Yin J, Michalick L, Tang C, et al. Role of transient receptor potential vanilloid 4 in neutrophil activation and acute lung injury. Am J Respir Cell Mol Biol 2016;54: 370–83.

14. Dalsgaard T, Sonkusare SK, Teuscher C, et al. Pharmacological inhibitors of TRPV4 channels reduce cytokine production, restore endothelial function and increase survival in septic mice. Sci Rep 2016;6:33841.

15. Rhodes A, Evans LE, Alhazzani W, et al. Surviving Sepsis Campaign: international guidelines for management of sepsis and septic shock: 2016. Crit Care Med 2017;45:486–552.

16. Mehta S, Granton J, Gordon AC, et al. Cardiac ischemia in patients with septic shock randomized to vasopressin or norepinephrine. Crit Care 2013;17:R117.

17. Stolk RF, van der Poll T, Angus DC, et al. Potentially inadvertent immunomodulation: norepinephrine use in sepsis. Am J Respir Crit Care Med 2016;194: 550–8.

18. Myburgh JA, Higgins A, Jovanovska A, et al. A comparison of epinephrine and norepinephrine in critically ill patients. Intensive Care Med 2008;34:2226–34.

19. Annane D, Vignon P, Renault A, et al. Norepinephrine plus dobutamine versus epinephrine alone for management of septic shock: a randomised trial. Lancet 2007;370:676–84.

20. Vail E, Gershengorn HB, Hua M, et al. Association between US norepinephrine shortage and mortality among patients with septic shock. JAMA 2017;317: 1433–42.

21. Bellomo R, Chapman M, Finfer S, et al. Low-dose dopamine in patients with early renal dysfunction: a placebo-controlled randomised trial. Lancet 2000; 356:2139–43.

22. De Backer D, Creteur J, Dubois MJ, et al. The effects of dobutamine on microcirculatory alterations in patients with septic shock are independent of its systemic effects. Crit Care Med 2006;34:403–8.

23. Aguilera G, Rabadan-Diehl C. Vasopressinergic regulation of the hypothalamic-pituitary-adrenal axis: implications for stress adaptation. Regul Pept 2000;96: 23–9.

24. Yamamoto K, Ikeda U, Okada K, et al. Arginine vasopressin increases nitric oxide synthesis in cytokine-stimulated rat cardiac myocytes. Hypertension 1997; 30:1112–20.

25. Rudichenko VM, Beierwaltes WH. Arginine vasopressin-induced renal vasodilation mediated by nitric oxide. J Vasc Res 1995;32:100–5.

26. Holmes CL, Walley KR, Chittock DR, et al. The effects of vasopressin on hemodynamics and renal function in severe septic shock: a case series. Intensive Care Med 2001;27:1416–21.

27. Malay MB, Ashton RC Jr, Landry DW, et al. Low-dose vasopressin in the treatment of vasodilatory septic shock. J Trauma 1999;47:699–703 [discussion: 703–5].

28. Patel BM, Chittock DR, Russell JA, et al. Beneficial effects of short-term vasopressin infusion during severe septic shock. Anesthesiology 2002;96:576–82.

29. Russell JA, Walley KR, Singer J, et al. Vasopressin versus norepinephrine infusion in patients with septic shock. N Engl J Med 2008;358:877–87.

30. Russell JA, Fjell C, Hsu JL, et al. Vasopressin compared with norepinephrine augments the decline of plasma cytokine levels in septic shock. Am J Respir Crit Care Med 2013;188:356–64.

31. Russell JA, Walley KR, Gordon AC, et al. Interaction of vasopressin infusion, corticosteroid treatment, and mortality of septic shock. Crit Care Med 2009; 37:811–8.

32. Gordon AC, Russell JA, Walley KR, et al. The effects of vasopressin on acute kidney injury in septic shock. Intensive Care Med 2010;36:83–91.

33. Gordon AC, Mason AJ, Thirunavukkarasu N, et al. Effect of early vasopressin vs norepinephrine on kidney failure in patients with septic shock: the VANISH randomized clinical trial. JAMA 2016;316:509–18.

34. Asfar P, Russell JA, Tuckermann J, et al. Selepressin in septic shock: a step toward decatecholaminization? Crit Care Med 2016;44:234–6.

35. He X, Su F, Taccone FS, et al. A selective V1a receptor agonist, selepressin, is superior to arginine vasopressin and to norepinephrine in ovine septic shock. Crit Care Med 2016;44:23–31.

36. Marks JA, Pascual JL. Selepressin in septic shock: sharpening the VASST effects of vasopressin? Crit Care Med 2014;42:1747–8.

37. Maybauer MO, Maybauer DM, Enkhbaatar P, et al. The selective vasopressin type 1a receptor agonist selepressin (FE 202158) blocks vascular leak in ovine severe sepsis. Crit Care Med 2014;42:e525–533.

38. Russell JA, Vincent JL, Kjolbye A, et al. Selepressin, a novel selective V1a agonist, reduces norepinephrine requirements and shortens duration of organ dysfunction in septic shock patients. Crit Care Med 2012;40:1.

39. Mayer B, Brunner F, Schmidt K. Inhibition of nitric oxide synthesis by methylene blue. Biochem Pharmacol 1993;45:367–74.

40. Marczin N, Ryan US, Catravas JD. Methylene blue inhibits nitrovasodilator- and endothelium-derived relaxing factor-induced cyclic GMP accumulation in cultured pulmonary arterial smooth muscle cells via generation of superoxide anion. J Pharmacol Exp Ther 1992;263:170–9.

41. Lopez A, Lorente JA, Steingrub J, et al. Multiple-center, randomized, placebo-controlled, double-blind study of the nitric oxide synthase inhibitor 546c88: effect on survival in patients with septic shock. Crit Care Med 2004;32:21–30.

42. Paciullo CA, McMahon Horner D, Hatton KW, et al. Methylene blue for the treatment of septic shock. Pharmacotherapy 2010;30:702–15.

43. Chawla LS, Busse L, Brasha-Mitchell E, et al. Intravenous angiotensin II for the treatment of high-output shock (ATHOS trial): a pilot study. Crit Care 2014;18: 534.

44. Correa TD, Takala J, Jakob SM. Angiotensin II in septic shock. Crit Care 2015; 19:98.

45. Nakada TA, Russell JA, Boyd JH, et al. Association of angiotensin II type 1 receptor-associated protein gene polymorphism with increased mortality in septic shock. Crit Care Med 2011;39:1641–8.

46. Khanna A, English SW, Wang XS, et al. Angiotensin ii for the treatment of vasodilatory shock. N Engl J Med 2017. http://dx.doi.org/10.1056/NEJMoa1704154.

47. Gordon AC, Wang N, Walley KR, et al. The cardiopulmonary effects of vasopressin compared with norepinephrine in septic shock. Chest 2012;142: 593–605.

48. D'Orio V, Wahlen C, Rodriguez LM, et al. Effects of intravascular volume expansion on lung fluid balance in a canine model of septic shock. Crit Care Med 1987;15:863–8.
49. Brooks HF, Moss RF, Davies NA, et al. Caecal ligation and puncture induced sepsis in the rat results in increased brain water content and perimicrovessel oedema. Metab Brain Dis 2014;29:837–43.
50. Goddard CM, Allard MF, Hogg JC, et al. Myocardial morphometric changes related to decreased contractility after endotoxin. Am J Physiol 1996;270: H1446–52.
51. Xu S, Chen YH, Tan ZX, et al. Vitamin D3 pretreatment alleviates renal oxidative stress in lipopolysaccharide-induced acute kidney injury. J Steroid Biochem Mol Biol 2015;152:133–41.
52. Prowle JR, Kirwan CJ, Bellomo R. Fluid management for the prevention and attenuation of acute kidney injury. Nat Rev Nephrol 2014;10:37–47.
53. Payen D, de Pont A, Sakr Y, et al. A positive fluid balance is associated with a worse outcome in patients with acute renal failure. Crit Care 2008;12:R74.
54. Iacobone EE. Sepsis-associated encephalopathy and its differential diagnosis. Crit Care Med 2009;37:S331–6.
55. Vincent JL, Moreno R, Takala J, et al. The SOFA (sepsis-related organ failure assessment) score to describe organ dysfunction/failure. Intensive Care Med 1996;22:707–10.
56. Khakpour S, Wilhelmsen K, Hellman J. Vascular endothelial cell Toll-like receptor pathways in sepsis. Innate Immun 2015;21:827–46.
57. Bruegger D, Schwartz L, Chappell D, et al. Release of atrial natriuretic peptide precedes shedding of the endothelial glycocalyx equally in patients undergoing on- and off-pump coronary artery bypass surgery. Basic Res Cardiol 2011;106: 1111–21.
58. Lin SM, Wang YM, Lin HC, et al. Serum thrombomodulin level relates to the clinical course of disseminated intravascular coagulation, multiorgan dysfunction syndrome, and mortality in patients with sepsis. Crit Care Med 2008;36:683–9.
59. Linder A, Christensson B, Herwald H, et al. Heparin-binding protein: an early marker of circulatory failure in sepsis. Clin Infect Dis 2009;49:1044–50.
60. Ziegler T, Horstkotte J, Schwab C, et al. Angiopoietin 2 mediates microvascular and hemodynamic alterations in sepsis. J Clin Invest 2013;123:3436–45.
61. Caironi P, Tognoni G, Masson S, et al. Albumin replacement in patients with severe sepsis or septic shock. N Engl J Med 2014;370:1412–21.
62. Lee WL, Slutsky AS. Sepsis and endothelial permeability. N Engl J Med 2010; 363:689–91.
63. Bentzer P, Fisher J, Kong HJ, et al. Heparin-binding protein is important for vascular leak in sepsis. Intensive Care Med Exp 2016;4:33.
64. Fisher J, Russell JA, Bentzer P, et al. Heparin-binding protein (HBP): a causative marker and potential target for heparin treatment of human sepsis-induced acute kidney injury. Shock 2017. http://dx.doi.org/10.1097/SHK.0000000000000862.
65. Linder A, Akesson P, Inghammar M, et al. Elevated plasma levels of heparin-binding protein in intensive care unit patients with severe sepsis and septic shock. Crit Care 2012;16:R90.
66. Mikacenic C, Hahn WO, Price BL, et al. Biomarkers of endothelial activation are associated with poor outcome in critical illness. PLoS One 2015;10:e0141251.
67. London NR, Zhu W, Bozza FA, et al. Targeting Robo4-dependent Slit signaling to survive the cytokine storm in sepsis and influenza. Sci Transl Med 2010;2: 23ra19.

68. Gamble JR, Drew J, Trezise L, et al. Angiopoietin-1 is an antipermeability and anti-inflammatory agent in vitro and targets cell junctions. Circ Res 2000;87: 603–7.
69. Roviezzo F, Tsigkos S, Kotanidou A, et al. Angiopoietin-2 causes inflammation in vivo by promoting vascular leakage. J Pharmacol Exp Ther 2005;314:738–44.
70. Fisher J, Douglas JJ, Linder A, et al. Elevated plasma angiopoietin-2 levels are associated with fluid overload, organ dysfunction, and mortality in human septic shock. Crit Care Med 2016;44:2018–27.
71. Bohn KA, Adkins CE, Nounou MI, et al. Inhibition of VEGF and angiopoietin-2 to reduce brain metastases of breast cancer burden. Front Pharmacol 2017;8:193.
72. Wu FT, Man S, Xu P, et al. Efficacy of cotargeting angiopoietin-2 and the VEGF pathway in the adjuvant postsurgical setting for early breast, colorectal, and renal cancers. Cancer Res 2016;76:6988–7000.
73. Natarajan V, Dudek SM, Jacobson JR, et al. Sphingosine-1-phosphate, FTY 720, and sphingosine-1-phosphate receptors in the pathobiology of acute lung injury. Am J Respir Cell Mol Biol 2013;49:6–17.
74. Frej C, Linder A, Happonen KE, et al. Sphingosine 1-phosphate and its carrier Apolipoprotein M in human sepsis and in Escherichia coli sepsis in baboons. J Cell Mol Med 2016;20:1170–81.
75. Kumaraswamy SB, Linder A, Akesson P, et al. Decreased plasma concentrations of Apolipoprotein M in sepsis and systemic inflammatory response syndromes. Crit Care 2012;16:R60.
76. Sun X, Ma SF, Wade MS, et al. Functional promoter variants in sphingosine 1-phosphate receptor 3 associate with susceptibility to sepsis-associated acute respiratory distress syndrome. Am J Physiol Lung Cell Mol Physiol 2013;305: L467–77.
77. Edmonds Y, Milstien S, Spiegel S. Development of small-molecule inhibitors of sphingosine-1-phosphate signaling. Pharmacol Ther 2011;132:352–60.
78. Camp SM, Chiang ET, Sun C, et al. Pulmonary endothelial cell barrier enhancement by novel fty720 analogs: methoxy-fty720, fluoro-fty720, and beta-glucuronide-fty720. Chem Phys Lipids 2015;191:16–24.
79. Wang Z, Sims CR, Patil NK, et al. Pharmacologic targeting of Sphingosine-1-Phosphate Receptor 1 improves the renal microcirculation during sepsis in the mouse. J Pharmacol Exp Ther 2015;352:61–6.
80. Murch O, Abdelrahman M, Collino M, et al. Sphingosylphosphorylcholine reduces the organ injury/dysfunction and inflammation caused by endotoxemia in the rat. Crit Care Med 2008;36:550–9.
81. Feistritzer C, Schuepbach RA, Mosnier LO, et al. Protective signaling by activated protein c is mechanistically linked to protein c activation on endothelial cells. J Biol Chem 2006;281:20077–84.
82. Finigan JH, Dudek SM, Singleton PA, et al. Activated protein c mediates novel lung endothelial barrier enhancement: role of sphingosine 1-phosphate receptor transactivation. J Biol Chem 2005;280:17286–93.
83. Bernard GR, Vincent JL, Laterre PF, et al. Efficacy and safety of recombinant human activated protein c for severe sepsis. N Engl J Med 2001;344:699–709.
84. Ranieri VM, Thompson BT, Barie PS, et al. Drotrecogin alfa (activated) in adults with septic shock. N Engl J Med 2012;366:2055–64.
85. Rehberg S, Ertmer C, Vincent JL, et al. Role of selective V1a receptor agonism in ovine septic shock. Crit Care Med 2011;39:119–25.
86. Laporte R, Kohan A, Heitzmann J, et al. Pharmacological characterization of FE 202158, a novel, potent, selective, and short-acting peptidic vasopressin v1a

receptor full agonist for the treatment of vasodilatory hypotension. J Pharmacol Exp Ther 2011;337:786–96.

87. Boucheix OB, Milano SP, Henriksson M, et al. Selepressin, a new V1a receptor agonist: hemodynamic comparison to vasopressin in dogs. Shock 2013;39: 533–8.

88. Statkevicius S, Bonnevier J, Bark BP, et al. The importance of albumin infusion rate for plasma volume expansion following major abdominal surgery - AIR: study protocol for a randomised controlled trial. Trials 2016;17:578.

89. MacRedmond R, Hollohan K, Stenstrom R, et al. Introduction of a comprehensive management protocol for severe sepsis is associated with sustained improvements in timeliness of care and survival. Qual Saf Health Care 2010; 19:e46.

90. Peake SL, Delaney A, Bailey M, et al. Goal-directed resuscitation for patients with early septic shock. N Engl J Med 2014;371:1496–506.

91. Yealy DM, Kellum JA, Huang DT, et al. A randomized trial of protocol-based care for early septic shock. N Engl J Med 2014;370:1683–93.

92. Mouncey PR, Osborn TM, Power GS, et al. Trial of early, goal-directed resuscitation for septic shock. N Engl J Med 2015;372:1301–11.

93. Boyd JH, Forbes J, Nakada TA, et al. Fluid resuscitation in septic shock: a positive fluid balance and elevated central venous pressure are associated with increased mortality. Crit Care Med 2011;39:259–65.

94. Murphy CV, Schramm GE, Doherty JA, et al. The importance of fluid management in acute lung injury secondary to septic shock. Chest 2009;136:102–9.

95. Genga K, Russell JA. Early liberal fluids for sepsis patients are harmful. Crit Care Med 2016;44:2258–62.

96. Genga KR, Russell JA. How much excess fluid impairs outcome of sepsis? Intensive Care Med 2017;43:680–2.

97. Myburgh JA, Finfer S, Bellomo R, et al. Hydroxyethyl starch or saline for fluid resuscitation in intensive care. N Engl J Med 2012;367:1901–11.

98. Perner A, Haase N, Guttormsen AB, et al. Hydroxyethyl starch 130/0.42 versus ringer's acetate in severe sepsis. N Engl J Med 2012;367:124–34.

99. Goddard CM, Poon BY, Klut ME, et al. Leukocyte activation does not mediate myocardial leukocyte retention during endotoxemia in rabbits. Am J Physiol 1998;275:H1548–57.

100. Granton JT, Goddard CM, Allard MF, et al. Leukocytes and decreased left-ventricular contractility during endotoxemia in rabbits. Am J Respir Crit Care Med 1977;155:1977–83.

101. Herbertson MJ, Werner HA, Goddard CM, et al. Anti-tumor necrosis factor-alpha prevents decreased ventricular contractility in endotoxemic pigs. Am J Respir Crit Care Med 1995;152:480–8.

102. Herbertson MJ, Werner HA, Russell JA, et al. Myocardial oxygen extraction ratio is decreased during endotoxemia in pigs. J Appl Physiol 1995;79:479–86.

103. Herbertson MJ, Werner HA, Studer W, et al. Decreased left ventricular contractility during porcine endotoxemia is not prevented by ibuprofen. Crit Care Med 1996;24:815–9.

104. Herbertson MJ, Werner HA, Walley KR. Nitric oxide synthase inhibition partially prevents decreased lv contractility during endotoxemia. Am J Physiol 1996;270: H1979–84.

105. McDonald TE, Grinman MN, Carthy CM, et al. Endotoxin infusion in rats induces apoptotic and survival pathways in hearts. Am J Physiol Heart Circ Physiol 2000; 279:H2053–61.

106. Simms MG, Walley KR. Activated macrophages decrease rat cardiac myocyte contractility: importance of ICAM-1-dependent adhesion. Am J Physiol 1999; 277:H253–60.

107. Walley KR. Mechanics and energetics of tumor necrosis factor-alpha in the left ventricle. Crit Care Med 1999;27:29–30.

108. Walley KR, Hebert PC, Wakai Y, et al. Decrease in left ventricular contractility after tumor necrosis factor-alpha infusion in dogs. J Appl Physiol 1994;76:1060–7.

109. Davani EY, Dorscheid DR, Lee CH, et al. Novel regulatory mechanism of cardiomyocyte contractility involving ICAM-1 and the cytoskeleton. Am J Physiol Heart Circ Physiol 2004;287:H1013–22.

110. Brown MA, Jones WK. NF-kappaB action in sepsis: the innate immune system and the heart. Front Biosci 2004;9:1201–17.

111. Madorin WS, Rui T, Sugimoto N, et al. Cardiac myocytes activated by septic plasma promote neutrophil transendothelial migration: role of platelet-activating factor and the chemokines LIX and KC. Circ Res 2004;94:944–51.

112. Massey KD, Strieter RM, Kunkel SL, et al. Cardiac myocytes release leukocyte-stimulating factors. Am J Physiol 1995;269:H980–7.

113. Hattori Y, Kasai K. Induction of mRNAs for ICAM-1, VCAM-1, and ELAM-1 in cultured rat cardiac myocytes and myocardium in vivo. Biochem Mol Biol Int 1997;41:979–86.

114. Niessen HW, Lagrand WK, Visser CA, et al. Upregulation of ICAM-1 on cardiomyocytes in jeopardized human myocardium during infarction. Cardiovasc Res 1999;41:603–10.

115. Niessen HW, Krijnen PA, Visser CA, et al. Intercellular adhesion molecule-1 in the heart. Ann N Y Acad Sci 2002;973:573–85.

116. Raeburn CD, Dinarello CA, Zimmerman MA, et al. Neutralization of IL-18 attenuates lipopolysaccharide-induced myocardial dysfunction. Am J Physiol Heart Circ Physiol 2002;283:H650–7.

117. Raeburn CD, Calkins CM, Zimmerman MA, et al. ICAM-1 and VCAM-1 mediate endotoxemic myocardial dysfunction independent of neutrophil accumulation. Am J Physiol Regul Integr Comp Physiol 2002;283:R477–86.

118. Boyd JH, Kan B, Roberts H, et al. S100A8 and S100A9 mediate endotoxin-induced cardiomyocyte dysfunction via the receptor for advanced glycation end products. Circ Res 2008;102:1239–46.

119. Parker MM, Shelhamer JH, Bacharach SL, et al. Profound but reversible myocardial depression in patients with septic shock. Ann Intern Med 1984;100:483–90.

120. Walley KR. Use of central venous oxygen saturation to guide therapy. Am J Respir Crit Care Med 2011;184:514–20.

121. Gattinoni L, Brazzi L, Pelosi P, et al. A trial of goal-oriented hemodynamic therapy in critically ill patients. SvO₂ collaborative group. N Engl J Med 1995;333: 1025–32.

122. Sandham JD, Hull RD, Brant RF, et al. A randomized, controlled trial of the use of pulmonary-artery catheters in high-risk surgical patients. N Engl J Med 2003; 348:5–14.

123. Stetz CW, Miller RG, Kelly GE, et al. Reliability of the thermodilution method in the determination of cardiac output in clinical practice. Am Rev Respir Dis 1982;126:1001–4.

124. Hamzaoui O, Georger JF, Monnet X, et al. Early administration of norepinephrine increases cardiac preload and cardiac output in septic patients with life-threatening hypotension. Crit Care 2010;14:R142.

125. Kanji HD, McCallum J, Sirounis D, et al. Limited echocardiography-guided therapy in subacute shock is associated with change in management and improved outcomes. J Crit Care 2014;29:700–5.
126. De Backer D, Biston P, Devriendt J, et al. Comparison of dopamine and norepinephrine in the treatment of shock. N Engl J Med 2010;362:779–89.
127. De Backer D, Creteur J, Silva E, et al. Effects of dopamine, norepinephrine, and epinephrine on the splanchnic circulation in septic shock: which is best? Crit Care Med 2003;31:1659–67.
128. Morelli A, Ertmer C, Westphal M, et al. Effect of heart rate control with esmolol on hemodynamic and clinical outcomes in patients with septic shock: a randomized clinical trial. JAMA 2013;310:1683–91.
129. Gordon AC, Perkins GD, Singer M, et al. Levosimendan for the prevention of acute organ dysfunction in sepsis. N Engl J Med 2016;375:1638–48.
130. Wittstein IS, Thiemann DR, Lima JA, et al. Neurohumoral features of myocardial stunning due to sudden emotional stress. N Engl J Med 2005;352:539–48.
131. Beloeil H, Mazoit JX, Benhamou D, et al. Norepinephrine kinetics and dynamics in septic shock and trauma patients. Br J Anaesth 2005;95:782–8.
132. Yancy CW, Jessup M, Bozkurt B, et al. 2016 ACC/AHA/HFSA focused update on new pharmacological therapy for heart failure: an update of the 2013 ACCF/AHA guideline for the management of heart failure. J Am Coll Cardiol 2016;68:1476–88.
133. Scheruebel S, Koyani CN, Hallstrom S, et al. I$_f$ blocking potency of ivabradine is preserved under elevated endotoxin levels in human atrial myocytes. J Mol Cell Cardiol 2014;72:64–73.
134. Miranda ML, Balarini MM, Balthazar DS, et al. Ivabradine attenuates the microcirculatory derangements evoked by experimental sepsis. Anesthesiology 2017;126:140–9.

Mechanisms of Organ Dysfunction in Sepsis

Rachel Pool, MD[a], Hernando Gomez, MD, MPH[b],*, John A. Kellum, MD, MCCM[b]

KEYWORDS

- Sepsis • Organ dysfunction • Microcirculation • Mitochondria • Metabolism
- Inflammation

KEY POINTS

- Organ dysfunction in sepsis involves multiple mechanisms, including endothelial and microvascular dysfunction, immune and autonomic dysregulation, and cellular metabolic reprogramming.
- Both adaptive and pathogenic responses result in decreased organ function; the clinical phenotype involves a mixture of these responses in a complex, time-dependent way.
- The concept of resistance is well engrained in medicine; but tolerance is less well understood and potentially as important, especially for the critically ill and injured.
- Multiple forms of organ crosstalk have been identified, helping to explain the multiple organ dysfunction that is characteristic of sepsis.

INTRODUCTION

Development of organ dysfunction is the most important clinical event during sepsis, as it directly relates to mortality and morbidity. Although the new definition of sepsis captures this concept, centering the clinical essence of sepsis on the development of a *'life-threatening organ dysfunction caused by a dysregulated host response to infection,'*[1] our understanding of the mechanisms by which sepsis induces organ dysfunction remains incomplete. This knowledge gap is not trivial because mortality from sepsis continues to be very high,[2] therapeutic options are limited and nonspecific, and morbidity after sepsis remains a significant burden for patients after hospital discharge.[3]

Disclosure Statement: The authors have no disclosures.
[a] Department of Anesthesiology, University of Pittsburgh Medical Center, 200 Lothrop Street, Pittsburgh, PA 15213, USA; [b] Center for Critical Care Nephrology, The CRISMA (Clinical Research, Investigation, and Systems Modeling of Acute Illness) Center, Department of Critical Care Medicine, University of Pittsburgh, 3347 Forbes Avenue, Suite 220, Pittsburgh, PA 15213, USA
* Corresponding author. Center for Critical Care Nephrology, Department of Critical Care Medicine, University of Pittsburgh School of Medicine, 3347 Forbes Avenue, Suite 220, Room 207, Pittsburgh, PA 15213.
E-mail address: gomezh@upmc.edu

Crit Care Clin 34 (2018) 63–80
http://dx.doi.org/10.1016/j.ccc.2017.08.003
0749-0704/18/© 2017 Elsevier Inc. All rights reserved.

In the past 15 years, several new concepts have shifted our understanding of what organ dysfunction means in the context of critical illness, and framed the study of possible mechanisms leading to organ dysfunction. Three of these disruptive ideas are of particular relevance here. The first is that organs can develop dysfunction during sepsis in the absence of decreased oxygen delivery,[4,5] suggesting that tissue hypoxia may not be an isolated mechanism. This explains why perfusion-targeted therapeutic efforts may surmount only to partial or to no benefit.[6] The second is that organ dysfunction can occur in the absence of significant cell death,[7–9] suggesting the lack of function is not due to structural damage but, rather, to a shut-down of usual cellular activities. This has fueled speculation that early on, organ dysfunction may be an adaptive strategy to overwhelming inflammatory injury.[10] Of course, should this process become sustained it will become maladaptive and carry the known association with poor prognosis. The third concept is the recognition that the action of the immune system against invading pathogens (also known as resistance capacity) is only part of the body's defense mechanisms against infection. Only recently was the mechanism known as Tolerance in the fields of plant ecology and biology, and defined as the capacity of the host to limit cellular and tissue injury derived from immune or pathogen action, described in mammals.[11] Findings from experimental studies demonstrating that Tolerance mechanisms can confer organ protection and a survival advantage independent of the ability of the host to control the infection (ie, Resistance), provides a framework to investigate organ dysfunction and pathways leading to adaptation versus pathology.

Re-establishing tissue perfusion has been a cornerstone of early therapeutic rescue for patients with septic shock. Microvascular and endothelial dysfunction, autonomic failure, and characteristic bioenergetic and metabolic responses at the cellular level have been observed in multiple studies. Thus, many investigators propose targeting one or more of these mechanisms to reduce the development of sepsis-induced organ dysfunction. Interestingly, some investigators, citing the potential for adaptation (albeit resulting in transient loss of function), have speculated that some of these 'pathologic' alterations (eg, bioenergetic responses) may protect organs and tissues in the long run. Therefore, the aim of this review is to examine the current understanding of these various mechanisms in sepsis and their relation to organ dysfunction. Our goals will be to explore explanatory mechanisms as well as potential therapeutic targets.

MICROVASCULAR DYSFUNCTION

An early study by De Backer and colleagues[12] demonstrated that septic patients had altered microcirculatory flow by monitoring the sublingual microcirculation with a hand-held orthogonal polarization spectral imaging technique. The characteristic findings were a decrease in the proportion of perfused vessels, an increase in the proportion of vessels with poor flow (ie, intermittent or stopped flow), capillary drop-out (a decrease in total vessel density), and an increase in the heterogeneity of blood flow distribution.[12] These findings have now been reported by multiple independent studies, and have been demonstrated in the stomach, small intestine, colon, liver and kidney in animal models.[13] Importantly, altered sublingual microcirculatory flow has been linked to organ failure and poor outcome in septic shock.[14] What is less well understood is whether these alterations represent the cause or consequence of sepsis-associated organ failure.

Mechanisms of Microvascular Dysfunction: Endothelial Injury and Loss of Autoregulation

Although the mechanisms leading to microcirculatory dysfunction in sepsis are still incompletely understood, **Fig. 1** summarizes the current conceptual framework.

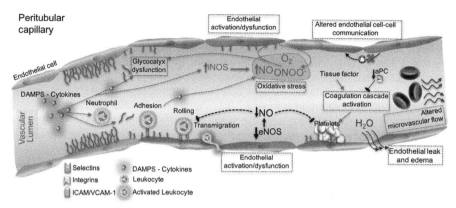

Fig. 1. Mechanisms leading to microcirculatory dysfunction: damage- and pathogen-associated molecular patterns (DAMPs and PAMPs), oxidative stress, and altered nitric oxide production contribute to endothelial dysfunction. As a result, glycocalyx denudation alters the colloid osmotic gradient between the capillary lumen and protein-rich area protected by the glycocalyx layer, leading to increased capillary leak and to increased adhesion of platelets and neutrophils. An inducible nitric oxide synthase (iNOS)–dependent decrease in endothelial nitric oxide synthase (eNOS)–derived nitric oxide production results in loss of endothelial protection via loss of direct vasodilation and loss of platelet aggregation and leukocyte activation inhibition and platelet adhesion and coagulation cascade activation in the setting of endothelial dysfunction. VCAM-1, vascular cell adhesion protein 1. (*Adapted from* Gómez H, Kellum JA. Sepsis-induced acute kidney injury. Curr Opin Crit Care 2016;22(6):546–53.)

Such mechanisms revolve around the loss of autoregulation secondary to endothelial cell injury and altered retrograde endothelial cell-cell communication[15]; impaired red blood cell deformability[16] and increased blood viscosity[17]; denudation of the glycocalyx (an organized layer of glycosaminoglycans that covers the luminal surface of the endothelium and has key biomechanical activities, including maintenance of blood flow and protection of the barrier function)[18]; platelet activation; leukocyte adhesion and rolling; and activation of the coagulation and complement systems.[19] Nitric oxide (NO) may also contribute to microcirculatory dysfunction. Sepsis is characterized by a global increase in NO production; however, the expression of one of the key catalysts of NO production, inducible NO synthase (iNOS), is heterogeneously distributed.[20] Such a distribution may parallel the heterogeneous flow patterns characteristic of septic microvascular dysfunction. Notably, selective inhibition of iNOS in sepsis has been associated with improvement in renal microcirculatory derangements and a decrease in functional renal impairment.[21] In addition, endothelial NO synthase–derived NO, which is protective of the endothelium by inhibiting cell aggregation and promoting local vasodilatation, is decreased in sepsis, contributing to microcirculatory dysfunction.[22]

Disrupted endothelial cell/glycocalyx lining results in interstitial edema, which is directly related to sepsis-induced organ failure.[23] The renal glomerular capillary endothelial cell glycocalyx seems to be particularly vulnerable to degradation in sepsis. In a cecal ligation and puncture (CLP) murine study, an increase in urinary albumin and ultrastructural changes of the glomerular filtration barrier were observed with decreased expression of syndecan-1, hyaluronic acid, and sialic acid, all significant glomerular glycocalyx components.[24] The cause of these barrier changes was linked to tumor necrosis factor (TNF)-α, as TNF administration to mice resulted in damage similar to lipopolysaccharide (LPS)-associated glomerular ultrastructural changes, whereas mice without TNF receptor-1 seemed resistant to LPS-induced changes in glomerular permeability.[25] A similar pathway of glycocalyx destruction has been observed in the lung, suggesting a common injury pathway.[26] In the lung, destruction of the alveolar endothelial glycocalyx stimulates increased endothelial cell fluid conductivity and results in pulmonary edema and sepsis-induced lung injury.[27] In the liver, sinusoidal endothelial architecture alterations have been linked to sepsis-induced hepatocellular injury and liver dysfunction. In a mouse LPS model, LPS injection resulted in loss of sieve-plate architecture of the hepatic sinusoidal endothelium, with resulting decrease in flow velocities, increase in leukocyte adhesion and sequestration, and increase in flow heterogeneity with supply/demand mismatch.[28]

Consequences of Altered Microvascular Flow

Altered microvascular flow potentially compromises tissue perfusion. Tissue perfusion depends on 2 essential characteristics: diffusion and convection. Diffusion is contingent on vessel density; as vessel density increases, the distance oxygen will need to diffuse to reach target cells decreases and vice versa. Convection depends on red blood cell velocity and hemoglobin saturation.[29] Thus, a decrease in capillary density (ie, capillary dropout) will induce tissue hypoxia by a diffusion-related mechanism, whereas a decline in the proportion of vessels with adequate flow (ie, increase in proportion of vessels with intermittent and stop flow) will induce tissue hypoxia by a convection-related mechanism. Functional capillary density (FCD), estimated as the perfused vessel density (PVD), reflects the number of small vessels (less than 20 μm) that are perfused continuously in a given area.[30] It provides a collective estimate of the derangements due to both diffusion (capillary density) and convection (capillary flow). Physiologically, a reduction in FCD/PVD reduces the surface area for capillary exchange, decreases the available oxygen for diffusion, and increases oxygen and nutrient diffusion distance.

An additional characteristic of the altered microcirculation in sepsis is the increased heterogeneity of blood flow distribution. Although heterogeneity is expected to occur in healthy individuals due to blood flow–metabolic demand coupling, sepsis induces a significant increase in the heterogeneity of flow, presumably uncoupling oxygen delivery from demand and, thus, making oxygen and nutrient delivery less efficient.[31] **Fig. 2** describes the decreased efficiency of increased heterogeneous flow relative to normal or homogeneously decreased flow conditions, specifically, the impact of cells with capillary flow in excess of demand (luxury flow) relative to cells with capillary flow too distant from perfused vessels (ie, hypoxic). The capillary oxygen saturation of perfused vessels that match metabolic demand is low in sepsis, suggesting sustained tissue uptake of delivered oxygen.[32] Because extraction is determined by metabolic demand, capillaries providing luxury flow will contribute to increased venous oxygen saturation (SvO_2). The decrease in capillary oxygen tension with an observed preservation or elevation in SvO_2 is termed the oxygen partial pressure gap; this indicates both a regional deficiency in oxygen supply and the presence of functional shunting.[33] Insufficient blood flow to match the local tissue metabolic demands is also characterized by a decrease in carbon dioxide (CO_2) washout with an increase in venous CO_2 content and partial pressure (Pco_2), resulting in an increase in the venoarterial difference of Pco_2 (Pco_2 gap). During sepsis, high Pco_2 gaps have been documented and an inverse relationship between Pco_2 gap and microcirculatory flow has been observed,[34] suggesting the presence of areas of stagnant flow with lack of removal of CO_2 or, alternatively, at risk of tissue hypoxia. Additionally, capillary leak in sepsis secondary to endothelial and glycocalyx damage limits the potential of crystalloid and colloid administration to reestablish intravascular volume and promotes interstitial

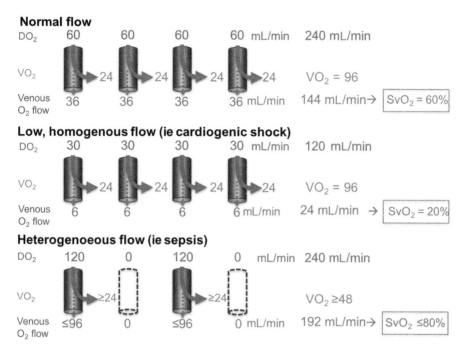

Fig. 2. Decreased efficiency of oxygen delivery with heterogeneous flow. In normal microcirculatory flow, cells extract oxygen to meet oxygen consumption (Vo_2) requirements. Homogenously decreased flow results in decreased oxygen delivery (DO_2) but preserved extraction and Vo_2, with a resulting decrease in venous oxygen saturation (SvO_2). In the presence of heterogeneous flow, despite preservation of total oxygen delivery, only a portion of capillaries is perfused. Cells too distant from perfused vessels do not receive enough oxygen to meet metabolic requirements and become hypoxic. Therefore, provided no changes in Vo_2, hypoxic regions could be found in the presence of an elevated SvO_2. (*Modified from* De Backer D, Ospina-Tascon G, Salgado D, et al. Monitoring the microcirculation in the critically ill patient: current methods and future approaches. Intensive Care Med 2010;36:1813–25; with permission.)

edema. Furthermore, interstitial edema may impair blood flow by increasing venous pressure, resulting in areas of microvascular stasis and decreased PVD.[35]

In addition to the risk of hypoxia, decreased local blood flow velocity may be associated with an amplification of the inflammation signal. In a porcine model of endotoxemia, decreased leukocyte velocity and increased leukocyte transit time were observed in areas of sluggish flow in myocardial capillaries.[36] As a prolonged transit is inherently accompanied by an increased time of exposure to cytokine-secreting leukocytes and the associated pathogen- and damage-associated molecular patterns, areas of sluggish flow show increased signs of focal oxidative stress and cellular injury. In a murine CLP model, an increase in reactive oxygen (ROS) and reactive nitrogen species (RNS) was observed within 4 hours of pathogen exposure and predominantly localized to areas of decreased or no blood flow.[37]

METABOLIC REPROGRAMING
Resistance and Tolerance

The host response against infection has been traditionally attributed to the capacity of the host's immune system to recognize, target, and eliminate foreign microbial agents with the aim to control pathogen load, a process known as resistance.[38] However, an alternative approach to pathogen defense, first described in plants but later described in mammals, is the capacity of the host to limit injury derived either from the infectious agent or from its own immune response. This process is known as tolerance and is characteristically independent of resistance.[38] For example, heme oxygenase-1 (HO-1) expression in the setting of malaria infection protects against cell-free hemoglobin-induced organ dysfunction and has been shown to improve survival independent of a persistent parasite burden.[39] Expression of HO-1 during sepsis has a similar effect, decreasing sepsis-induced acute kidney injury (AKI) and improving survival, independent of the capacity of the host to control the bacterial burden.[40] Although little is known about the specific tolerance pathways triggered to protect a host in response to different threats, this concept lends a framework to understand the potential effect of metabolic adaptations on cell and organ protection and portrays the trade-off in terms of organ dysfunction.[41]

Metabolic Reprogramming as a Cell Survival Strategy

The cellular metabolic downregulation observed in early sepsis is proposed to be adaptive with the aim to reprioritize energy consumption to limit additional injury, maintain energy balance, prevent DNA damage, and preserve cellular composition.[10,42] Hochachka and Guppy[43] proposed that cells exposed to persistent hypoxic conditions responded by decreasing O_2 demand, a mechanism called oxygen conformance. Buck and Hochachka[44] confirmed this by demonstrating that sea turtle hepatocytes downregulated energy consumption up to 10-fold in response to hypoxia, by following a hierarchical shutdown of high-energy consumptive processes, including protein synthesis, while maintaining life-sustaining processes, such as preservation of membrane potentials. Schumacker and colleagues[45] demonstrated a similar mechanism in rodent hepatocytes that, in response to chronic (but not acute) hypoxia, suppressed their respiratory rate up to 40% to 60%, demonstrating this is a conserved mechanism across species.

Therefore, transient loss of function seems to be a conserved cellular adaptive mechanism that may explain early organ dysfunction in response to sepsis. In the heart, sepsis induces a loss of contractility without cardiomyocyte death. This loss has been associated with protein downregulation and decreased activity of mitochondrial cytochrome c oxidase.[46,47] Improvement of cytochrome c oxidase activity by exogenous cytochrome c restored cardiac contractility,[47] suggesting a direct relationship between mitochondrial alterations and loss of organ function. In the lung, energy sinks, such as the sodium and chloride transporters and ATPase-linked transmembrane pumps, are inactivated and internalized during sepsis, avoiding the overtaxing use of energy, while hindering the ability of the alveolar epithelium to clear fluid from the alveolar space and resulting in pulmonary edema (**Fig. 3**).[48] In the kidney, inflammation induced by LPS or proinflammatory cytokines results in downregulation of chloride and sodium channels, the most relevant energy sinks in the tubular epithelial cell (see **Fig. 3**).[49] This mechanism has been suggested to link tubular injury and glomerular filtration in ischemia reperfusion,[50] as an increase in tubular chloride concentration (not reabsorbed because of downregulation of channels) beyond the proximal tubule activates tubuloglomerular feedback at the level of the macula densa,[51] resulting in reduced glomerular filtration rate by constriction of the afferent arteriole. However, this mechanism has yet to be demonstrated in the context of sepsis.[52] In the liver, decreased synthesis of excreted proteins and impaired transformation of exogenous and

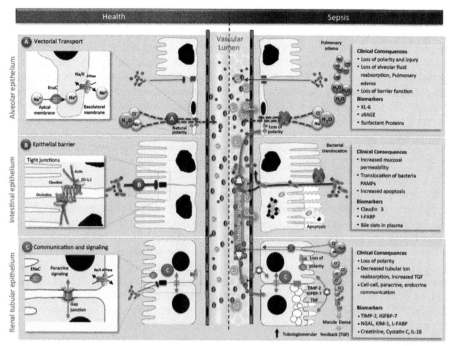

Fig. 3. Common epithelial functions in health and in sepsis. Vectorial transport in the lung becomes altered in sepsis causing loss of polarity and barrier function (*A*); epithelial barrier function in the intestine becomes impaired in sepsis causing increased permeability and bacterial translocation (*B*); and communication and signaling in the kidney becomes associated with cell-cell, paracrine, and endocrine communication in sepsis (*C*). Cl, chloride; H_2O, water; I-FABP, intestinal-fatty acid binding protein; IGFBP-7, insulinlike growth factor binding protein-7; IL-18, interleukin-18; K, potassium; KIM-1, kidney injury molecule-1; KL-6, Krebs Von den Lungen-6; Na, sodium; NGAL, neutrophil gelatinase–associated lipocalin; PAMPs, pathogen-associated molecular patterns; sRAGE, soluble receptor of advanced glycation end products; TGF, transforming growth factor; TIMP-2, tissue inhibitor of metalloproteinases-2; ZO, zonula occludens. (*From* Acute dialysis quality initiative 14. Available at: www.adqi.org. Accessed June 7, 2017; with permission.)

endogenous toxins is observed in sepsis.[53] Hotchkiss and colleagues[7] have shown that human sepsis is characterized by a paucity of cell death in several organs, with the exception of the gut, the immune system, and the spleen, where more apoptosis was found to occur relative to other organs. During sepsis, the barrier function of the gut epithelia is altered because of increased epithelial apoptosis[54] and decreased crypt proliferation,[55] which results in an increase in mucosal permeability and bacterial translocation (see **Fig. 3**).[56] Although the role of energy regulation in the induction of intestinal epithelial apoptosis is unclear, there is evidence to suggest that T CD4[+] lymphocytes confer protection from apoptosis[57]; thus, T CD4[+] apoptosis during sepsis may contribute to intestinal epithelial apoptosis. Finally, cellular metabolic reprogramming in response to sepsis may be orchestrated by several coordinated programs, including shifts in metabolic ATP generation (between oxidative phosphorylation [OXPHOS] and glycolysis), inhibition of mitochondrial respiration, activation of quality-control mitochondrial processes, and induction of cell cycle arrest.

Metabolic Reprogramming: From Oxidative Phosphorylation to Aerobic Glycolysis

The preferential oxidation of glucose through glycolysis despite the availability of oxygen (ie, aerobic glycolysis), a phenomenon known as the Warburg effect, is of particular interest. Although largely observed in cancer cells, immune cells also use this mechanism in response to inflammatory stimulation.[58] Using this mechanism, immune cells reprogram the pathways of energy generation such that housekeeping functions are sustained through OXPHOS, whereas the energy required for activation is derived from aerobic glycolysis. Furthermore, experimental models of sepsis have shown an early response characterized by a metabolic shift toward aerobic glycolysis in renal tissue of rodents exposed to CLP.[59] Despite being less energetically efficient than OXPHOS, there are at least 2 advantages of using glycolysis for activation roles. First, it allows for the production of essential structural components, such as fatty acids, amino acids, and nucleotides, while producing sufficient energy for cell survival.[60] Second, because of shunting of glycolytic intermediaries through the pentose phosphate pathway, increased glycolysis results in an increase in nicotinamide adenine dinucleotide phosphate (NADPH),[61] which is key to reducing oxidative damage from the production of mitochondrial ROS. On the other hand, failure to restore OXPHOS at later stages of experimental sepsis has been shown to perpetuate a proinflammatory state that limits organ function and survival.[62] Accordingly, multiple studies have shown that the stimulation of OXPHOS promoters in experimental sepsis was protective against organ damage and improved survival.[62–64] The shifts in cellular metabolism in inflammatory cells have been shown to be secondary to the complex interaction of important cellular regulation nodes that include the Akt/mammalian target of rapamycin complex 1 (mTORC1)/hypoxia inducible factor 1 alpha (HIF-1α) pathway driving the initial shift toward glycolysis,[65] and sirtuins (particularly Sirt1 and 6) driving the switch back to OXPHOS at a later stage (**Fig. 4**).[66]

Respiratory Electron Transport Chain Inhibition

The effect of sepsis on mitochondrial respiration and on specific electron transport chain complexes has been documented in both animal models[42] and human sepsis.[67] Complex I and IV activity of the mitochondrial electron transport chain was significantly reduced in skeletal muscle biopsies of critically ill patients, with nonsurvivors demonstrating a more profound reduction in activity and a concomitantly greater reduction in tissue ATP.[67,68] These events have also been documented in the liver in rodent models of sepsis,[42] suggesting this is not specific to skeletal muscle but rather a potentially universal mechanism. Mitochondrial complexes I and IV are susceptible to persistent inhibition by nitrosylation, a reaction facilitated by RNS, that is elevated in the setting of sepsis,[69,70] limits cell death, and, importantly, is reversible to reestablish normal organ function.

Cellular Regulation of Mitochondria: Mitophagy and Biogenesis

Increased autophagy, the cellular digestion of unnecessary or dysfunctional components, has been observed in multiple organs during the early stages of experimental sepsis[71–73] and has been documented in human sepsis.[71] Autophagy occurs during sepsis in response to Toll-like receptor 4 (TLR-4)–mediated inflammation,[74] oxidative stress,[75] and mitochondrial membrane depolarization due to uncoupled respiration from ATP production in the electron transport chain.[76] In this context, sepsis-induced inhibition of electron transport chain complexes may serve as a signaling mechanism to activate autophagy. Activation of autophagy is clinically relevant because lack of initiation of the autophagic response is associated with prolonged critical illness and lack of recovery from organ dysfunction.[77] Furthermore, pharmacologic enhancement of

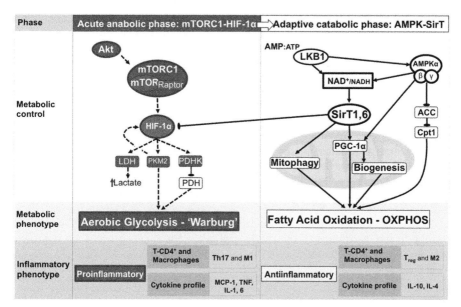

Fig. 4. Inflammation-induced metabolic shift from OXPHOS to aerobic glycolysis. In mono-cytes, the shift toward aerobic glycolysis has been attributed to the activation of HIF-1 α. This shift results in increased expression of cytoplasm glucose transporters, enhanced activity of glycolytic enzymes, expression of pyruvate kinase isoform M2 (PKM2, slows conversion of phos-phoenolpyruvate to pyruvate), and expression of pyruvate dehydrogenase kinase (PDHK, limits pyruvate entrance into Krebs cycle). A shift back to OXPHOS has been attributed to the nicotin-amide adenine dinucleotide (NAD)–dependent deacetylases (sirtuins) SirT1 and SirT6, which blocks the HIF-1α axis. ACC, acetyl CoA carboxylase; Akt, serine/threonine-specific protein ki-nase; AMP, adenosine monophosphate; ATP, adenosine triphosphate; cpt1, carnitine palmitoyl transferase; HIF-1a, hypoxia inducible factor-1 alpha; IL, interleukin; IL-1, IL-4, IL-6, and IL-10, interleukin 1, 4, 6 and 10, respectively; LDH, lactate dehydrogenase; M1, macrophage activa-tion phenotype with inflammatory functions; M2, macrophage activation phenotype with anti-inflammatory functions; MCP-1, monocyte chemoattractant protein-1; mTOR, mamma-lian target of rapamicin; mTORC1, mammalian target of rapamicin complex; NAD+/NADH, oxidized/reduced nicotinamide adenine dinucleotide; PDH, pyruvate dehydrogenase; PGC-1a, Peroxisome proliferator-activated receptor gamma coactivator 1-alpha; Sirt1,6, sirtuin 1 and 6; T-CD4+, T lymphocyte-cluster of differentiation 4; Th17, T helper 17 cell; TNF, tumor necrosis factor; Treg, regulatory T cell. (*Adapted from* Gómez H, Kellum JA, Ronco C, et al. Metabolic reprogramming and tolerance during sepsis-induced AKI. Nat Rev Nephrol 2017;13(3):143–51.)

autophagy by inhibiting mTOR with temsirolimus or epirubicin results in protection from AKI[78] and in improved survival,[79] respectively, in murine models of LPS-induced sepsis. By contrast, inhibition of autophagy by blocking vacuolar sorting protein 34 (VPS34), a central protein in promoting autophagic signaling, resulted in increased liver dysfunc-tion.[72] The autophagic response has also been suggested to be an integral mechanism of metabolic reprogramming in response to inflammation because removing dysfunc-tional mitochondria and decreasing mitochondrial mass can decrease ROS-induced injury and OXPHOS, particularly in the acute shift toward aerobic glycolysis.[41]

Mitophagy is coupled to mitochondrial biogenesis by redox pathways and TLR-9–dependent mechanisms.[80] Replenishment of the mitochondrial pool may be integral in recovery from sepsis. Accordingly, Peroxisome proliferator-activated receptor gamma coactivator 1-α (PGC-1α), a transcriptional coactivator of mitochondrial biogenesis, was shown to be increased in muscle biopsies of sepsis survivors as compared with nosurvivors.[68] Furthermore, exogenous activation of mitochondrial biogenesis with inhaled carbon monoxide during experimental sepsis was protective from hepatic injury.[81,82]

Regulation of the Cell Cycle

Mitochondria are also involved in regulation of the cell cycle[76] and may induce cell cycle arrest as a protective mechanism. In its simplest terms, the cell cycle is the progression of the cell through specific phases in preparation for cell division (including G0, G1, S, G2, and M for mitosis). During this progression, the cell seems to use specific checkpoints to verify it is ready to advance to the next stage. The G1-S checkpoint seems to be important from an energy standpoint because it is at this stage that mitochondria coalesce into a giant mesh,[83] presumably to increase energy availability for replication of DNA during G2. During these checkpoints, the cell seems to verify if it is ready to advance to the next stage. If not ready, cell cycle arrest can prevent the energetic cost of replication but can also prevent cell death in the setting of cell injury (**Fig. 5**).

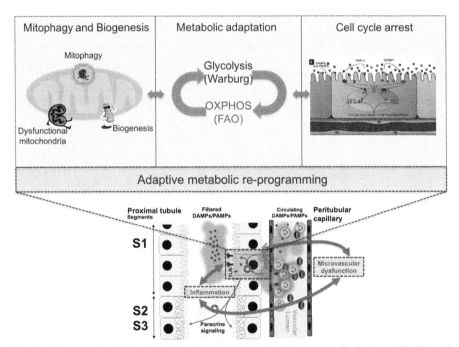

Fig. 5. Inflammation-induced metabolic reprogramming. Exposure of tubular epithelial cells to damage-associated molecular patterns (DAMPs) and pathogen-associated molecular patterns (PAMPs) leads to changes in metabolic regulation within the cell that can impact cell survival, organ function and, possibly, repair events after injury subsides. The image shows 3 possible domains of acute-phase metabolic regulation, including triggering of mitochondrial quality control processes including mitophagy and biogenesis, shifting metabolism from OXPHOS toward glycolysis, and inducing cell cycle arrest. FAO, fatty acid oxidation; IGFBP7, insulinlike growth factor-binding protein 7; OXPHOS, oxidative phosphorylation; TIMP-2, tissue inhibitor of metalloproteinases-2; TLR-4, toll-like receptor-4. (*Adapted from* Gómez H, Kellum JA. Sepsis-induced acute kidney injury. Curr Opin Crit Care 2016;22(6):546–53.)

This prevention is supported by the findings of Yang and colleagues[84] who demonstrated that G1-S cell cycle arrest was associated with AKI after CLP-induced sepsis, and recovery, with progression to G2. Interestingly, the recently approved AKI biomarkers, tissue inhibitor of metalloproteinases-2 and insulinlike growth factor-binding protein 7, are known to induce G1 cell cycle arrest. These biomarkers were superior to other markers for identifying the risk of AKI during critical illness, including sepsis.[85]

ORGAN CROSSTALK

Dysfunctional organs may impact other remote organs through complex, and incompletely understood, biological communication processes known as organ crosstalk. Kidney-brain crosstalk was observed in animal models of AKI in which local renal inflammation secondary to TNFα administration was associated with a disrupted, more permeable blood-brain barrier and activation of brain astrocytes.[86] Glial fibrillary acidic protein, a cellular marker of brain inflammation, was elevated in animal models of AKI but was not elevated in animal models of liver injury, suggesting specificity for AKI.[86] In other animal models, AKI has been associated with alterations in cerebral neurotransmitter concentrations and depletion of brain catecholamine concentrations.[87,88] Lung-brain crosstalk occurs in patients following lung injury with subsequent development of brain damage despite otherwise normal prior neurologic function.[89] This neuropathology was shown to be independent of hypoxia in a porcine model of acute lung injury in which similar levels of hypoxemia were achieved by pulmonary lavage and decreased fraction inspired oxygen, with lavage animals ultimately showing greater brain damage.[90]

Differentiating crosstalk from other inflammatory syndromes is difficult. For example, LPS-challenged rats subjected to moderate positive end expiratory pressure (7 cm H_2O) and low tidal volume ventilation showed decreased lung injury and systemic inflammation compared with rats ventilated with high tidal volumes; yet, expression of c-Fos, an early marker of neuronal activation in the brain, was similarly elevated in the same regions of the brain in both LPS and high tidal volume groups.[91,92] Inflammatory crosstalk via systemic cytokines between the kidney and lungs has been observed in preclinical and clinical studies with ventilator-induced lung injury (VILI) associated with high tidal volume mechanical ventilation contributing to the development of AKI.[93] There seems to be a unique pattern of renal inflammation in kidney-lung crosstalk. A mouse model of AKI with subgroups exposed to CLP, VILI, and sham demonstrated an elevation in vascular endothelial growth factor, an angiogenic and endothelium activating protein, and vascular cell adhesion protein 1, a leukocyte adhesion molecule, in only those animals within the VILI subgroup.[94] In a murine model of AKI and bacterial pneumonia, AKI alone did not cause clinically significant acute lung injury; however, in the setting of bacterial pneumonia, AKI did attenuate pulmonary neutrophil recruitment and increase bacterial load with resulting compromised oxygenation.[95]

Although not solid organs, the coagulation and complement systems influence each other through interrelated pathways in the setting of sepsis. This relationship is observed in early sepsis with coinciding robust complement activation and the potential for disseminated intravascular coagulation. Complement end products increase thrombogenicity of the blood, induce procoagulant and antifibrinolytic proteins, and inhibit anticoagulant pathways.[96,97] C3 convertase inhibition in bacteria-induced sepsis in baboons prevented sepsis-induced complement activation, decreased thrombocytopenia and coagulopathy, and preserved endothelial anticoagulant properties.[98] Coagulation factors also impact complement activation. Thrombin and coagulation factor Xa directly activate components of the complement cascade[99]; protein C inhibits complement activation,[100] and coagulation factor XIIa directly activates the classic complement pathway.[101]

Autonomic Nervous System

A conceptual extension of this crosstalk involves communication between the autonomic nervous system and immune system in the setting of inflammation. Increased circulating catecholamines in early sepsis enhances the initial inflammatory response. In addition to autonomic neurons, leukocytes can synthesize catecholamines[102] and express adrenergic receptors, demonstrating neurotransmitter-influenced lymphocytic trafficking, vascular perfusion, and immune cellular proliferation and apoptosis.[103] Furthermore, portal venous drainage of gut-derived catecholamines can alter the functional state of the liver Kupffer cells and hepatocytes through α_2-adrenergic receptor signaling.[104,105]

Vagus afferents stimulated by cytokines and inflammatory molecules promote vagal nerve efferent cholinergic signaling, inhibiting the excessive release of TNF and other proinflammatory cytokines.[106] This cholinergic signaling is communicated via α-7 nicotinic acetylcholine receptors found on macrophages and other immune cells.[107] This inflammatory reflex for excessive proinflammatory signaling also extends to efferent vagal communication with the splenic nerve.[108] Vagal nerve stimulation 24 hours after CLP-induced sepsis in a murine model improved survival.[109] On the other hand, vagotomy was associated with increased proinflammatory cytokine levels in endotoxemic animals.[106]

SUMMARY

Sepsis is a complex syndrome characterized by significant clinical heterogeneity, in which morbidity and mortality are driven by organ dysfunction. Importantly, organ dysfunction in sepsis is now recognized to be more than just the consequence of decreased tissue oxygen delivery and instead involves multiple responses to inflammation, including endothelial and microvascular dysfunction, immune and autonomic dysregulation, and cellular metabolic reprogramming. Experimental data suggest that targeting these mechanisms may result in organ protection and offer survival advantage. However, it also underscores that the effect of targeting these mechanistic pathways on short- and long-term outcomes depends highly on the timing of therapeutic intervention. In moving forward, efforts to understand the adaptive or maladaptive character of these mechanisms, to discover phase-specific biomarkers to guide therapy and to conceptualize these mechanisms in terms of resistance and tolerance will provide a structured research platform, a translational gateway, and an opportunity to improve patient outcomes.

REFERENCES

1. Singer M, Deutschman CS, Seymour CW, et al. The third international consensus definitions for sepsis and septic shock (sepsis-3). JAMA 2016;315: 801–10.
2. Angus DC, van der Poll T. Severe sepsis and septic shock. N Engl J Med 2013; 369:840–51.
3. Yende S, Iwashyna TJ, Angus DC. Interplay between sepsis and chronic health. Trends Mol Med 2014;20:234–8.
4. Langenberg C, Wan L, Egi M, et al. Renal blood flow in experimental septic acute renal failure. Kidney Int 2006;69:1996–2002.

5. Prowle JR, Ishikawa K, May CN, et al. Renal blood flow during acute renal failure in man. Blood Purif 2009;28:216–25.
6. The ProCESS Investigators. A randomized trial of protocol-based care for early septic shock. N Engl J Med 2014;370:1683–93.
7. Hotchkiss RS, Swanson PE, Freeman BD, et al. Apoptotic cell death in patients with sepsis, shock, and multiple organ dysfunction. Crit Care Med 1999;27: 1230–51.
8. Takasu O, Gaut JP, Watanabe E, et al. Mechanisms of cardiac and renal dysfunction in patients dying of sepsis. Am J Respir Crit Care Med 2013;187: 509–17.
9. Lerolle N, Nochy D, Guerot E, et al. Histopathology of septic shock induced acute kidney injury: apoptosis and leukocytic infiltration. Intensive Care Med 2010;36:471–80.
10. Singer M, De Santis V, Vitale D, et al. Multiorgan failure is an adaptive, endocrine-mediated, metabolic response to overwhelming systemic inflammation. Lancet 2004;364:545–8.
11. Råberg L, Sim D, Read AF. Disentangling genetic variation for resistance and tolerance to infectious diseases in animals. Science 2007;318:812–4.
12. De Backer D, Creteur J, Preiser JC, et al. Microvascular blood flow is altered in patients with sepsis. Am J Respir Crit Care Med 2002;166:98–104.
13. Krejci V, Hiltebrand L, Banic A, et al. Continuous measurements of microcirculatory blood flow in gastrointestinal organs during acute haemorrhage. Br J Anaesth 2000;84:468–75.
14. Sakr Y, Dubois MJ, De Backer D, et al. Persistent microcirculatory alterations are associated with organ failure and death in patients with septic shock. Crit Care Med 2004;32:1825–31.
15. Tyml K, Wang X, Lidington D, et al. Lipopolysaccharide reduces intercellular coupling in vitro and arteriolar conducted response in vivo. Am J Physiol Heart Circ Physiol 2001;281:H1397–406.
16. Katz SD, Khan T, Zeballos GA, et al. Decreased activity of the N-arginine–nitric oxide metabolic pathway in patients with congestive heart failure. Circulation 1999;99:2113–7.
17. Astiz ME, DeGent GE, Lin RY, et al. Microvascular function and rheologic changes in hyperdynamic sepsis. Crit Care Med 1995;23:265–71.
18. Weinbaum S, Tarbell JM, Damiano ER. The structure and function of the endothelial glycocalyx layer. Annu Rev Biomed Eng 2007;9:121–67.
19. De Backer D, Donadello K, Taccone FS, et al. Microcirculatory alterations: potential mechanisms and implications for therapy. Ann Intensive Care 2011;1:27.
20. Cunha FQ, Assreuy J, Moss DW, et al. Differential induction of nitric oxide synthase in various organs of the mouse during endotoxaemia: role of TNF-alpha and IL-1-beta. Immunology 1994;81:211–5.
21. Tiwari MM, Brock RW, Megyesi JK, et al. Disruption of renal peritubular blood flow in lipopolysaccharide-induced renal failure: role of nitric oxide and caspases. Am J Physiol Renal Physiol 2005;289:F1324–32.
22. Ince C, Mayeux PR, Nguyen T, et al. The endothelium in sepsis. Shock 2016;45: 259–70.
23. Rubio-Gayosso I, Platts SH, Duling BR. Reactive oxygen species mediate modification of glycocalyx during ischemia-reperfusion injury. Am J Physiol Heart Circ Physiol 2006;290:H2247–56.

24. Adembri C, Sgambati E, Vitali L, et al. Sepsis induces albuminuria and alterations in the glomerular filtration barrier: a morphofunctional study in the rat. Crit Care 2011;15:R277.
25. Xu C, Chang A, Hack BK, et al. TNF-mediated damage to glomerular endothelium is an important determinant of acute kidney injury in sepsis. Kidney Int 2014;85:72–81.
26. Schmidt EP, Yang Y, Janssen WJ, et al. The pulmonary endothelial glycocalyx regulates neutrophil adhesion and lung injury during experimental sepsis. Nat Med 2012;18:1217–23.
27. Maniatis NA, Orfanos SE. The endothelium in acute lung injury/acute respiratory distress syndrome. Curr Opin Crit Care 2008;14:22–30.
28. Ito Y, Abril ER, Bethea NW, et al. Mechanisms and pathophysiological implications of sinusoidal endothelial cell gap formation following treatment with galactosamine/endotoxin in mice. Am J Physiol Gastrointest Liver Physiol 2006;291: G211–8.
29. Ince C. The rationale for microcirculatory-guided fluid therapy. Curr Opin Crit Care 2014;20:301–8.
30. De Backer D, Hollenberg S, Boerma C, et al. How to evaluate the microcirculation: report of a round table conference. Crit Care 2007;11(5):R101.
31. Goldman D, Bateman RM, Ellis CG. Effect of decreased O2 supply on skeletal muscle oxygenation and O2 consumption during sepsis: role of heterogeneous capillary spacing and blood flow. Am J Physiol Heart Circ Physiol 2006;290: H2277–85.
32. Ellis CG, Bateman RM, Sharpe MD, et al. Effect of a maldistribution of microvascular blood flow on capillary O_2 extraction in sepsis. Am J Physiol Heart Circ Physiol 2002;282:H156–64.
33. Ince C, Sinaasappel M. Microcirculatory oxygenation and shunting in sepsis and shock. Crit Care Med 1999;27:1369–77.
34. De Backer D, Creteur J, Dubois MJ, et al. The effects of dobutamine on microcirculatory alterations in patients with septic shock are independent of its systemic effects. Crit Care Med 2006;34:403–8.
35. Rajendram R, Prowle JR. Venous congestion: are we adding insult to kidney injury in sepsis? Crit Care 2014;18:104.
36. Goddard CM, Allard MF, Hogg JC, et al. Prolonged leukocyte transit time in coronary microcirculation of endotoxemic pigs. Am J Physiol 1995;269(4 Pt 2): H1389–97.
37. Wang Z, Holthoff JH, Seely KA, et al. Development of oxidative stress in the peritubular capillary microenvironment mediates sepsis-induced renal microcirculatory failure and acute kidney injury. Am J Pathol 2012;180:505–16.
38. Schneider DS, Ayres JS. Two ways to survive infection: what resistance and tolerance can teach us about treating infectious diseases. Nat Rev Immunol 2008;8:889–95.
39. Ferreira A, Balla J, Jeney V, et al. A central role for free heme in the pathogenesis of severe malaria: the missing link? J Mol Med 2008;86:1097–111.
40. Larsen R, Gozzelino R, Jeney V, et al. A central role for free heme in the pathogenesis of severe sepsis. Sci Transl Med 2010;2:51ra71.
41. Gomez H, Kellum JA, Ronco C. Metabolic reprogramming and tolerance during sepsis-induced AKI. Nat Rev Nephrol 2017;13:143–51.
42. Brealey D, Karyampudi S, Jacques TS, et al. Mitochondrial dysfunction in a long-term rodent model of sepsis and organ failure. Am J Physiol Regul Integr Comp Physiol 2004;286:R491–7.

43. Hochachka PW, Guppy M. Animal anaerobes. In: Hochachka PW, Guppy M, editors. Metabolic arrest and the control of biological time. Cambridge (MA): Harvard Univ Press; 1987. p. 10–35.

44. Buck LT, Hochachka PW. Anoxic suppression of Na^+-K^+-ATPase and constant membrane potential in hepatocytes: support for channel arrest. Am J Physiol 1993;265(5 Pt 2):R1020–5.

45. Schumacker PT, Chandel N, Agusti AG. Oxygen conformance of cellular respiration in hepatocytes. Am J Physiol 1993;265(4 Pt 1):L395–402.

46. Levy RJ, Piel DA, Acton PD, et al. Evidence of myocardial hibernation in the septic heart. Crit Care Med 2005;33:2752–6.

47. Piel DA, Gruber PJ, Weinheimer CJ, et al. Mitochondrial resuscitation with exogenous cytochrome c in the septic heart. Crit Care Med 2007;35:2120–7.

48. Vadasz I, Dada LA, Briva A, et al. AMP-activated protein kinase regulates CO2-induced alveolar epithelial dysfunction in rats and humans by promoting Na,K-ATPase endocytosis. J Clin Invest 2008;118:752–62.

49. Schmidt C, Hocherl K, Schweda F, et al. Proinflammatory cytokines cause downregulation of renal chloride entry pathways during sepsis. Crit Care Med 2007; 35:2110–9.

50. Singh P, Blantz RC, Rosenberger C, et al. Aberrant tubuloglomerular feedback and HIF-1a confer resistance to ischemia after subtotal nephrectomy. J Am Soc Nephrol 2012;23:483–93.

51. Schnermann J, Ploth DW, Hermle M. Activation of tubule-glomerular feedback by chloride transport. Pflugers Arch 1976;362:229–40.

52. Matejovic M, Ince C, Chawla LS, et al. Renal hemodynamics in AKI: in search of new treatment targets. J Am Soc Nephrol 2016;27:49–58.

53. Kim PK, Chen J, Andrejko KM, et al. Intraabdominal sepsis down-regulates transcription of sodium taurocholate cotransporter and multidrug resistance-associated protein in rats. Shock 2000;14:176–81.

54. Perrone EE, Jung E, Breed E, et al. Mechanisms of methicillin-resistant Staphylococcus aureus pneumonia-induced intestinal epithelial apoptosis. Shock 2012;38:68–75.

55. Coopersmith CM, Stromberg PE, Davis CG, et al. Sepsis from Pseudomonas aeruginosa pneumonia decreases intestinal proliferation and induces gut epithelial cell cycle arrest. Crit Care Med 2003;31:1630–7.

56. Meng M, Klingensmith NJ, Coopersmith CM. New insights into the gut as the driver of critical illness and organ failure. Curr Opin Crit Care 2017;23:143–8.

57. Stromberg PE, Woolsey CA, Clark AT, et al. CD4+ lymphocytes control gut epithelial apoptosis and mediate survival in sepsis. FASEB J 2009;23:1817–25.

58. Frauwirth KA, Riley JL, Harris MH, et al. The CD28 signaling pathway regulates glucose metabolism. Immunity 2002;16:769–77.

59. Waltz P, Carchman E, Gomez H, et al. Sepsis results in an altered renal metabolic and osmolyte profile. J Surg Res 2016;202:8–12.

60. Vander Heiden MG, Cantley LC, Thompson CB. Understanding the Warburg effect: the metabolic requirements of cell proliferation. Science 2009;324: 1029–33.

61. Patra KC, Hay N. The pentose phosphate pathway and cancer. Trends Biochem Sci 2014;39:347–54.

62. Yang L, Xie M, Yang M, et al. PKM2 regulates the Warburg effect and promotes HMGB1 release in sepsis. Nat Commun 2014;5:4436.

63. Opal S, Ellis JL, Suri V, et al. Sirt1 activation markedly alters transcription profiles and improves outcome in experimental sepsis. Shock 2016;45:411–8.

64. Vachharajani VT, Liu T, Brown CM, et al. SIRT1 inhibition during the hypoinflammatory phenotype of sepsis enhances immunity and improves outcome. J Leukoc Biol 2014;96:785–96.
65. Cheng SC, Quintin J, Cramer RA, et al. mTOR- and HIF-1-mediated aerobic glycolysis as metabolic basis for trained immunity. Science 2014;345:1250684.
66. Liu TF, Vachharajani VT, Yoza BK, et al. NAD$^+$ dependent Sirtuin 1 and 6 proteins coordinate a switch from glucose to fatty acid oxidation during the acute inflammatory response. J Biol Chem 2012;287:25758–69.
67. Brealey D, Brand M, Hargreaves I, et al. Association between mitochondrial dysfunction and severity and outcome of septic shock. Lancet 2002;360:219–23.
68. Carré JE, Orban JC, Re L, et al. Survival in critical illness is associated with early activation of mitochondrial biogenesis. Am J Respir Crit Care Med 2010;182:745–51.
69. Cuzzocrea S, Mazzon E, Di Paola R, et al. A role for nitric oxide-mediated peroxynitrite formation in a model of endotoxin-induced shock. J Pharmacol Exp Ther 2006;319:73–81.
70. Beltran B, Orsi A, Clementi E, et al. Oxidative stress and S-nitrosylation of proteins in cells. Br J Pharmacol 2000;129:953–60.
71. Watanabe E, Muenzer JT, Hawkins WG, et al. Sepsis induces extensive autophagic vacuolization in hepatocytes: a clinical and laboratory-based study. Lab Invest 2009;89:549–61.
72. Carchman EH, Rao J, Loughran PA, et al. Heme oxygenase-1-mediated autophagy protects against hepatocyte cell death and hepatic injury from infection/sepsis in mice. Hepatology 2011;53:2053–62.
73. Hsiao HW, Tsai KL, Wang LF, et al. The decline of autophagy contributes to proximal tubular dysfunction during sepsis. Shock 2012;37:289–96.
74. Waltz P, Carchman EH, Young AC, et al. Lipopolysaccharide induces autophagic signaling in macrophages via a TLR4, heme oxygenase-1 dependent pathway. Autophagy 2011;7:315–20.
75. Frank M, Duvezin-Caubet S, Koob S, et al. Mitophagy is triggered by mild oxidative stress in a mitochondrial fission dependent manner. Biochim Biophys Acta 2012;1823:2297–310.
76. Green DR, Galluzzi L, Kroemer G. Mitochondria and the autophagy-inflammation-cell death axis in organismal aging. Science 2011;333:1109–12.
77. Vanhorebeek I, Gunst J, Derde S, et al. Insufficient activation of autophagy allows cellular damage to accumulate in critically ill patients. J Clin Endocrinol Metab 2011;96:E633–45.
78. Howell GM, Gomez H, Collage RD, et al. Augmenting autophagy to treat acute kidney injury during endotoxemia in mice. PLoS One 2013;8:e69520.
79. Figueiredo N, Chora A, Raquel H, et al. Anthracyclines induce DNA damage response-mediated protection against severe sepsis. Immunity 2013;39:874–84.
80. Carchman EH, Whelan S, Loughran P, et al. Experimental sepsis-induced mitochondrial biogenesis is dependent on autophagy, TLR4, and TLR9 signaling in liver. FASEB J 2013;27:4703–11.
81. Fredriksson K, Hammarqvist F, Strigard K, et al. Derangements in mitochondrial metabolism in intercostal and leg muscle of critically ill patients with sepsis-induced multiple organ failure. Am J Physiol 2006;291:E1044–50.
82. MacGarvey NC, Suliman HB, Bartz RR, et al. Activation of mitochondrial biogenesis by heme oxygenase-1-mediated NF-E2-related factor-2 induction rescues

mice from lethal Staphylococcus aureus sepsis. Am J Respir Crit Care Med 2012;185(8):851–61.

83. Mitra K, Wunder C, Roysam B, et al. A hyperfused mitochondrial state achieved at G1-S regulates cyclin E buildup and entry into S phase. Proc Natl Acad Sci U S A 2009;106:11960–5.

84. Yang QH, Liu DW, Long Y, et al. Acute renal failure during sepsis: potential role of cell cycle regulation. J Infect 2009;58:459–64.

85. Kashani K, Al-Khafaji A, Ardiles T, et al. Discovery and validation of cell cycle arrest biomarkers in human acute kidney injury. Crit Care 2013;17:R25.

86. Liu M, Liang Y, Chigurupati S, et al. Acute kidney injury leads to inflammation and functional changes in the brain. J Am Soc Nephrol 2008;19:1360–70.

87. Palkovits M, Sebekova K, Gallatz K, et al. Neuronal activation in the CNS during different forms of acute renal failure in rats. Neuroscience 2009;159:862–82.

88. Haase-Fielitz A, Haase M, Bellomo R. Decreased catecholamine degradation associates with shock and kidney injury after cardiac surgery. J Am Soc Nephrol 2009;20:1393–403.

89. Capuron L, Miller AH. Immune system to brain signaling: neuropsychopharma-cological implications. Pharmacol Ther 2011;130:226–38.

90. Fries M, Bickenbach J, Henzler D, et al. S-100 protein and neurohistopathologic changes in a porcine model of acute lung injury. Anesthesiology 2005;102: 761–7.

91. Markiewski MM, Nilsson B, Ekdahl KN, et al. Complement and coagulation: strangers or partners in crime? Trends Immunol 2007;28:184–92.

92. Ritis K, Doumas M, Mastellos D, et al. A novel C5a receptor-tissue factor cross-talk in neutrophils links innate immunity to coagulation pathways. J Immunol 2006;177:4794–802.

93. Silasi-Mansat R, Zhu H, Popescu NI, et al. Complement inhibition decreases the procoagulant response and confers organ protection in a baboon model of Escherichia coli sepsis. Blood 2010;116:1002–10.

94. Huber-Lang M, Sarma JV, Zetoune FS, et al. Generation of C5a in the absence of C3: a new complement activation pathway. Nat Med 2006;12:682–7.

95. Conway EM. Thrombomodulin and its role in inflammation. Semin Immunopathol 2012;34:107–25.

96. Ghebrehiwet B, Randazzo BP, Dunn JT, et al. Mechanisms of activation of the classical pathway of complement by Hageman factor fragment. J Clin Invest 1983;71:1450–6.

97. Quilez ME, Fuster G, Villar J, et al. Injurious mechanical ventilation affects neuronal activation in ventilated rats. Crit Care 2011;15:R124.

98. Quilez ME, Rodríguez-González R, Turon M, et al. Moderate PEEP after tracheal lipopolysaccharide instillation prevents inflammation and modifies the pattern of brain neuronal activation. Shock 2015;44:601–8.

99. Kuiper JW, Vaschetto R, Della Corte F, et al. Bench-to-bedside review: ventilation-induced renal injury through systemic mediator release–just theory or a causal relationship? Crit Care 2011;15:228.

100. Hepokoski M, Englert JA, Baron R. Ventilator-induced lung injury increases expression of endothelial inflammatory mediators in the kidney. Am J Physiol Renal Physiol 2016;312:F654–60.

101. Singbartl K, Bishop JV, Wen X, et al. Differential effects of kidney-lung cross talk during acute kidney injury and bacterial pneumonia. Kidney Int 2011;80:633–44.

102. Flierl MA, Rittirsch D, Nadeau BA, et al. Phagocyte-derived catecholamines enhance acute inflammatory injury. Nature 2007;449:721–5.

103. Kradin R, Rodberg G, Zhao LH, et al. Epinephrine yields translocation of lymphocytes to the lung. Exp Mol Pathol 2001;70:1–6.

104. Zhou M, Das P, Simms HH, et al. Gut- derived norepinephrine plays an important role in up-regulating IL-1b and IL-10. Biochim Biophys Acta 2005;1740: 446–52.

105. Yang S, Zhou M, Chaudry IH, et al. Norepinephrine-induced hepatocellular dysfunction in early sepsis is mediated by activation of α2-adrenoceptors. Am J Physiol Gastrointest Liver Physiol 2001;281:G1014–21.

106. Borovikova LV, Ivanova S, Zhang M, et al. Vagus nerve stimulation attenuates the systemic inflammatory response to endotoxin. Nature 2000;405:458–62.

107. Wang H, Yu M, Ochani M, et al. Nicotinic acetylcholine receptor alpha7 subunit is an essential regulator of inflammation. Nature 2003;421:384–8.

108. Rosas-Ballina M, Ochani M, Parrish WR, et al. Splenic nerve is required for cholinergic antiinflammatory pathway control of TNF in endotoxemia. Proc Natl Acad Sci U S A 2008;105:11008–110013.

109. Huston JM, Gallowitsch-Puerta M, Ochani M, et al. Transcutaneous vagus nerve stimulation reduces serum high mobility group box 1 levels and improves survival in murine sepsis. Crit Care Med 2007;35:2762–8.

Endocrine and Metabolic Alterations in Sepsis and Implications for Treatment

Catherine Ingels, MD, PhD, Jan Gunst, MD, PhD,
Greet Van den Berghe, MD, PhD*

KEYWORDS

- Sepsis • Growth hormone • Thyroid hormone • Cortisol • Hyperglycemia • Insulin
- Nutrition • Endocrine

KEY POINTS

- The neuroendocrine response to sepsis and other critical illnesses follows a biphasic pattern; although acute changes are probably adaptive, they may become maladaptive in a later phase.
- In corticosteroid-naive patients with sepsis, cortisol supplementation should only be considered in patients with fluid-resistant and vasopressor-resistant refractory shock.
- The optimal blood glucose target in patients with sepsis remains unclear and may depend on diabetes status, the available equipment and treatment protocols, and the feeding strategy.
- In the acute phase of sepsis, current evidence supports accepting a low macronutrient intake and does not support the use of early parenteral nutrition.

INTRODUCTION

Sepsis is one of the most stressful conditions encountered by humans and animals.[1] The stereotypical neuroendocrine response to any form of stress, first described in 1878 by Claude Bernard,[2] is a complex constellation of alterations and interactions between the autonomic, endocrine, metabolic, and immune systems. This response is assumed to provide a survival advantage because it works to restore homeostasis.

Conflicts of Interest: The authors have no conflicts of interest.
Funding sources: This work was supported by the Clinical Research Foundation of UZ Leuven, Belgium (C. Ingels and J. Gunst). G. Van den Berghe receives research grants from the Research Foundation Flanders, the Methusalem Program funded by the Flemish Government (METH/14/06), and from the European Research Council under the European Union's Seventh Framework Program (FP7/2013-2018 ERC Advanced Grant Agreement no. 321670).
Clinical Division and Laboratory of Intensive Care Medicine, Department of Cellular and Molecular Medicine, KU Leuven, Herestraat 49, Leuven 3000, Belgium
* Corresponding author.
E-mail address: greet.vandenberghe@kuleuven.be

Crit Care Clin 34 (2018) 81–96
http://dx.doi.org/10.1016/j.ccc.2017.08.006
0749-0704/18/© 2017 Elsevier Inc. All rights reserved.

The central nervous system (CNS) is able to recognize major threats to survival and induces specific physiologic responses, whereas the innate immune system is activated by pathogenic invaders. Crosstalk between both systems is essential to mount an adequate response to sepsis.[1,3] The innate immune system acts as a sensory organ, capable of detecting the presence of pathogens and signaling this invasion to the nervous system.[4] In sepsis, afferent signals to the brain arise from different origins, such as vagus nerve stimulation, the presence of bacterial products, and the production of cytokines and other inflammatory and neurotoxic mediators.[1,5] In this respect, it has been postulated that proinflammatory cytokines such as tumor necrosis factor alpha (TNF-α), interleukin (IL)-1, IL-6, IL-12, and IL-18 are involved in regulation of the acute stress response.[6] As an example, IL-6 is a cytokine that functions as an activator of the hypothalamic-pituitary-adrenal axis. IL-6 is also a potent pyrogen that interacts with hypothalamic centers to induce fever.[3] The generated afferent signals are thus capable of triggering efferent CNS responses that lead to activation of the autonomic nervous system and of the different neurohormonal axes, comprising the hypothalamopituitary-adrenal (HPA) axis, the hypothalamopituitary-thyroid (HPT) axis, the somatotropic axis, and the gonadal axis.

Critical illness is characterized by dysregulation of all hypothalamopituitary axes, and this is associated with an increased risk of morbidity and mortality.[7] As intensive care medicine evolved, more patients have been able to survive acute, life-threatening stress, entering a phase of protracted critical illness. It has become obvious that the neuroendocrine responses to acute and prolonged critical illness differ (**Table 1**) and may necessitate a different management approach. In the past, endocrine treatments have been advocated based on the erroneous extrapolation of changes

Table 1 Neuroendocrine changes in acute and prolonged critical illness		
Hormone	**Acute Phase**	**Protracted Phase**
1. HPA Axis		
ACTH	↑ =	↓
Cortisol	↑ ↑	↑ (= ↓)
2. HPT Axis		
Pulsatile TSH release	↑ =	↓
T4	↑ =	↓
T3	↓	↓ ↓
rT3	↑	↑ =
3. Somatotropic Axis		
Pulsatile GH release	↑	↓
IGF-1	↓	↓ ↓
ALS	↓	↓ ↓
IGFBP-3	↓	↓ ↓
4. Male Gonadal Axis and Prolactin		
Pulsatile LH release	↑ =	↓
Testosterone	↓	↓ ↓
Pulsatile PRL release	↑	↓

Abbreviations: ACTH, adrenocorticotropic hormone; ALS, acid-labile subunit; GH, growth hormone; IGF-I, insulinlike growth factor-I; IGFBP, insulinlike growth factor binding protein; LH, luteinizing hormone; PRL, prolactin; TSH, thyroid-stimulating hormone (thyrotropin).

occurring in the acute phase of illness to the more protracted phase. This error may explain the unexpected increase in mortality found with some of these treatments.

Sepsis-related endocrine and inflammatory changes lead to hyperglycemia. This response was traditionally considered to be adaptive, in order to ensure sufficient nutrient availability to immune cells and other cells not relying on insulin for glucose uptake. Concomitantly, patients develop anorexia and/or cannot engage in oral feeding. The ensuing development of a caloric and protein deficit has been associated with the development of muscle weakness and poor outcome.[8] Therefore, experts advocate administration of early nutritional support to septic and other severely ill patients.[9] However, randomized controlled trials (RCTs) have shown that prolonged hyperglycemia and early aggressive nutritional support may induce harm.[10–14] This article highlights the most recent insights in the neuroendocrine and metabolic responses to sepsis, and the potential implications for treatment.

THE NEUROENDOCRINE RESPONSES TO SEPSIS
The Hypothalamic-Pituitary-Adrenal Axis

Activation of the HPA axis is one of the most essential responses to acute stress, and illness in general.[15] Many decades ago, the importance of glucocorticoid production for surviving life-threatening stress was highlighted by Selye.[16] Moreover, earlier work by Addison revealed that the adrenal cortex is essential for survival, because adrenalectomy was inevitably linked to death of the test animals.[15,17]

In normal physiologic conditions, the hypothalamus secretes corticotropin-releasing hormone (CRH) in a pulsatile manner. This hormone induces pulsatile secretion of adrenocorticotropic hormone (ACTH; also known as corticotrophin) by the anterior pituitary gland, which in turn regulates the adrenal production of cortisol and dehydroepiandrosterone (DHEA). Moreover, aldosterone, which is primarily regulated by the renin-angiotensin system, is also influenced by ACTH secretion. Cortisol, and exogenously administered corticosteroids, exert a negative feedback on CRH and ACTH production.[15,18] IL-6 is a major immune stimulator of the HPA axis. Vasopressin produced by the hypothalamus also stimulates ACTH secretion when CRH is present. Cortisol is thought to have an essential role for survival because of its effects, among other things, on gluconeogenesis, inflammation, maintenance of fluid homeostasis, and vascular tone, and via its stimulatory effect on vascular sensitivity to catecholamines.[15,19]

In acute critical illness, the HPA axis is activated by both neuronal circuits and by the massive release of inflammatory cytokines (particularly IL-6, TNF-α, and IL-1), which stimulate CRH and ACTH secretion.[19] Different cytokine receptors have been detected within the neurohumoral organs.[19,20] Vasopressin, endothelin, and atrial-natriuretic factor (ANF) also emerge as stimulators of cortisol secretion. In particular, in septic shock, macrophage-inhibiting factor secretion, triggered by excessive inflammation, modulates the HPA axis. All these additive effects expectedly result in a highly activated HPA axis with increased levels of ACTH and total and free cortisol. However, plasma ACTH concentrations are often low. Besides increased production of cortisol by the adrenal glands, impaired glucocorticoid clearance also contributes to the very high cortisol levels seen in critical illness,[21] that are far in excess of those encountered in many patients with Cushing syndrome. Moreover, corticosteroid binding globulin (CBG) levels are usually suppressed as part of the acute-phase response, especially in patients with impaired hepatic function, and there is enhanced elastase cleavage of CBG,[22] thus contributing to increased free cortisol availability.[15] The biological effects of cortisol may be further amplified by an increase in glucocorticoid receptor (GR) number and sensitivity,[23] although suppression of the GR has also been observed.[24] In cases of severe sepsis or septic shock, excessive or disproportionate cytokine production may have the ability to reduce the number and binding affinity of GRs.[24] This reduction could lead to the state of glucocorticoid resistance that is sometimes encountered in these conditions, a possibility that requires further investigation. The suppressed cortisol metabolism in the liver and kidney may specifically accentuate cortisol availability in these tissues and contribute to increased plasma levels.[21] The normal diurnal variation of cortisol secretion is lost during critical illness.[7,25] Another feature of enhanced cortisol availability during acute stress is its poor suppressibility by the administration of exogenous steroids.[26]

A substantial proportion of patients survive the acute threat of sepsis or critical illness, providing an adequate and immediate HPA axis response. However, when patients enter the chronic, protracted phase of critical illness, this exposes them to other threats. During this chronic phase, circulating cortisol levels remain increased, but this seems not to be induced by corticotrophin-mediated increases in cortisol production,[7] because high cortisol levels are dissociated from low ACTH levels.[27] Putative factors that drive cortisol secretion apart from CRH include cytokines, ANF, endothelin, and substance P.[27] However, the cortisol production rate is only moderately increased beyond the very acute phase in septic patients treated in the intensive care unit (ICU), whereas the role of suppressed cortisol breakdown becomes more prominent.[21] Whatever the exact mechanism underlying the increase in plasma cortisol, persisting hypercortisolism observed in protracted critical illness may confer certain advantages by providing energy from gluconeogenesis, minimizing excessive inflammation, and preserving vascular tone. It may also mediate some harmful complications such as hyperglycemia, myopathy, and increased susceptibility to infection.[15]

The degree of the increase in circulating cortisol reflects the severity of illness.[28] However, several events may hamper an adequately increased cortisol availability, such as the direct damage to the hypothalamus or the pituitary gland with head injuries, adrenal hemorrhage, inflammatory mediators, and the use of certain pharmacologic agents (etomidate, azoles, phenytoin, and opioids).[27,29] Moreover, there is an important interindividual variation in cortisol levels after a stressful event, as well as variation related to age. An important unresolved issue is how to assess whether the cortisol availability in a given patient is sufficient or insufficient. The clinical term relative or functional adrenal insufficiency, also referred to as critical illness-related corticosteroid insufficiency, has been proposed to denote those patients with septic shock for whom corticosteroid treatment brings about improvement of hemodynamic status. Although sepsis holds a risk of absolute adrenal failure, for several reasons, there is still much controversy regarding the definition of relative adrenal insufficiency, its diagnosis, and its treatment.[27,30]

At present, experts still advise to use the cosyntropin stimulation test to detect relative adrenal insufficiency in critically ill patients. After injection of 250 μg of cosyntropin, a synthetic ACTH analogue, plasma cortisol is measured repeatedly over 1 hour. However, because 250 μg of cosyntropin induces supraphysiologic ACTH activity, some experts therefore advise to use a lower dose (1 μg) instead.[31] There is no consensus at present as to which cosyntropin dose should be used, what plasma level should assess the cortisol response to cosyntropin (cortisol peak level or incremental cortisol response), or which cutoff reference should be used to diagnose this condition. Hence, there is even more uncertainty on which patients may potentially benefit from corticosteroid treatment of such presumed relative adrenal insufficiency. A further rationale for using corticosteroids in such patients, mostly those with sepsis or septic shock, is based on their potent antiinflammatory properties and their effect on the vasopressor response and thus on blood pressure. It is postulated that cortico-steroids are capable of preventing sepsis-induced catecholamine receptor desensiti-zation.[15] Corticosteroid treatment of patients with sepsis or septic shock has evolved from the use of very high doses to lower daily doses (200 mg), although the latter are still the equivalent of 6-fold to 10-fold greater than the normal daily cortisol production rate.[21] More than 15 years ago, following several smaller studies that showed earlier shock reversal with hydrocortisone treatment, a multicenter RCT showed that 200 mg daily of intravenous (IV) hydrocortisone plus 50 μg of fludrocortisone admin-istered enterally for 7 days reduced mortality in those patients with septic shock who showed an incremental cortisol response of less than 9 μg/dL to 250 μg of cosyn-tropin.[32] However, this RCT has been criticized for the high mortality in the control group and the use of an inappropriate statistical test to assess a mortality differ-ence.[33,34] Moreover, a subsequent RCT could not confirm these results in patients with septic shock who received 200 mg of IV hydrocortisone per day for 5 days.[35] It has been suggested that the absence of a benefit in the latter RCT was explained by the omission of fludrocortisone. However, an RCT randomizing patients with septic shock to administration of hydrocortisone or hydrocortisone plus fludrocortisone found no difference between the two strategies.[36] A more recent trial could also not detect a benefit from hydrocortisone when administered to patients with severe sepsis.[37] Current Surviving Sepsis guidelines recommend administration of 200 mg of hydrocortisone per day only to patients with fluid-resistant and vasopressor-resistant septic shock (weak recommendation).[38] The guidelines also advise dose tapering as quickly as clinically tolerated.

The Hypothalamic-Pituitary-Thyroid Axis

Thyroid hormone is essential for regulation of energy metabolism in virtually all tissues and plays an essential role in many physiologic processes of cell differentiation, growth, and metabolism.[39] In health, the production and release of thyrotropin (thy-roid-stimulating hormone [TSH]) by the pituitary is controlled by hypothalamic thyrotropin-releasing hormone (TRH). TSH, released in bursts that are superimposed on basal, nonpulsatile secretion, activates the thyroid gland to produce T4. T4 is peripherally converted into the active hormone T3 and the metabolic inactive rT3 by deiodinases. T4 and T3 both exert negative feedback on TRH and TSH.

During critical illness, profound alterations occur within the HPT axis. After a stress-ful event, such as the onset of sepsis, circulating levels of T3 immediately decrease and rT3 levels increase. The degree of these changes reflects the severity of illness. These alterations are predominantly brought about by altered peripheral conversion of T4. Thyrotropin and T4 levels increase briefly and return to normal, although occa-sionally, in very severe acute disease, T4 levels can decrease. Although TSH levels quickly decrease within the normal range, the normal nocturnal TSH surge is absent. Because low T3 levels persist despite normalization of TSH, this condition has been referred to as the low T3 syndrome, sick euthyroid syndrome, or more recently non-thyroidal illness (NTI). From an evolutionary point of view, NTI can be interpreted as an attempt to protect the organism by reducing energy consumption and catabolism, and may thus be beneficial in the acute setting. The changes encountered in NTI resemble those induced by starvation, with decreased peripheral activation and increased inactivation of thyroid hormone. In addition, reduced concentrations of thy-roid hormone binding proteins, inhibition of hormone binding, and changes in hormone transport are further hallmarks of the low T3 syndrome of critical illness.[6,40]

In the acute phase of critical illness, such peripheral changes in thyroid hormone action and metabolism dominate. In contrast, the chronic phase of critical illness is characterized by a combination of peripheral and central adaptations. After several days of critical illness, levels of T3 further decline and T4 levels are also reduced. Moreover, pulsatile TSH secretion is suppressed and this correlates with suppressed hypothalamic TRH gene expression.[6] The combination of low peripheral thyroid hormone levels together with low TSH and TRH levels suggests a major change in the central regulation of the HPT axis. Several findings support such a resetting of the hypothalamic set point for feedback inhibition, including increasing TSH levels as a marker of recovery onset, and the ability of an infusion of TRH (particularly in combination with growth hormone [GH] secretagogues) to restore normal levels of TSH, T4, and T3.[6,40,41] The triggers of these changes in the HPT axis during protracted illness remain unclear, but possible players are cytokines, sustained hypercortisolism, neuropeptide Y, and alterations in hypothalamic deiodinase activity and thyroid hormone transporter expression. In addition, iatrogenic factors such as treatment with dopamine and corticosteroids could play a role.[6,40,42]

Because low levels of thyroid hormone and low T3/rT3 ratios have been associated with risk of death, the question arises whether these low levels should be treated. Are these low levels merely a reflection of the severity of illness, and could they be adaptive and protective against hypercatabolism, or do they represent a maladaptive response that should be treated? Because the acute changes that occur uniformly immediately after the onset of critical illness are comparable with, and coincide with, a fasting response, it is likely that these represent a neuroendocrine beneficial evolutionary conserved adaptation; an attempt to reduce energy consumption and protein catabolism.[43] Therefore, it seems common sense to not treat this acute NTI. However, the central and peripheral changes that occur in the prolonged phase of critical illness, when patients are usually fully fed, are different and may be maladaptive. The protracted phase of illness with ongoing dependency on intensive care represents an unnatural condition to which evolutionary adaptation has not been possible. Whether the low circulating and tissue thyroid hormone levels in the chronic phase of illness should be treated is still a matter of debate. Studies on this topic have used either substitution doses or high doses of the peripheral hormones T4 or T3 and did not reveal any benefit. However, during critical illness, substitution doses of T4 and T3 are unable to increase the circulating plasma levels of thyroid hormones, and supraphysiologic doses lead to a risk of overtreatment with further TSH suppression as a consequence. Because the chronic phase of illness is characterized by hypothalamic suppression, a more logical approach would be to infuse TRH, because this also respects normal feedback mechanisms and hence prevents overtreatment. Infusion of the combination of TRH (together with a GH secretagogue) restored the pulsatile secretion of TSH and reestablished normal physiologic levels of peripheral hormones in prolonged critical illness.[44] Although this intervention, when continued for 5 days, also elicited an anabolic/anticatabolic response, no RCTs exist that have investigated the impact on patient-centered, clinically relevant outcomes.[43]

The Somatotropic Axis

GH, secreted by the somatotropic cells, is the most abundant pituitary hormone.[45] Besides its well-known essential role in linear growth in childhood, GH also supports many important functions throughout the lifespan.[45] In adults, GH deficiency is associated with a distinct clinical syndrome comprising physical and psychological defects, such as altered body composition with increased fat and decreased lean body mass, relative hypercortisolism (caused by increased conversion of cortisone to cortisol), increased loss of water and sodium, loss of skeletal muscle mass, impairment of cardiovascular function, and reduced exercise capacity.[45] Under normal conditions, the synthesis and secretion of GH is regulated by hypothalamic GH-releasing hormone (GHRH), the gut hormone ghrelin, and the inhibitory somato-statin.[7,45] GH is secreted in a typical pulsatile pattern, which seems to be essential for its metabolic effects[7] and responds to physiologic stimuli like stress, food intake, and circadian rhythms.[45] Moreover, synthetic releasing peptides and nonpeptide GH-secretagogues interact with the ghrelin receptor and, in synergy with GHRH, stimulate pulsatile GH secretion.[7,45] GH has direct and indirect effects that are mediated by insulinlike growth factor-I (IGF-I) and insulinlike growth factor binding proteins (IGFBPs).[7]

In response to acute stress, the typical pattern of GH secretion is altered, with higher pulse frequency, amplitude, and interpulse levels, in the presence of peripheral GH resistance in tissues such as the liver; this is reflected by decreased serum concentrations of IGF-I, IGFBP-3, and the acid-labile subunit (ALS).[46] Enhanced GH secretion may contribute to lipolysis and insulin antagonism, thereby providing valuable fatty acids and glucose, whereas the indirect anabolic effects that are brought about by IGF-I, which at that time are not essential for survival, are suppressed.[7] Particularly in patients with sepsis and severe sepsis, low IGF-I and IGFBP-3 levels have been reported, further decreasing in septic shock. Moreover, IGF-I levels were related to IGFBP-3, T3, and T4, and were inversely related to cortisol, the severity of sepsis, CRP, and IL-6.[47] Normalization of the altered somatotropic axis components precedes clinical recovery, whereas failure to do so was associated with worse clinical outcomes from sepsis-induced multiorgan dysfunction syndrome.[48] However, in the prolonged phase of critical illnesses, a dramatic reduction in GH pulsatile secretion and further reduction of IGF-I and IGFBP-3 levels are present, which may contribute to hypercatabolism, an inability to rebuild tissues, and to the so-called wasting syndrome.[48,49]

Recent research has highlighted the role of ghrelin in sepsis. This enteric hormone is produced by the stomach and, when adequately acetylated, acts on the brain to stimulate the somatotropic axis. Ghrelin is a strong stimulator of GH secretion as well as a potent vasodilatory peptide.[50,51] Moreover, ghrelin has been reported to downregulate inflammatory cytokines[50] and to attenuate age-related immunosuppression in septic rats.[52] Acetylated ghrelin levels were significantly decreased in an animal model of endotoxemia,[53] suggesting that ghrelin or ghrelin receptor agonists could provide therapeutic benefit in sepsis. Previous attempts to restore GH action with the use of recombinant GH gave conflicting results. A large multicenter RCT by Takala and colleagues[54] showed that treatment with GH, given in high doses with the intention of overcoming GH resistance, resulted in a striking increase in mortality, in longer ICU stays, and in longer durations of mechanical ventilation. In contrast, earlier studies had indicated that GH has the ability to reduce catabolism and improve nitrogen balance in selected patient populations.[48,55,56] The high doses used in the Takala and colleagues[54] study may have been relevant in mediating the harm. Infusion of releasing factors, such as GHRH and the GH-releasing peptide-2 (GHRP-2), produces a more physiologic reactivation of endogenous pulsatile GH secretion; respecting normal feedback loops, overtreatment was also prevented.[7] Furthermore, coinfusion of GHRP-2 with TRH for 5 days was effective in restoring pulsatile secretion of GH and TSH, with increases of IGF-I and thyroid hormone levels within the low-normal ranges, suppressing breakdown of muscle and increasing bone anabolism.[41] Experimental, animal, and in vitro studies have supported a role for ghrelin in improving hemodynamics, reducing catabolism, attenuating immunosuppression, and enhancing autophagic repair mechanisms in sepsis models.[48,53,57,58] However, there are currently no large RCTs that have investigated the potential clinical relevance and safety of these experimental findings.

The Male Gonadal Axis and Prolactin

The gonadal axis is hallmarked by pulsatile secretion of the hypothalamic gonado-tropin releasing hormone (GnRH), in response to which luteinizing hormone (LH) and follicle-stimulating hormone (FSH) are secreted by the pituitary. In men, LH mediates production of androgens and, in concert with FSH, stimulates spermatogenesis. In women, LH causes ovarian androgen production and FSH aromatizes androgens to estrogens.[7] Sex steroids exert a negative feedback inhibition on gonadotropins and GnRH. Prolactin (PRL) is secreted in a pulsatile manner by a distinct cell type in the anterior pituitary, under a tight negative control by dopamine. PRL is a stress hormone with immune-enhancing properties.[7]

In the acute phase of critical illness in men, plasma testosterone concentrations are immediately suppressed in the presence of increased or maintained LH levels. In the prolonged phase of critical illness, suppressed LH secretion further contributes to the low circulating levels of testosterone in men. In addition, increased aromatization of testosterone to estrogen occurs.[59,60] Because testosterone is a powerful anabolic hormone, low testosterone levels during critical illness may contribute to the catabolic wasting syndrome. Also, PRL levels increase rapidly after onset of critical illness; this may be interpreted as an attempt to activate the immune system. However, in the pro-longed phase, PRL secretion is blunted, possibly adding to immune suppression in prolonged illness.[7,59]

In protracted critical illness, pulsatile GnRH treatment can increase pulsatile LH secretion. However, when only LH is reactivated, only a transient increase in circu-lating testosterone level followed. In contrast, pulsatile administration of GnRH com-bined with infusion of GHRP-2 and TRH induced an increase in testosterone and a clear anabolic response in target tissues.[61] The clinical relevance of these findings has not yet been investigated in large RCTs.

Summary of the Neuroendocrine Responses to Sepsis

The acute neuroendocrine response to sepsis and other critical illnesses consists pri-marily of an activated hypothalamopituitary function with inactivated peripheral (anabolic) pathways. This response is thought to be adaptive, because it temporarily shuts down anabolic processes to provide metabolic substrates for essential survival functions. As patients survive this acute phase and enter a more protracted critical illness, another pattern of changes can be discerned. Here, a uniformly reduced pul-satile secretion of ACTH, TSH, GH, PRL, and LH is observed, which may be related to a reduced availability of hypothalamic and peripheral releasing hormones. The pulsa-tile secretion of TSH, GH, and LH can be reestablished by relevant combinations of releasing factors. This process offers an important safety aspect because active feed-back inhibition mechanisms prevent the target organs and cells from being overstimu-lated. Administration of a combination of GHRP-2, TRH, and GnRH can positively affect metabolism.[61] Further research is needed to address the therapeutic potential in large RCTs.

METABOLIC RESPONSES TO SEPSIS

The neuroendocrine and inflammatory alterations in response to a life-threatening insult also induce metabolic changes.

Stress Hyperglycemia

The development of hyperglycemia is a universal metabolic response to severe phys-ical stress, including sepsis. Hyperglycemia is induced by stress hormones (cortisol,

GH, glucagon, and catecholamines) and proinflammatory cytokines, leading to gluco-neogenesis and peripheral insulin resistance. Drugs such as catecholamines and corticosteroids that increase insulin resistance, as well (parenteral) nutrition, may further aggravate the degree of hyperglycemia.[62] The hyperglycemic response to severe stress, first described by Selye,[16] used to be interpreted as a desirable, adaptive process, hypothesized to provide a survival advantage by providing sufficient nutrients to cells that do not rely on insulin for glucose uptake, including neurons and leukocytes.[62] However, several studies have associated the degree of hyperglycemia with an increased mortality risk.[63,64] Whether hyperglycemia merely reflects severity of illness or causally relates to outcome has been a matter of ongoing debate.

Three RCTs from Leuven[10-12] have shown that strictly normalizing blood glucose concentrations to the healthy fasting range with insulin therapy (80–110 mg/dL for adults, 70–100 mg/dL for children older than 1 year, and 50–80 mg/dL for infants) reduced morbidity and mortality of critically ill patients compared with tolerating hyperglycemia up to 215 mg/dL, with the clinical benefit maintained up to 4 years after randomization.[10-12,65,66] All studied patient subgroups benefited from tight blood glucose control (TGC), with the potential exception of patients with preadmission diabetes mellitus, in whom there was only a nonsignificant trend toward benefit.[67] Mechanistic animal studies identified the avoidance of glucose toxicity to cells with insulin-independent glucose uptake as a mediator of organ protection, rather than the insulin treatment.[68-72] These beneficial effects of reducing glucose level included a beneficial impact on immune function.[68-70] Post hoc observational studies suggested a dose-dependent effect of glucose reduction on mortality risk, with the greatest mortality reduction achieved by targeting strict normoglycemia.[67]

Although several implementation studies and smaller RCTs subsequently confirmed a clinical benefit from implementing TGC, in part by preventing infections, multicenter RCTs did not confirm this, with the largest multicenter RCT even finding an excess mortality with TGC.[36,73-80] The investigators of that trial subsequently attributed the increased mortality risk to an increased incidence of hypoglycaemia.[81] However, in the Leuven studies, hypoglycaemia also occurred more frequently with TGC and, in this context, a nested case-control study could not detect a harmful impact (including long term) of a short-lasting episode of iatrogenic hypoglycemia.[66,82] Several methodological differences may explain the opposite effects of TGC on outcomes in these trials. First, the multicenter RCTs targeted a lower glucose target in the control group than the Leuven trials, in general less than 180 mg/dL, which decreases any potential benefit of such an intervention.[67] Second, in contrast with Leuven, the largest multicenter RCT did not focus on standardization, because it was designed as a pragmatic study in order to maximize external validity.[80] As a consequence, glucometers and capillary glucose measurements were allowed, which were shown to be too inaccurate to target a narrow glycemic range.[83] This inaccuracy may have led to an increased incidence of prolonged and undetected hypoglycaemia, which may have increased the mortality risk. The feeding protocol was also not standardized in these pragmatic multicenter studies, in contrast with the Leuven studies, in which early parenteral nutrition was administered as a standard of care to all patients. However, because this feeding strategy was afterward shown to be harmful in 2 multicenter RCTs, it remains unknown whether TGC remains beneficial in the absence of early parenteral nutrition.

Hence, the optimal blood glucose target remains unclear. This target may depend on the patient population, the equipment and protocols used, and the feeding regimen. Until new evidence becomes available, it seems prudent to avoid severe hyperglycemia in all critically ill patients, including patients with sepsis.

Anorexia and Artificial Feeding

Anorexia accompanies any form of acute physical stress. In response to an infection, it is at least partially mediated via both central neural and peripheral effects of proinflammatory cytokines.[84] In addition, a poor general condition often precludes any volitional intake. From an evolutionary point of view, anorexia may have conferred some survival benefit, helping the host to recover from illness or to combat an infection.[85] However, prolonged underfeeding is associated with ongoing catabolism, an increased risk of infections, and mortality.[8,86] Therefore, clinical practice guidelines have recommended early, full enteral nutrition, eventually supplemented by parenteral nutrition, although the recommended timing to add parenteral nutrition has differed.[9,87] Because of the lack of sufficiently powered RCTs, these recommendations were mainly based on expert opinion. However, several large RCTs have recently challenged these guidelines. Early, full nutritional support did not deliver the hypothesized benefit and may harm critically ill patients, including patients with sepsis.[88] Two large multicenter RCTs found no benefit from normocaloric enteral feeding compared with so-called trophic hypocaloric feeding during the first weeks of ICU stay.[89,90] One of these RCTs also restricted protein calories in the hypocaloric feeding arm,[90] whereas the other administered isonitrogenous feeding to both groups, thereby only restricting nonprotein calories in the hypocaloric group.[89] Both studies found a neutral impact on clinical outcome and did not identify any subgroup in which the effect of the intervention was different. The results from these 2 RCTs were recently corroborated by 2 meta-analyses, which investigated the impact of normocaloric versus hypocaloric enteral feeding in critically ill patients.[91,92] Neither of these meta-analyses, with slightly different inclusion criteria, detected a benefit from normocaloric enteral feeding. One meta-analysis even suggested potential harm, with increased rates of bloodstream infections and renal replacement therapy.[91]

Likewise, recent RCTs have not confirmed the hypothesized benefit from early supplementation of insufficient enteral nutrition with parenteral nutrition; the 2 largest multicenter RCTs even found significant harm.[13,14,93] Compared with withholding supplemental parenteral nutrition for 1 week, early supplemental parenteral nutrition increased the ICU dependency of both critically ill adults and children, with a prolonged need for vital organ support and an increased incidence of new infections. Importantly, in these 2 multicenter studies, both randomization groups received sufficient micronutrients and vitamins in the acute phase, to prevent refeeding syndrome.[13,14] The harmful effect of early parenteral nutrition was present in all studied subgroups, including patients with sepsis on admission and patients with the highest nutritional risk scores. In the adult population, in contrast with expectations, early parenteral nutrition also increased the incidence of muscle weakness and hampered recovery.[94] Mechanistic research attributed the harmful impact of early parenteral nutrition to nutrient-induced suppression of autophagy, a crucial cellular repair process that removes damaged organelles, toxic protein aggregates, and intracellular or macrophage-engulfed microorganisms.[94,95] However, restricting macronutrient intake may come at a price, and may only be tolerated for a limited period of time. The optimal timing when parenteral nutrition can be initiated safely and effectively remains unclear.

Small studies have suggested that certain specialized nutritional formulae may have immune-modulating properties that could improve outcomes. These formulations contain mixtures enriched in glutamine, omega-3 fatty acids, and/or pharmacologic amounts of micronutrients and vitamins such as vitamin C, vitamin E, beta-carotene, selenium, and zinc. However, large, multicenter RCTs have not confirmed the hypothesized benefit of administering these formulations, with several RCTs even suggesting harm, especially for glutamine supplementation.[96–99] Hence, the authors do not recommend the use of these so-called immunonutrients.

SUMMARY AND FUTURE DIRECTIONS

In conclusion, the neuroendocrine response to any form of stress, including sepsis, follows a distinct biphasic pattern. The acute neuroendocrine changes are probably adaptive and directed toward restoring homeostasis and limiting unnecessary energy consumption. These changes may become maladaptive in the prolonged phase of critical illness, in which a there is a central suppression of the neuroendocrine axes. Further research is needed to establish whether hypothalamic release factors improve the outcomes of these patients.[61] In the acute phase, hydrocortisone treatment can be considered in patients with fluid-resistant and vasopressor-resistant refractory septic shock, although this recommendation is based on a low level of evidence.

The optimal blood glucose target in patients with sepsis remains to be studied and may depend on diabetic status, available equipment, and the blood glucose control algorithm and feeding regimen being used. Strict blood glucose control requires accurate monitoring tools and a validated (computerized) insulin infusion protocol, which minimizes the risk of hypoglycemia.[100] Until new evidence from RCTs becomes available, preventing severe hyperglycemia is recommended for all critically ill patients. In the acute phase of sepsis, current evidence supports tolerating low macronutrient intake and does not support the use of early parenteral nutrition.

REFERENCES

1. Gheorghiţă V, Barbu AE, Gheorghiu ML, et al. Endocrine dysfunction in sepsis: a beneficial or deleterious host response? Germs 2015;5:17–25.
2. Bernard C. Leçons sur les phénomènes de la vie communs aux animaux et aux végétaux. Paris: JB Baillière et fils; 1878.
3. Munford RS, Tracey KJ. Is severe sepsis a neuroendocrine disease? Mol Med 2002;8:437–42.
4. Sharshar T, Hopkinson NS, Orlikowski D, et al. Science review: the brain in sepsis - culprit and victim. Crit Care 2005;9:37–44.
5. Akrout N, Sharshar T, Annane D. Mechanisms of brain signaling during sepsis. Curr Neuropharmacol 2009;7:296–301.
6. Peeters RP, Debaveye Y, Fliers E, et al. Changes within the thyroid axis during critical illness. Crit Care Clin 2006;22:41–55.
7. Langouche L, Van den Berghe G. The dynamic neuroendocrine response to critical illness. Endocrinol Metab Clin North Am 2006;35:777–91.
8. Alberda C, Gramlich L, Jones N, et al. The relationship between nutritional intake and clinical outcomes in critically ill patients: results of an international multicenter observational study. Intensive Care Med 2009;35:1728–37.
9. Singer P, Berger MM, Van den Berghe G, et al. ESPEN guidelines on parenteral nutrition: intensive care. Clin Nutr 2009;28:387–400.
10. Van den Berghe G, Wouters P, Weekers F, et al. Intensive insulin therapy in critically ill patients. N Engl J Med 2001;345:1359–67.
11. Van den Berghe G, Wilmer A, Hermans G, et al. Intensive insulin therapy in the medical ICU. N Engl J Med 2006;354:449–61.
12. Vlasselaers D, Milants I, Desmet L, et al. Intensive insulin therapy for patients in paediatric intensive care: a prospective, randomised controlled study. Lancet 2009;373:547–56.

13. Casaer MP, Mesotten D, Hermans G, et al. Early versus late parenteral nutrition in critically ill adults. N Engl J Med 2011;36:506–17.
14. Fivez T, Kerklaan D, Mesotten D, et al. Early versus late parenteral nutrition in critically ill children. N Engl J Med 2016;374:1111–22.
15. Arafah BM. Hypothalamic pituitary adrenal function during critical illness: limitations of current assessment methods. J Clin Endocrinol Metab 2006;91: 3725–45.
16. Selye H. What is stress? Metabolism 1956;5:525–30.
17. Biedl A. The internal secretory organs: their physiology and pathology. London: Bale and Danielsson; 1912.
18. Chrousos GP. The hypothalamic-pituitary-adrenal axis and immune-mediated inflammation. N Engl J Med 1995;332:1351–62.
19. Mastorakos G, Chrousos GP, Weber JS. Recombinant interleukin-6 activates the hypothalamic-pituitary-adrenal axis in humans. J Clin Endocrinol Metab 1993; 77:1690–4.
20. Tsigos C, Papanicolaou DA, Defensor R, et al. Dose effects of recombinant human interleukin-6 on pituitary hormone secretion and energy expenditure. Neuroendocrinology 1997;66:54–62.
21. Boonen E, Vervenne H, Meersseman P, et al. Reduced cortisol metabolism during critical illness. N Engl J Med 2013;368:1477–88.
22. Pemberton PA, Stein PE, Pepys MB, et al. Hormone binding globulins undergo serpin conformational change in inflammation. Nature 1988;336:257–8.
23. Beishuizen A, Thijs LG, Vermes I. Patterns of corticosteroid-binding globulin and the free cortisol index during septic shock and multitrauma. Intensive Care Med 2001;27:1584–91.
24. Molijn GJ, Spek JJ, van Uffelen JC, et al. Differential adaptation of glucocorticoid sensitivity of peripheral blood mononuclear leukocytes in patients with sepsis or septic shock. J Clin Endocrinol Metab 1995;80:1799–803.
25. Vanhorebeek I, Peeters RP, Vander Perre S, et al. Cortisol response to critical illness: effect of intensive insulin therapy. J Clin Endocrinol Metab 2006;91: 3803–13.
26. Perrot D, Bonneton A, Dechaud H, et al. Hypercortisolism in septic shock is not suppressible by dexamethasone infusion. Crit Care Med 1993;21:396–401.
27. Schuetz P, Müller B. The hypothalamic-pituitary-adrenal axis in critical illness. Endocrinol Metab Clin North Am 2006;35:823–38, x.
28. Annane D, Sébille V, Troché G, et al. 3-level prognostic classification in septic shock based on cortisol levels and cortisol response to corticotropin. JAMA 2000;283:1038–45.
29. Peeters B, Güiza F, Boonen E, et al. Drug-induced HPA axis alterations during acute critical illness: a multivariable association study. Clin Endocrinol (Oxf) 2017;86:26–36.
30. Boonen E, Van den Berghe G. Mechanisms in endocrinology: new concepts to further unravel adrenal insufficiency during critical illness. Eur J Endocrinol 2016;175:R1–9.
31. Dickstein G, Saiegh L. Low-dose and high-dose adrenocorticotropin testing: indications and shortcomings. Curr Opin Endocrinol Diabetes Obes 2008;15: 244–9.
32. Annane D, Sébille V, Charpentier C, et al. Effect of treatment with low doses of hydrocortisone and fludrocortisone on mortality in patients with septic shock. JAMA 2002;288:862–71.

33. Cooke CR, Rubenfeld GD. Epoetin alfa in critically ill patients. N Engl J Med 2007;357:2516.
34. Rubenfeld GD. When survival is not the same as mortality. Crit Care Alert 2003; 10:113–5.
35. Sprung CL, Annane D, Keh D, et al. Hydrocortisone therapy for patients with septic shock. N Engl J Med 2008;358:111–24.
36. Annane D, Cariou A, Maxime V, et al. Corticosteroid treatment and intensive insulin therapy for septic shock in adults. A randomized controlled trial. JAMA 2010;303:341–8.
37. Keh D, Trips E, Marx G, et al. Effect of hydrocortisone on development of shock among patients with severe sepsis: the HYPRESS randomized clinical trial. JAMA 2016;316:1775–85.
38. Rhodes A, Evans LE, Alhazzani W, et al. Surviving Sepsis Campaign: international guidelines for management of sepsis and septic shock: 2016. Intensive Care Med 2017;43:304–77.
39. Mebis L, Debaveye Y, Visser TJ, et al. Changes within the thyroid axis during the course of critical illness. Endocrinol Metab Clin North Am 2006;35:807–21.
40. Van den Berghe G. Non-thyroidal illness in the ICU: a syndrome with different faces. Thyroid 2014;24:1456–65.
41. Van den Berghe G, Wouters P, Weekers F, et al. Reactivation of pituitary hormone release and metabolic improvement by infusion of growth hormone-releasing peptide and thyrotropin-releasing hormone in patients with protracted critical illness. J Clin Endocrinol Metab 1999;84:1311–23.
42. Fliers E, Alkemade A, Wiersinga WM. The hypothalamic-pituitary-thyroid axis in critical illness. Best Pract Res Clin Endocrinol Metab 2001;15:453–64.
43. Van den Berghe G. On the neuroendocrinopathy of critical illness. Perspectives for feeding and novel treatments. Am J Respir Crit Care Med 2016;194:1337–48.
44. Van den Berghe G, de Zegher F, Baxter RC, et al. Neuroendocrinology of prolonged critical illness: effects of exogenous thyrotropin-releasing hormone and its combination with growth hormone secretagogues. J Clin Endocrinol Metab 1998;83:309–19.
45. Cummings DE, Merriam GR. Growth hormone therapy in adults. Annu Rev Med 2003;54:513–33.
46. Baxter RC, Hawker FH, To C, et al. Thirty-day monitoring of insulin-like growth factors and their binding proteins in intensive care unit patients. Growth Horm IGF Res 1998;8:455–63.
47. Papastathi C, Mavrommatis A, Mentzelopoulos S, et al. Insulin-like growth factor I and its binding protein 3 in sepsis. Growth Horm IGF Res 2013;23:98–104.
48. Marquardt DJ, Knatz NL, Wetterau LA, et al. Failure to recover somatotropic axis function is associated with mortality from pediatric sepsis-induced multiple organ dysfunction syndrome. Pediatr Crit Care Med 2010;11:18–25.
49. Van den Berghe G. Dynamic neuroendocrine responses to critical illness. Front Neuroendocrinol 2002;23:370–91.
50. Jacob A, Wu R, Zhou M, et al. Mechanism of the inhibitory effect of ghrelin in sepsis. Hepat Med 2010;2:33–8.
51. Wiley KE, Davenport AP. Comparison of vasodilators in human internal mammary artery: ghrelin is a potent physiological antagonist of endothelin-1. Br J Pharmacol 2002;136:1146–52.
52. Zhou M, Yang WL, Aziz M, et al. Therapeutic effect of human ghrelin and growth hormone: attenuation of immunosuppression in septic aged rats. Biochim Biophys Acta 2017 [pii:S0925-4439(17) 30027–3].

53. Chang L, Zhao J, Yang J, et al. Therapeutic effects of ghrelin on endotoxic shock in rats. Eur J Pharmacol 2003;473:171–6.

54. Takala J, Ruokonen E, Webster NR, et al. Increased mortality associated with growth hormone treatment in critically ill adults. N Engl J Med 1999;341:785–92.

55. Duska F, Fric M, Waldauf P, et al. Frequent intravenous pulses of growth hormone together with glutamine supplementation in prolonged critical illness after multiple trauma: effects on nitrogen balance, insulin resistance, and substrate oxidation. Crit Care Med 2008;36:1707–13.

56. Jeschke MG, Finnerty CC, Kulp GA, et al. Combination of recombinant human growth hormone and propranolol decreases hypermetabolism and inflammation in severely burned children. Pediatr Crit Care Med 2008;9:209–16.

57. Waseem T, Duxbury M, Ito H, et al. Exogenous ghrelin modulates release of pro-inflammatory and anti-inflammatory cytokines in LPS-stimulated macrophages through distinct signaling pathways. Surgery 2008;143:334–42.

58. Wan SX, Shi B, Lou XL, et al. Ghrelin protects small intestinal epithelium against sepsis-induced injury by enhancing the autophagy of intestinal epithelial cells. Biomed Pharmacother 2016;83:1315–20.

59. Mechanick JI, Nierman DM. Gonadal steroids in critical illness. Crit Care Clin 2006;22:87–103.

60. Spratt DI. Altered gonadal steroidogenesis in critical illness: is treatment with anabolic steroids indicated? Best Pract Res Clin Endocrinol Metab 2001;15:479–94.

61. Van den Berghe G, Baxter RC, Weekers F, et al. The combined administration of GH-releasing peptide-2 (GHRP-2), TRH and GnRH to men with prolonged critical illness evokes superior endocrine and metabolic effects compared to treatment with GHRP-2 alone. Clin Endocrinol (Oxf) 2002;56:655–69.

62. Ingels C, Vanhorebeek I, Van den Berghe G. Glucose homeostasis, nutrition and infections during critical illness. Clin Microbiol Infect 2017 [pii:S1198-S1743X(17)30004-6].

63. Falciglia M, Freyberg RW, Almenoff PL, et al. Hyperglycemia-related mortality in critically ill patients varies with admission diagnosis. Crit Care Med 2009;37:3001–9.

64. Kosiborod M, Rathore SS, Inzucchi SE, et al. Admission glucose and mortality in elderly patients hospitalized with acute myocardial infarction: implications for patients with and without recognized diabetes. Circulation 2005;111:3078–86.

65. Ingels C, Debaveye Y, Milants I, et al. Strict blood glucose control with insulin during intensive care after cardiac surgery: impact on 4-years survival, dependency on medical care, and quality-of-life. Eur Heart J 2006;27(22):2716–24.

66. Mesotten D, Gielen M, Sterken C, et al. Neurocognitive development of children 4 years after critical illness and treatment with tight glucose control a randomized controlled trial. JAMA 2012;308:1641–50.

67. Van den Berghe G, Wilmer A, Milants I, et al. Intensive insulin therapy in mixed medical/surgical intensive care units - benefit versus harm. Diabetes 2006;55:3151–9.

68. Ellger B, Debaveye Y, Vanhorebeek I, et al. Survival benefits of intensive insulin therapy in critical illness - impact of maintaining normoglycemia versus glycemia-independent actions of insulin. Diabetes 2006;55:1096–105.

69. Gunst J, Van den Berghe G. Blood glucose control in the ICU: don't throw out the baby with the bathwater! Intensive Care Med 2016;42:1478–81.

70. Weekers F, Giulietti AP, Michalaki M, et al. Metabolic, endocrine, and immune effects of stress hyperglycemia in a rabbit model of prolonged critical illness. Endocrinology 2003;144:5329–38.
71. Vanhorebeek I, Gunst J, Ellger B, et al. Hyperglycemic kidney damage in an animal model of prolonged critical illness. Kidney Int 2009;76:512–20.
72. Vanhorebeek I, Ellger B, De Vos R, et al. Tissue-specific glucose toxicity induces mitochondrial damage in a burn injury model of critical illness. Crit Care Med 2009;37:1355–64.
73. Krinsley JS. Effect of an intensive glucose management protocol on the mortality of critically ill adult patients. Mayo Clin Proc 2004;79:992–1000.
74. Lecomte P, Van Vlem B, Coddens J, et al. Tight perioperative glucose control is associated with a reduction in renal impairment and renal failure in non-diabetic cardiac surgical patients. Crit Care 2008;12:R154.
75. Bilotta F, Spinelli A, Giovannini F, et al. The effect of intensive insulin therapy on infection rate, vasospasm, neurologic outcome, and mortality in neurointensive care unit after intracranial aneurysm clipping in patients with acute subarachnoid hemorrhage: a randomized prospective pilot trial. J Neurosurg Anesthesiol 2007;19:156–60.
76. Bilotta F, Caramia R, Paoloni FP, et al. Safety and efficacy of intensive insulin therapy in critical neurosurgical patients. Anesthesiology 2009;110:611–9.
77. Jeschke MG, Kulp GA, Kraft R, et al. Intensive insulin therapy in severely burned pediatric patients a prospective randomized trial. Am J Respir Crit Care Med 2010;182:351–9.
78. Preiser JC, Devos P, Ruiz-Santana S, et al. A prospective randomised multicentre controlled trial on tight glucose control by intensive insulin therapy in adult intensive care units: the Glucontrol study. Intensive Care Med 2009;35:1738–48.
79. Kalfon P, Giraudeau B, Ichai C, et al. Tight computerized versus conventional glucose control in the ICU: a randomized controlled trial. Intensive Care Med 2014;40:171–81.
80. Finfer S, Blair D, Bellomo R, et al. Intensive versus conventional glucose control in critically ill patients. N Engl J Med 2009;360:1283–97.
81. Finfer S, Liu B, Chittock DR, et al. Hypoglycemia and risk of death in critically ill patients. N Engl J Med 2012;367:1108–18.
82. Vanhorebeek I, Gielen M, Boussemaere M, et al. Glucose dysregulation and neurological injury biomarkers in critically ill children. J Clin Endocrinol Metab 2010;95:4669–79.
83. Scott MG, Bruns DE, Boyd JC, et al. Tight glucose control in the intensive care unit: are glucose meters up to the task? Clin Chem 2009;55:18–20.
84. Langhans W. Anorexia of infection: current prospects. Nutrition 2000;16:996–1005.
85. Murray MJ, Murray AB. Anorexia of infection as a mechanism of host defense. Am J Clin Nutr 1979;32:593–6.
86. Dvir D, Cohen J, Singer P. Computerized energy balance and complications in critically ill patients: an observational study. Clin Nutr 2006;25:37–44.
87. McClave SA, Martindale RG, Vanek VW, et al. Guidelines for the provision and assessment of nutrition support therapy in the adult critically ill patient: Society of Critical Care Medicine (SCCM) and American Society for Parenteral and Enteral Nutrition (ASPEN). JPEN J Parenter Enteral Nutr 2009;33:277–316.
88. Gunst J, Van den Berghe G. Parenteral nutrition in the critically ill. Curr Opin Crit Care 2017;23:149–58.

89. Arabi YM, Aldawood AS, Haddad SH, et al. Permissive underfeeding or standard enteral feeding in critically ill adults. N Engl J Med 2015;372:2398–408.

90. Rice TW, Wheeler AP, Thompson BT, et al. Initial trophic vs full enteral feeding in patients with acute lung injury: the EDEN randomized trial. JAMA 2012;307: 795–803.

91. Al-Dorzi HM, Albarrak A, Ferwana M, et al. Lower versus higher dose of enteral caloric intake in adult critically ill patients: a systematic review and meta-analysis. Crit Care 2016;20:358.

92. Marik PE, Hooper MH. Normocaloric versus hypocaloric feeding on the outcomes of ICU patients: a systematic review and meta-analysis. Intensive Care Med 2016;42:316–23.

93. Casaer MP, Van den Berghe G. Nutrition in the acute phase of critical illness. N Engl J Med 2014;370:1227–36.

94. Hermans G, Casaer MP, Clerckx B, et al. Effect of tolerating macronutrient deficit on the development of intensive-care unit acquired weakness: a subanalysis of the EPaNIC trial. Lancet Respir Med 2013;1:621–9.

95. Derde S, Vanhorebeek I, Guiza F, et al. Early parenteral nutrition evokes a phenotype of autophagy deficiency in liver and skeletal muscle of critically ill rabbits. Endocrinology 2012;153:2267–76.

96. van Zanten ARH, Sztark F, Kaisers UX, et al. High-protein enteral nutrition enriched with immune-modulating nutrients vs standard high-protein enteral nutrition and nosocomial infections in the ICU. A randomized clinical trial. JAMA 2014;312:514–24.

97. Heyland D, Muscedere J, Wischmeyer PE, et al. A randomized trial of glutamine and antioxidants in critically ill patients. N Engl J Med 2013;368:1489–97.

98. Bloos F, Trips E, Nierhaus A, et al. Effect of sodium selenite administration and procalcitonin-guided therapy on mortality in patients with severe sepsis or septic shock. A randomized clinical trial. JAMA Intern Med 2016;176:1266–76.

99. Andrews PJD, Avenell A, Noble DW, et al. Randomised trial of glutamine, selenium, or both, to supplement parenteral nutrition for critically ill patients. BMJ 2011;342:d1542.

100. Van Herpe T, Mesotten D, Wouters PJ, et al. LOGIC-Insulin algorithm-guided versus nurse-directed blood glucose control during critical illness the LOGIC-1 single-center, randomized, controlled clinical trial. Diabetes Care 2013;36: 188–94.

Management of Sepsis-Induced Immunosuppression

Fabienne Venet, PharmD, PhD[a,b], Thomas Rimmelé, MD, PhD[b,c],
Guillaume Monneret, PharmD, PhD[a,b,d],*

KEYWORDS

- Sepsis • Septic shock • Immunosuppression • HLA-DR • Immunostimulation • IL-7
- GM-CSF • Lymphopenia

KEY POINTS

- Profound acquired immunosuppression develops within a few days after septic shock in patients.
- Magnitude and/or persistence of sepsis-induced immunosuppression are associated with increased occurrence of nosocomial infections and mortality.
- In animal models, immunostimulation is associated with clinical improvement.
- Results from clinical trials based on interleukin 7 and granulocyte macrophage colony-stimulating factor immunoadjuvant therapies in septic shock patients are expected for 2018.

INTRODUCTION: THE PROCESS OF SEPSIS-INDUCED IMMUNOSUPPRESSION

Although sepsis has been frequently described as solely inducing a tremendous systemic inflammation, current data indicate that it leads to a more complex immune response that evolves over time, with the simultaneous implication of both proinflammatory and anti-inflammatory mechanisms.[1] As a result, after a short unbridled proinflammatory phase, an important subgroup of septic patients presents with profound

Disclosure Statement: The authors declare they do not have any conflicts of interest regarding this article.
[a] Laboratoire d'Immunologie, Cellular Immunology Laboratory, Hospices Civils de Lyon, Hôpital Edouard Herriot, Pavillon E - 5 place d'Arsonval, Lyon Cedex 03 69437, France; [b] EA 7426 PI3 "Pathophysiology of Injury-induced Immunosuppression", Université Claude Bernard Lyon I, Hospices Civils de Lyon, bioMérieux, Hôpital Edouard Herriot, Place d'Arsonval, Lyon Cedex 03 69437, France; [c] Departement of Anesthesiology, Hospices Civils de Lyon, Hôpital Edouard Herriot, Pavillon E - 5 place d'Arsonval, Lyon Cedex 03 69437, France; [d] TRIGGERSEP (TRIal Group for Global Evaluation and Research in SEPsis), F-CRIN Network, France
* Corresponding author. Cellular Immunology Laboratory, Hôpital Edouard Herriot, Hospices Civils de Lyon, Pavillon E - 5 place d'Arsonval, Lyon Cedex 03 69437, France.
E-mail address: guillaume.monneret@chu-lyon.fr

Crit Care Clin 34 (2018) 97–106
http://dx.doi.org/10.1016/j.ccc.2017.08.007
0749-0704/18/© 2017 Elsevier Inc. All rights reserved.

acquired immunosuppression, which could be associated with difficulties to efficiently eradicate the primary infection despite adequate antibiotic treatment.[1–3] Such immune deficiency is also proposed to predispose patients to reactivation of latent viruses (cytomegalovirus or herpes simplex virus) or nosocomial infections due to pathogens, including fungi usually held in abeyance by a functional immune system.[4–7] In addition, it likely contributes to delayed excess mortality (over weeks and years) for which infectious etiologies are frequently involved.[8] Collectively, these immune alterations are believed responsible for worsening outcome in septic patients who survived initial resuscitation.[9]

Consequently, new therapeutic options based on adjunctive immunostimulation (interferon gamma [IFN]-γ, granulocyte macrophage colony-stimulating factor [GM-CSF], interleukin [IL-7], anti–programmed cell death 1 protein [PD1]/anti–PD1–ligand [L]1 antibodies) are emerging.[9,10] Recent data have shown that most aspects of immune responses are modulated in septic patients. Neutrophils lose their anti-infectious properties and shift toward an immature profile and cells with immunosuppressive functions. Monocytes and dendritic cells lose their capacity to produce inflammatory cytokines and to appropriately present antigens to lymphocytes (due to the loss of major histocompatibility complex class II expression [eg, HLA-DR]). The few effector lymphocytes surviving intense apoptotic process occurring after sepsis present with an exhausted phenotype (loss of major effector functions: proliferation, cytokine production, and increased coinhibitory receptor expression) whereas regulatory T- cell and B-cell subpopulations are expanding.[1] Consequently, treatments able to rejuvenate immune functions represent interesting therapeutic candidates in sepsis.[1,8,10] Nevertheless, because there is no clinical sign of immune dysfunctions, such therapeutic intervention must rely on biomarkers[11] for identifying the patients who could benefit from immunostimulation (ie, those presenting with profound and/or long-lasting immune dysfunctions).

MANAGEMENT GOALS AND STRATEGIES
Is There Still Room for Anti-inflammatory Strategies in Sepsis?

Although the main focus of this review is on immunostimulatory therapies in sepsis, there is likely still room for anti-inflammatory treatments in the very first hours of the syndrome. As discussed previously for immunostimulation, however, a major challenge is to identify patients who could benefit from such treatments (ie, in this case, patients who are still on ascending curve of the proinflammatory response). To date, despite a few promising reports,[12] data are still missing regarding this approach.

Extracorporeal Therapies

Several extracorporeal blood purification therapies can potentially positively interfere with the host immune response by removing both inflammatory and anti-inflammatory mediators and consequently preventing forthcoming immunosuppression. In a porcine model, high-volume hemofiltration could prevent endotoxin hyporesponsiveness. CD14 expression on monocytes, oxidative burst, and phagocytosis capacity of granulocytes were also improved by the technique.[13] The IVOIRE multicenter randomized controlled trial (RCT), however, comparing ultrafiltration flow rates of 35 mL/kg/h versus 70 mL/kg/h in patients with septic shock and acute kidney injury, did not show any survival benefit.[14] Hemoperfusion is based on the interaction between a sorbent and molecules targeted for removal via adsorption. In a recent meta-analysis, the beneficial effect of blood purification on mortality was mainly driven by the results of studies assessing hemoperfusion with polymyxin B.[15] Because it targets the endotoxin, polymyxin B hemoperfusion is proposed for the treatment of gram-negative infections. In addition to hemodynamic and respiratory improvements, the EUPHAS trial suggested a survival benefit for septic patients receiving this therapy.[16] Nevertheless, the recent ABDO-MIX study did not confirm these findings.[17] Potential effects on preventing secondary immunosuppression are not reported yet. Additional information will be soon available with the release of the results of the EUPHRATES trial (NCT01046669). Coupled plasma filtration adsorption may also be able to have an impact on the host response due to cytokine adsorption on a specific resin. In a pilot study on septic patients, coupled plasma filtration adsorption was more efficient than high-volume hemofiltration to reverse immunoparalysis (increased expression of monocyte HLA-DR and lipopolysaccharide [LPS]-induced TNF production).[18] Finally, renal replacement therapy membranes used for kidney support in case of acute kidney injury can be modified to serve as a blood purification device. For example, adding a positively charged polymer to a standard polyacrylonitrile membrane enhances its adsorption capacities of LPS and cytokines.[19] Other aspects of the membrane can also be modified, such as the cutoff (increase of the pore size), allowing for the removal of a larger spectrum of (anti)-inflammatory mediators.

All these extracorporeal blood purification therapies should be considered under scientific investigation. Experts who recently updated the Surviving Sepsis Campaign guidelines could not make any recommendation concerning their use in daily clinical practice.[20] Further research, therefore, is urgently warranted in this field.

Intravenous Immunoglobulin

In patients with septic shock, low levels of circulating immunoglobulins are detected in association with predisposition to recurrent infections.[21] The administration of intravenous immunoglobulins (IVIG) was thus proposed as an effective adjunctive therapy in sepsis through improvement of bacterial clearance and immunomodulation.[22] Clinical trials evaluated the effects of IVIG as adjunctive treatments in patients with sepsis, the results of which are still under debate.[23] A meta-analysis reported a general reduction in mortality (approximately 21%) in adult patients with sepsis and septic shock who received polyclonal immunoglobulins and a more evident effect on mortality in the subgroup receiving IgM-enriched immunoglobulin.[24] A more recent meta-analysis by Cochrane showed a reduction in mortality in patients who received polyclonal IVIG, although this positive effect disappeared when analyzing only trials with low bias.[23] A large retrospective study in 8264 patients in Japan evaluated the effect of IVIG as an adjunctive treatment in patients with septic shock due to pneumonia.[25] No benefit was found in terms of mortality in the group of patients receiving the immunoglobulins.

Thus the most recent guidelines of the Surviving Sepsis Campaign suggest against the use of IVIG in patients with sepsis.[20] Only toxin-mediated bacterial diseases, such as severe *Staphylococcus* and *Streptococcus* infections, are currently given as examples of indications for IVIG therapy in infection.

Interferon Gamma

IFN-γ is a prototypical type 1 helper T-cell cytokine and a major activator of monocytes that increases their antigen-presentation capacity and primes these cells for LPS-induced production of cytokines. The beneficial effect of IFN-γ on monocyte deactivation in septic patients was first described in 1997 by Docke and colleagues[26] in a limited open-label study. In 2002, Nakos and colleagues[27] confirmed these results in trauma patients by showing that inhaled IFN-γ treatment led to HLA-DR expression recovery in alveolar macrophages and decreased incidence of ventilator-associated pneumonia. After these 2 seminal studies, the use of IFN-γ in severely infected patients was only reported in clinical cases.[28,29] These case reports systematically showed the association between this immune-adjuvant treatment and improved immune functions, including increased HLA-DR expression. More recently, IFN-γ therapy was even proposed to improve outcome and immune dysfunctions in invasive fungal infections.[30] A recent case report in a woman with fungal sepsis (mucormycosis) unresponsive to conventional therapy showed the efficacy of IFN-γ therapy associated with nivolumab (anti-PD1 antibody) in restoring immune dysfunctions and clearing such invasive infection.[31] Despite these promising preliminary data, no RCT has been conducted yet in ICU patients with IFN-γ. Thus, the beneficial effect of such immunotherapy on clinical outcomes, such as mortality, secondary infection, or ICU length of stay remains elusive.

Granulocyte Macrophage Colony-Stimulating Factor

GM-CSF is a hematopoietic growth factor stimulating the production of neutrophils and monocytes by the bone marrow. This cytokine is also a potent stimulant of monocyte survival and functions. Whereas the use of GM-CSF as a prophylaxis of infections in neutropenic patients did not show any benefit,[32] this growth factor was subsequently evaluated as an immune-adjuvant therapy in sepsis. In an open-label RCT in non-neutropenic children admitted to a pediatric ICU with immunoparalysis (ie, reduced ex vivo TNF-α production), Hall and colleagues[33] showed that GM-CSF therapy facilitated recovery of TNF-α response and prevented nosocomial infections. In a report of 4 cases, Nelson[34] showed that GM-CSF therapy was associated with reversal of T-cell anergy and a significant decrease in infections in otherwise immunologically healthy children with recurrent infections. Finally, in 56 septic neonates, Drossou-Agakidou and colleauges[35] showed that GM-CSF treatment resulted in an earlier increase of the number of monocytes expressing HLA-DR after the onset of sepsis. In adults, 4 RCTs totaling 158 patients evaluated this therapeutic approach so far. GM-CSF treatment was associated with improved clinical outcomes, such as reduced rate of secondary infections and hospital length of stay,[36] up-regulation of functional markers on monocytes (HLA-DR expression),[37] and improved gas exchange.[38] An interesting approach used by Meisel and colleagues[39] was to restrict the administration of GM-CSF to patients with immune dysfunctions (decreased monocyte HLA-DR expression). The investigators observed that biomarker-guided GM-CSF therapy in sepsis was safe and effective for restoring monocytic immunocompetence. In addition, use of GM-CSF shortened the time of mechanical ventilation and hospital/ICU stay.

GM-CSF represents thus a promising immunoadjuvant therapy in sepsis although larger RCTs are now warranted to confirm these initial results. One clinical trial (GRID trial) evaluating this therapeutic approach in septic shock patients is soon to be completed (NCT02361528).

Interleukin 7

IL-7, produced by bone marrow and thymus cells, is an indispensable cytokine for growth, differentiation, and effector functions of T cells.[40] As a treatment, recombinant human (rh)IL-7 has been proposed in the therapeutic arsenal of patients with lymphopenia and lymphopenia-driven diseases. This cytokine is also currently undergoing clinical testing as an immune-enhancing agent in patients with cancer and progressive multifocal leukoencephalopathy.[40,41] Because septic patients present with severe lymphocyte alterations (in number, phenotype, and functions) associated with increased mortality, rhIL-7 is proposed in this clinical context and is even considered by experts as one of the most promising potential adjuvant treatments of sepsis-induced immunosuppression.[1,8] In septic mice, Unsinger and colleagues[42] showed that rhIL-7 was able to reduce T-cell apoptosis, restore IFN-γ production, improve leukocyte trafficking, and finally improve mice survival. Similar results were observed in a clinically relevant 2-hit model of fungal sepsis.[43] In an ex vivo study in septic patients' cells, T-lymphocyte functions were also enhanced with rhIL-7 (ie. proliferation, INF-γ production, STAT5 phosphorylation, and B-cell lymphoma 2 induction).[44] In addition, IL-7 has demonstrated positive effects in enhancing immune response during anti-PD1 treatment in cancer.[44] Based on these convincing preclinical results, a phase 2 multicenter RCT assessing rhIL-7 in patients with septic shock was designed (IRIS trial [NCT02640807]). Its primary aim was to confirm that rhIL-7 was safe and able to increase the absolute lymphocyte count in immunosuppressed septic patients. This clinical study has just been completed with patients enrolled in France and in the United States. Results are expected to be published in the near future. To date, rhIL-7 treatment seems a serious candidate to tackle sepsis-induced immunosuppression.

Immune Checkpoint Inhibitors

PD1 receptor system constitutes a potent immunoregulatory pathway that negatively controls immune responses. This system is composed of PD1 and its 2 ligands, PD-L1 and PD-L2. Immune checkpoint inhibitors are antibodies that target this key signaling pathway that are currently revolutionizing treatment of cancer.[45,46] Several observational studies described the increased expression of PD1-related molecules on circulating immune cells in septic patients in association with immune dysfunctions and deleterious outcomes.[47] In addition, ex vivo studies in septic patients' cells showed that PD1/PD-L1 pathway blockade decreased sepsis-induced immune dysfunctions.[48–50] No RCT evaluating immune checkpoint inhibitors in sepsis, however, has been published so far. Only 2 case reports describe the use of a single dose of nivolumab (anti-PD1 blocking monoclonal antibody) in combination with repeated IFN-γ treatment in a 30-year-old woman with invasive mucormycosis unresponsive to conventional therapy and presenting with immunosuppression.[31] After these treatments, the patient improved slowly, did not show persistent sign of immunosuppression or residual infection, and was finally discharged from the ICU on day 80. A phase 1 clinical study of nivolumab in the treatment of sepsis is ongoing (NCT02960854).

PERSPECTIVES
Novel Design for Randomized Controlled Trial in Sepsis

Because there is no clinical sign of immune dysfunctions, it is crucial to use appropriate biomarkers for patients' stratification according to their immune status.[11] Some patients spontaneously restore their immune functions overtime and, therefore, do not need to receive any immunoadjuvant intervention.[9] Most importantly, before treating patients with immunostimulatory therapies, clinicians have to ascertain that the first unbridled inflammatory phase is over because immunostimulatory molecules might putatively reactivate cytokine storm. Therefore, it is recommended not to treat patients with these drugs during the first 2 days after admission and this approach is thus restricted to patients who survived the first inflammatory hours/days after sepsis. To date, numerous biomarkers have been proposed to identify immunosuppression (immature neutrophils count, immune checkpoint inhibitor expression, and functional testing[11,51,52]). So far, the most consensually accepted parameter is the decreased expression of HLA-DR on monocytes.[1,52,53] Lowest values are regularly reported to be associated with increased mortality and nosocomial infections rates after severe injuries (eg, sepsis, trauma, and burns). Results are obtained thanks to standardized flow cytometry protocols.[54,55] Because flow cytometry facilities are not accessible everywhere, let alone 24/7, fully automated bedside cytometer is under evaluation. The other parameter usable in this context is total lymphocyte count because magnitude of lymphopenia has been reported to be associated with mortality.[56,57] Of major importance, current GM-CSF RCT is stratified based on monocyte HLA-DR values below 8000 AB/C (NCT02361528) whereas the IL-7 trial is stratified on lymphocyte count below 0.9 G/L (NCT02640807).

Another novelty regarding these trials is primary outcome that is evaluated. Mortality judged after 28 days is likely not appropriate because deleterious effects of sepsis are believed to last more than 1 month.[8,58] In addition, because secondary infections are mostly believed to be consequences of immunosuppression, the capacity of a given molecule to decrease the rate of nosocomial infections seems a clinically relevant endpoint to monitor. In addition, although secondary infections may only modestly contribute to overall mortality,[59] they augment ICU and hospital lengths of stay and number of days on ventilator and thus raise global costs related to sepsis. Similarly, in the first year after sepsis, the first cause of hospital readmission (and additional cost) is infection, suggesting that immune functions are still compromised.[60] Restoring immune functions may thus have a significant impact on public health economy. Considering the expending economic burden of sepsis, all these parameters deserve to be evaluated in next trials as well.

Beyond Sepsis: Broadening the Area of Application

Acquired immunosuppression in the ICU is not specific to sepsis. Similar mechanisms develop each time the body faces a systemic and potential lethal inflammatory response. Even if kinetics of occurrence and magnitude of immune dysfunctions may be somewhat different, severe burn and trauma, major surgery, and pancreatitis induce similar immune dysfunctions.[61–63] In each of these clinical conditions, an association between immune alterations and secondary infections has been reported. In other infectious contexts, such as severe flu, measles, Ebola infection, and septic shock in pediatrics, similar observations are also made.[64–67] Collectively, the monitoring of immune response in ICU patients thus appears of major interest in the better control of nosocomial/delayed infections.

The Future

In this brief review, only the most likely therapeutic possibilities for battling immunosuppression are detailed. This field is just opening and numerous molecules are potential candidates. Of them, a nonexhaustive list includes thymolysin-α, growth hormone, Toll-like receptor agonists, IL-3, IL-15, and Flt3 ligand. Importantly, in preclinical studies, next molecules should be evaluated in appropriate animal models. For instance, the cecal ligation and puncture procedure has been modified to better mimic the process of sepsis-induced immunosuppression. Punctures are smaller; animals are treated with antibiotics, analgesia, and fluid resuscitation to mimic clinical management received by patients and present with similar immune defects as those seen in patients. In this model, after a few days, animals become unable to fight a second infectious challenge by weak pathogenic germs whereas sham animals easily clear such infections.[43] Finally, sepsis and cancer share many similarities regarding weakened immune defense.[68] Considering that the use of immunotherapy in cancer is currently burgeoning with tremendous success, it is reasonable to plan that novel cancer biotherapies will rapidly translate to innovative therapeutic advances in ICU patients.

SUMMARY

The weight of sepsis-induced immunosuppression is now well established. Nevertheless, the demonstration of efficacy of immunostimulation in improving some or all deleterious outcomes remains to be made. That given, innovative immunomonitoring strategies characterizing the host immune response and thus permitting personalized immunostimulation seem a reasonable perspective. This would allow better taking into account the rapidly changing immune response overtime after initial infection, from exacerbated inflammation to severe immunosuppression. First results from an RCT (IL-7 and GM-CSF) in sepsis-induced immunosuppression should be soon released (end 2017 to early 2018). They would help in better delineate the way for efficient immunostimulation.

REFERENCES

1. Hotchkiss RS, Monneret G, Payen D. Sepsis-induced immunosuppression: from cellular dysfunctions to immunotherapy. Nat Rev Immunol 2013;13(12):862–74.
2. Torgersen C, Moser P, Luckner G, et al. Macroscopic postmortem findings in 235 surgical intensive care patients with sepsis. Anesth Analg 2009;108(6):1841–7.
3. Boomer JS, To K, Chang KC, et al. Immunosuppression in patients who die of sepsis and multiple organ failure. JAMA 2011;306(23):2594–605.
4. Landelle C, Lepape A, Voirin N, et al. Low monocyte human leukocyte antigen-DR is independently associated with nosocomial infections after septic shock. Intensive Care Med 2010;36(11):1859–66.
5. Monneret G, Venet F, Kullberg BJ, et al. ICU-acquired immunosuppression and the risk for secondary fungal infections. Med Mycol 2011;49(Suppl 1):S17–23.
6. Walton AH, Muenzer JT, Rasche D, et al. Reactivation of multiple viruses in patients with sepsis. PLoS One 2014;9(2):e98819.
7. Ong DSY, Bonten MJM, Spitoni C, et al. Epidemiology of multiple herpes viremia in previously immunocompetent patients with septic shock. Clin Infect Dis 2017; 64(9):1204–10.
8. Delano MJ, Ward PA. Sepsis-induced immune dysfunction: can immune therapies reduce mortality? J Clin Invest 2016;126(1):23–31.
9. Hotchkiss RS, Monneret G, Payen D. Immunosuppression in sepsis: a novel understanding of the disorder and a new therapeutic approach. Lancet Infect Dis 2013;13(3):260–8.
10. Hutchins NA, Unsinger J, Hotchkiss RS, et al. The new normal: immunomodulatory agents against sepsis immune suppression. Trends Mol Med 2014;20(4):224–33.
11. Venet F, Lukaszewicz AC, Payen D, et al. Monitoring the immune response in sepsis: a rational approach to administration of immunoadjuvant therapies. Curr Opin Immunol 2013;25(4):477–83.
12. Panacek EA, Marshall JC, Albertson TE, et al. Efficacy and safety of the monoclonal anti-tumor necrosis factor antibody F(ab')2 fragment afelimomab in patients with severe sepsis and elevated interleukin-6 levels. Crit Care Med 2004; 32(11):2173–82.
13. Yekebas EF, Eisenberger CF, Ohnesorge H, et al. Attenuation of sepsis-related immunoparalysis by continuous veno-venous hemofiltration in experimental porcine pancreatitis. Crit Care Med 2001;29(7):1423–30.
14. Joannes-Boyau O, Honore PM, Perez P, et al. High-volume versus standard-volume haemofiltration for septic shock patients with acute kidney injury (IVOIRE study): a multicentre randomized controlled trial. Intensive Care Med 2013;39(9):1535–46.

15. Zhou F, Peng Z, Murugan R, et al. Blood purification and mortality in sepsis: a meta-analysis of randomized trials. Crit Care Med 2013;41(9):2209–20.
16. Cruz DN, Antonelli M, Fumagalli R, et al. Early use of polymyxin B hemoperfusion in abdominal septic shock: the EUPHAS randomized controlled trial. JAMA 2009; 301(23):2445–52.
17. Payen DM, Guilhot J, Launey Y, et al. Early use of polymyxin B hemoperfusion in patients with septic shock due to peritonitis: a multicenter randomized control trial. Intensive Care Med 2015;41(6):975–84.
18. Mao HJ, Yu S, Yu XB, et al. Effects of coupled plasma filtration adsorption on immune function of patients with multiple organ dysfunction syndrome. Int J Artif Organs 2009;32(1):31–8.
19. Rimmele T, Assadi A, Cattenoz M, et al. High-volume haemofiltration with a new haemofiltration membrane having enhanced adsorption properties in septic pigs. Nephrol Dial Transplant 2009;24(2):421–7.
20. Rhodes A, Evans LE, Alhazzani W, et al. Surviving sepsis campaign: international guidelines for management of sepsis and septic shock: 2016. Intensive Care Med 2017;43(3):304–77.
21. Notarangelo LD, Fischer A, Geha RS, et al. Primary immunodeficiencies: 2009 update. J Allergy Clin Immunol 2009;124(6):1161–78.
22. Schwab I, Nimmerjahn F. Intravenous immunoglobulin therapy: how does IgG modulate the immune system? Nat Rev Immunol 2013;13(3):176–89.
23. Alejandria MM, Lansang MA, Dans LF, et al. Intravenous immunoglobulin for treating sepsis, severe sepsis and septic shock. Cochrane Database Syst Rev 2013;(9):CD001090.
24. Kreymann KG, de Heer G, Nierhaus A, et al. Use of polyclonal immunoglobulins as adjunctive therapy for sepsis or septic shock. Crit Care Med 2007;35(12): 2677–85.
25. Tagami T, Matsui H, Fushimi K, et al. Intravenous immunoglobulin and mortality in pneumonia patients with septic shock: an observational nationwide study. Clin Infect Dis 2015;61(3):385–92.
26. Docke WD, Randow F, Syrbe U, et al. Monocyte deactivation in septic patients: restoration by IFN-gamma treatment. Nat Med 1997;3(6):678–81.
27. Nakos G, Malamou-Mitsi VD, Lachana A, et al. Immunoparalysis in patients with severe trauma and the effect of inhaled interferon-gamma. Crit Care Med 2002; 30(7):1488–94.
28. Nalos M, Santner-Nanan B, Parnell G, et al. Immune effects of interferon gamma in persistent staphylococcal sepsis. Am J Respir Crit Care Med 2012;185(1):110–2.
29. Lukaszewicz AC, Faivre V, Payen D. Is monocyte HLA-DR expression monitoring a useful tool to predict the risk of secondary infection? Minerva Anestesiol 2010; 76(9):737–43.
30. Delsing CE, Gresnigt MS, Leentjens J, et al. Interferon-gamma as adjunctive immunotherapy for invasive fungal infections: a case series. BMC Infect Dis 2014;14:166.
31. Grimaldi D, Pradier O, Hotchkiss RS, et al. Nivolumab plus interferon-gamma in the treatment of intractable mucormycosis. Lancet Infect Dis 2017;17(1):18.
32. Bohlius J, Herbst C, Reiser M, et al. Granulopoiesis-stimulating factors to prevent adverse effects in the treatment of malignant lymphoma. Cochrane Database Syst Rev 2008;(4):CD003189.
33. Hall MW, Knatz NL, Vetterly C, et al. Immunoparalysis and nosocomial infection in children with multiple organ dysfunction syndrome. Intensive Care Med 2011; 37(3):525–32.

34. Nelson LA. Use of granulocyte-macrophage colony-stimulating factor to reverse anergy in otherwise immunologically healthy children. Ann Allergy Asthma Immunol 2007;98(4):373–82.

35. Drossou-Agakidou V, Kanakoudi-Tsakalidou F, Sarafidis K, et al. In vivo effect of rhGM-CSF and rhG-CSF on monocyte HLA-DR expression of septic neonates. Cytokine 2002;18(5):260–5.

36. Orozco H, Arch J, Medina-Franco H, et al. Molgramostim (GM-CSF) associated with antibiotic treatment in nontraumatic abdominal sepsis: a randomized, double-blind, placebo-controlled clinical trial. Arch Surg 2006;141(2):150–3 [discussion: 154].

37. Rosenbloom AJ, Linden PK, Dorrance A, et al. Effect of granulocyte-monocyte colony-stimulating factor therapy on leukocyte function and clearance of serious infection in nonneutropenic patients. Chest 2005;127(6):2139–50.

38. Presneill JJ, Harris T, Stewart AG, et al. A randomized phase II trial of granulocyte-macrophage colony-stimulating factor therapy in severe sepsis with respiratory dysfunction. Am J Respir Crit Care Med 2002;166(2):138–43.

39. Meisel C, Schefold JC, Pschowski R, et al. Granulocyte-macrophage colony-stimulating factor to reverse sepsis-associated immunosuppression: a double-blind, randomized, placebo-controlled multicenter trial. Am J Respir Crit Care Med 2009;180(7):640–8.

40. Mackall CL, Fry TJ, Gress RE. Harnessing the biology of IL-7 for therapeutic application. Nat Rev Immunol 2011;11(5):330–42.

41. Lundstrom W, Fewkes NM, Mackall CL. IL-7 in human health and disease. Semin Immunol 2012;24(3):218–24.

42. Unsinger JMM, Kasten KR, Hoekzema AS, et al. IL-7 promotes T cell viability, trafficking, and functionality and improves survival in sepsis. J Immunol 2010;184(7): 3768–79.

43. Unsinger J, Burnham CA, McDonough J, et al. Interleukin-7 ameliorates immune dysfunction and improves survival in a 2-hit model of fungal sepsis. J Infect Dis 2012;206(4):606–16.

44. Venet F, Foray AP, Villars-Mechin A, et al. IL-7 restores lymphocyte functions in septic patients. J Immunol 2012;189(10):5073–81.

45. Giroux Leprieur E, Dumenil C, Julie C, et al. Chinet T: immunotherapy revolutionises non-small-cell lung cancer therapy: results, perspectives and new challenges. Eur J Cancer 2017;78:16–23.

46. Yang Y. Cancer immunotherapy: harnessing the immune system to battle cancer. J Clin Invest 2015;125(9):3335–7.

47. Huang X, Venet F, Wang YL, et al. PD-1 expression by macrophages plays a pathologic role in altering microbial clearance and the innate inflammatory response to sepsis. Proc Natl Acad Sci U S A 2009;106(15):6303–8.

48. Chang KC, Burnham CA, Compton SM, et al. Blockade ofthe negative co-stimulatory molecules PD-1 and CTLA-4 improves survival in primary and secondary fungal sepsis. Crit Care 2013;17(3):R85.

49. Chang K, Svabek C, Vazquez-Guillamet C, et al. Targeting the programmed cell death 1: programmed cell death ligand 1 pathway reverses T cell exhaustion in patients with sepsis. Crit Care 2014;18(1):R3.

50. Zhang Y, Zhou Y, Lou J, et al. PD-L1 blockade improves survival in experimental sepsis by inhibiting lymphocyte apoptosis and reversing monocyte dysfunction. Crit Care 2010;14(6):R220.

51. Monneret G, Demaret J, Gossez M, et al. Novel approach in monocyte intracellular TNF measurement: application to sepsis-induced immune alterations. Shock 2016;47(3):318–22.
52. Monneret G, Venet F. Sepsis-induced immune alterations monitoring by flow cytometry as a promising tool for individualized therapy. Cytometry B Clin Cytom 2016;90(4):376–86.
53. Venet F, Lepape A, Monneret G. Clinical review: flow cytometry perspectives in the ICU : from diagnosis of infection to monitoring of injury-induced immune dysfunctions. Crit Care 2011;15(5):231.
54. Demaret J, Walencik A, Jacob MC, et al. Inter-laboratory assessment of flow cytometric monocyte HLA-DR expression in clinical samples. Cytometry B Clin Cytom 2013;84(1):59–62.
55. Docke WD, Hoflich C, Davis KA, et al. Monitoring temporary immunodepression by flow cytometric measurement of monocytic HLA-DR expression: a multicenter standardized study. Clin Chem 2005;51(12):2341–7.
56. Drewry AM, Samra N, Skrupky LP, et al. Persistent lymphopenia after diagnosis of sepsis predicts mortality. Shock 2014;42(5):383–91.
57. Girardot T, Rimmele T, Venet F, et al. Apoptosis-induced lymphopenia in sepsis and other severe injuries. Apoptosis 2016;22(2):295–305.
58. Arens C, Bajwa SA, Koch C, et al. Sepsis-induced long-term immune paralysis - results of a descriptive, explorative study. Crit Care 2016;20(1):93.
59. van Vught LA, Klein Klouwenberg PM, Spitoni C, et al. Incidence, risk factors, and attributable mortality of secondary infections in the intensive care unit after admission for sepsis. JAMA 2016;315(14):1469–79.
60. Kaur A, Levy MM. Role of sepsis in delayed mortality. Ann Transl Med 2016; 4(19):378.
61. Venet F, Tissot S, Debard AL, et al. Decreased monocyte human leukocyte antigen-DR expression after severe burn injury: correlation with severity and secondary septic shock. Crit Care Med 2007;35(8):1910–7.
62. Gouel-Cheron A, Allaouchiche B, Guignant C, et al. Early interleukin-6 and slope of monocyte human leukocyte antigen-DR: a powerful association to predict the development of sepsis after major trauma. PLoS One 2012;7(3):e33095.
63. Satoh A, Miura T, Satoh K, et al. Human leukocyte antigen-DR expression on peripheral monocytes as a predictive marker of sepsis during acute pancreatitis. Pancreas 2002;25(3):245–50.
64. Ruibal P, Oestereich L, Ludtke A, et al. Unique human immune signature of Ebola virus disease in Guinea. Nature 2016;533(7601):100–4.
65. Mina MJ, Metcalf CJ, de Swart RL, et al. Long-term measles-induced immunomodulation increases overall childhood infectious disease mortality. Science 2015; 348(6235):694–9.
66. Wu W, Shi Y, Gao H, et al. Immune derangement occurs in patients with H7N9 avian influenza. Crit Care 2014;18(2):R43.
67. Genel F, Atlihan F, Ozsu E, et al. Monocyte HLA-DR expression as predictor of poor outcome in neonates with late onset neonatal sepsis. J Infect 2010;60(3):224–8.
68. Hotchkiss RS, Moldawer LL. Parallels between cancer and infectious disease. N Engl J Med 2014;371(4):380–3.

Nutrition Therapy in Sepsis

Paul E. Wischmeyer, MD, EDIC

KEYWORDS

- Protein • Parenteral nutrition • Enteral nutrition • Calories • Lean body mass
- Lipids

KEY POINTS

- Sepsis is characterized by early massive catabolism, lean body mass (LBM) loss, and escalating hypermetabolism persisting for months to years.
- Early enteral nutrition should attempt to correct micronutrient/vitamin deficiencies, deliver adequate protein (~1.0 g/kg/d), and moderated nonprotein calories (~15 kcal/kg/d), as well-nourished patients can generate significant endogenous energy for a limited period.
- After resuscitation, increasing protein (1.5–2.0 g/kg/d) and calories is needed to attenuate LBM loss and promote early mobility and recovery.
- Following ICU, significant protein/calorie delivery for months to years is required to facilitate functional and LBM recovery, with high protein oral supplements being essential to achieve adequate nutrition (>3000 kcal/d and higher protein [>1.5 g/kg/d] likely needed).
- Screening for preillness malnutrition is essential, with supplemental parenteral nutrition added if the protein/calorie goals are not met with timeliness, depending on the preillness nutrition/LBM status.

INTRODUCTION

Sepsis, requiring care in the intensive care unit (ICU), is characterized by an acute catabolic response leading to rapid mobilization of energy stores, as muscle, glycogen, and lipid stores are broken down to drive glucose production.[1,2] This catabolism contributes to rapid loss of lean body mass (LBM) contributing to muscle wasting, weakness, and loss of physical function commonly known as ICU-acquired weakness (ICU-AW) or post-ICU syndrome (PICS).[3] This LBM loss is exacerbated by sepsis-induced anorexia

Disclosure Statement: P.E. Wischmeyer is an associate editor of *Clinical Nutrition* (Elsevier), has received grant funding related to this work from the NIH NHLBI R34 HL109369, Canadian Institutes of Health Research, Baxter, Fresenius, Lyric Pharmaceuticals, Isomark LLC, and Medtronics. He has served as a consultant to Nestle, Abbott, Fresenius, Baxter, Medtronics, Nutricia, Lyric Pharmaceuticals, and Takeda for research related to this work. He has limited ownership shares in Isomark for his consulting work with Isomark, which has otherwise been unpaid in nature. He has received honoraria or travel expenses for lectures on improving nutrition care in illness from Abbott, Fresenius, and Medtronics.

Department of Anesthesiology, Duke University School of Medicine, 2400 Pratt Street, Office: NP 7060, Durham, NC 27705, USA
E-mail address: Paul.Wischmeyer@Duke.edu

and the inability to take nutrients by mouth volitionally for days to months.[4] Unless nutrition therapy is provided via enteral or parenteral routes, patients also accumulate a rapidly evolving energy deficit, which further contributes to muscle wasting and worsened outcomes.[5–7] This illness and, unfortunately, iatrogenic starvation are superimposed on the marked inflammatory and endocrine-mediated acute-phase stress response. Critically ill (burns) patients can lose as much as 1 kg of LBM per day.[8] Other ICU patients also have significant LBM loss, much of it in the first 7 to 10 days of their ICU stay.[9] Patients often regain weight after the ICU stay, but much of this is only fat mass rather than functional LBM.[10] This finding is not surprising, as data from burn ICU patients demonstrate that catabolism and subsequent increasing hypermetabolism following injury can persist for up to 2 years following discharge from the hospital; this can markedly hinder recovery of LBM and function.[8]

This evolutionarily conserved stress response allows the injured or septic human to generate energy to escape an attacker and recover from initial illness in a period when food gathering and consumption would initially be limited. Before the relatively recent (evolutionarily) development of ICU and hospital care, this period of cachexia and catabolism was self-limited, likely to a few days. The injured or infected (septic) human escaped its attacker and then either improved and reinitiated volitional nutrition intake or death occurred. However, modern ICU care now allows prolonged survival from sepsis via the ability to provide vital organ support for extended periods of time, making previously unsurvivable septic insults now survivable. In fact, innovations in ICU care have recently led to an almost yearly reduction of hospital mortality from sepsis.[11] However, these same data reveal many patients with sepsis are not returning home to functional lives after ICU discharge but instead to rehabilitation settings where it is unclear if they ever returned to a meaningful quality of life (QoL). In fact, in the same period that in-hospital ICU mortality seems to be declining, there has been a tripling in the number of patients going to rehabilitation settings.[11] Up to 40% of mortality within the first year of ICU stay occurs following ICU discharge.[12] Unfortunately, for those who do survive, nearly half will not return to work in the first year after discharge,[13] often because of PICS and ICU-AW.[3]

A growing body of data indicates that persistent underfeeding throughout the ICU stay, particularly protein underfeeding, may significantly contribute to long-term mortality and QoL impairment months later.[5,14–16] If we are to optimize recovery from sepsis and critical care, we need to consider basic metabolism and a historic understanding of starvation and recovery to use targeted nutritional care to our critically ill patients with sepsis. The focus of modern ICU nutrition therapy and research efforts should emphasize the realization that nutritional needs change over the course of a septic illness, as catabolism persists and increasing hypermetabolism evolves and persists, often for months to years.[9] Finally, screening for preillness malnutrition and the presence of nutritional risk (as defined by scores, such as the NUTRIC (Nutrition Risk in the Critically Ill) score,[17,18] or computed tomography [CT] LBM analysis[19]) is essential at diagnosis of sepsis. In patients found to have preexisting sarcopenia or malnutrition, parenteral nutrition (PN), with adequate protein delivery and modern balanced lipids, can be safely added when enteral nutrition (EN) is failing.

MANAGEMENT GOALS FOR NUTRITION IN SEPSIS
Acute Catabolic Phase of Sepsis

Acute phase: adequate protein and moderated nonprotein calories
As stated earlier, the early or acute phase of sepsis is characterized by massive mobilization of the body's calorie reserves as muscle, glycogen, and lipid stores are broken

down to generate glucose to support ATP production (**Figs. 1** and **2**, **Table 1**A).[1,2] This metabolic response to stress can generate 50% to 75% of glucose needs during illness[2] and is not suppressed by feeding or intravenous glucose infusion.[16] Further, the early acute phase of sepsis and trauma are not hypermetabolic states; rather, patients have a total energy expenditure (TEE) to resting energy expenditure (REE) ratio of 1.0 and 1.1 for sepsis and trauma, respectively.[20] Thus, caloric need does not consistently increase in the early phases of sepsis. In fact, the more severe the septic shock, the lower the REE, as the body hibernates and reduces metabolism in response to severe sepsis.[21] This idea is shown in **Table 1** in the context of caloric needs from the World Health Organization in health and the landmark Minnesota Starvation Study.[7] Data from Uehara and colleagues[20] demonstrate that REE in the first 2 to 5 days (acute phase) in elderly patients with sepsis (mean age: 67 years) is approximately 1850 kcal/d with a TEE of approximately 1920 kcal/d (giving a TEE of 25 kcal/kg). These data and other recent trials[22] suggest we should consider feeding less nonprotein calories early in the acute phase (first 24–96 hours) of critical illness and markedly increase calorie delivery during recovery as illustrated in **Fig. 1**. At the same time, it is well known that protein losses increase 4-fold in the first 24 hours of critical illness[23] and health carers are exceedingly poor at meeting these needs.[23] Unfortunately, large international surveys indicate ICU practitioners deliver an average of 0.6 g/kg/d of protein for the first 2 weeks following ICU admission.[6] This amount is 33% to 50% of the latest ICU guideline-recommended protein delivery of 1.2 to 2.0 g/kg/d.[24] In contrast to conventional teaching, the delivery of additional nonprotein calories does not significantly improve nitrogen balance in illness beyond delivery of 50% of predicted REE.[16] A secondary analysis of the pediatric PEPANIC (Early versus Late Parenteral Nutrition in the Pediatric Intensive Care Unit) trial by the Vanhorebeek[25] group demonstrates that very early higher protein delivery may be associated with adverse outcomes, related possibly to inhibition of autophagy. Of note, increased lipid delivery early in critical illness was associated with earlier ICU

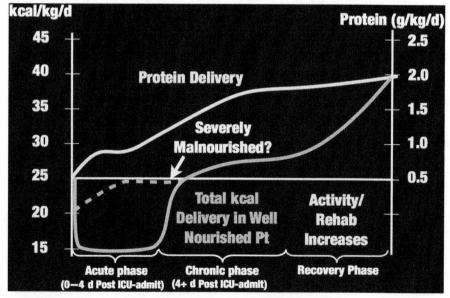

Fig. 1. Proposal for targeted nutrition delivery in sepsis. Pt, patient.

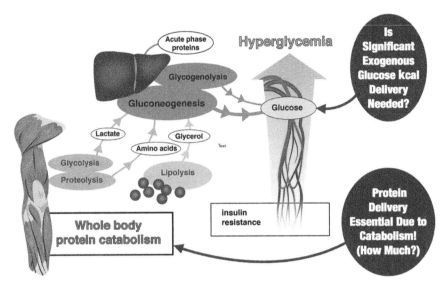

Body Can Generate 50%–75% of Pts Glucose Requirements Early!

Fig. 2. Early acute-phase catabolic response to sepsis. Pts, patients. (*Adapted from* Gillis C, Carli F. Promoting perioperative metabolic and nutritional care. Anesthesiology 2015;123(6): 1455–72.)

discharge. These hypothesis-generating findings from this study leave the clinician in a challenging position with an essential need to provide protein during ICU recovery, yet it remains unclear currently how much to give and when to escalate protein delivery to guideline goals. Thus, an ideal targeted feeding strategy may perhaps be approximately 15 kcal/kg/d of total energy needs during the early ICU stay (acute phase: day 1–4), while ensuring patients receive an optimal lower protein delivery (~1.0 g/kg/d) as early as possible after ICU admission (see **Fig. 1**). Reduced calorie/protein delivery during the acute phase may not, however, be applicable in severely malnourished patients (ie, patients with significant pre-ICU weight loss or NUTRIC score [without interleukin 6 (IL-6) levels] ≥5) who are unlikely to have the metabolic reserve to generate endogenous energy needs.[18,24] Ironically, the most recent guidelines from the Society of Critical Care Medicine (SCCM)/American Society for Parenteral and Enteral Nutrition (ASPEN) emphasize these points suggesting hypocaloric PN (≤20 kcal/kg/d or 80% of estimated energy needs) *with adequate protein* (≥1.2 g protein per kilogram per day) be considered in patients requiring PN over the first week in critical care.[24] In early sepsis, they suggest provision of trophic feeds (defined as 10–20 kcal/h, up to 500 kcal/d) for the initial phase of sepsis, advancing as tolerated after 24 to 48 hours to greater than 80% of the target energy needs with early delivery of *1.2 to 2.0 g of protein per kilogram per day*.[24] These data for moderated nonprotein calorie delivery are driven by recent large randomized controlled trials (RCTs) showing equivalent outcomes from trophic versus higher-energy feeding (nonprotein kilocalorie delivery).[26,27] The need for additional protein intake has been well described by Hoffer and Bistrian[14,15,28] in several recent publications questioning whether it is actually protein deficit and not calorie deficit that is important in improving outcomes in critical illness. Given the limited higher protein, lower kilocalorie EN options, total PN (TPN) or EN protein supplements may be required. TPN is now a significantly more viable option to achieve this goal, as 3 recent large trials of both

Table 1
Nutritional interventions in sepsis

Nutritional Intervention	Recommended Delivery/Dose	Rationale/Recent Evidence	References
A. Nutritional interventions in sepsis: acute phase (first 24–96 h in ICU until resuscitated)			
Early EN	Protein: ~1.0 g/kg/d Nonprotein kcal: ~15 kcal/kg/d (in well-nourished pts) • Benefit for key role of elevating lipid dose in nonprotein kcal delivery in day 1–4?	• Prevent LBM wasting, weakness, and infections to improve recovery • Concern for ↑↑ protein dose (>1.2–1.5 g/kg/d?) (day 1–4?) creating risk due to impaired autophagy	9,14,16,24–28
PN	• Well nourished: consider delay until day 3–7 if <60% EN protein/kcal goal • Malnourished pts: start at ICU admit goal: ~1.2 g/kg/d protein total kcal ~15–20 kcal/kg/d	• Prevent caloric deficit early to reduce LBM loss, enhance recovery, physical function, and QoL • Signal of benefit in pts failing EN, EN contraindications, or pre-ICU malnutrition • No increased risk of infection over EN or other IV fluid delivery from TPN	2,5,9,15–18,22,24,25,29–31
Prokinetics and/or postpyloric feeding	Consider metoclopramide or erythromycin for GRVs >500 or feeding intolerance symptoms Consider postpyloric feeding for GRVs >500, feeding intolerance symptoms; may reduce silent aspiration if the tube is past third portion of duodenum?	• Inconclusive: may be reduced aspiration with post-pyloric feeding in meta-analysis; however, postpyloric feeding equivalent to gastric feeding in recent RCT on aspiration risk and EN delivery • Need future new efficacious and low side-effect prokinetics	24,36–38

Supplemental parenteral feeding during first week in ICU	• Well nourished: consider a delay until day 3–7 if <60% EN protein/kcal goal
	• Malnourished pts:
	  Start at ICU admit goal: ~1.2 g/kg/d
	  ~15–20 kcal/kg/d
	  Start at ICU admit in malnourished pts with NUTRIC >5 (w/o IL-6) and/or NRS ≥5
		• Prevent caloric deficit early to enhance recovery
		• No clear benefit of higher kcal dosages (>25 kcal/kg/d) in well-nourished ICU pts receiving dextrose-predominant, low protein PN in first 3 d
		• Potential benefit in pts with contraindication to EN or failing EN, especially malnourished pts at ICU admit
			2,5,6,9,15–18,24,25,29–31

(continued on next page)

Table 1
(continued)

Nutritional Intervention	Recommended Delivery/Dose	Rationale/Recent Evidence	References
More protein (>1.2 g g/kg/d) early (day 1–4 in ICU)	Protein: ~ 1.0 g/kg/d Until further research is completed on effects of very early protein delivery	Key area of controversy • Spare endogenous protein to reduce LBM loss, facilitate early mobility, and enhance recovery • Concern for ↑↑ protein dose (>1.2–1.5 g/kg/d?) (day 1–4?) creating risk due to impaired autophagy	2,5,6,14,15,23–25,28,40
Thiamine	Strongly consider repletion all pts in septic shock requiring vasopressors: dosage: 200 mg IV thiamine twice daily for 7 d	• ~ 35% of pts with septic shock potentially thiamine deficient • In thiamine-deficient pts: mortality from septic shock reduced by thiamine replacement • Potential for thiamine, vitamin C, and low-dose steroids to reduce mortality	51–53
Vitamin D	• Vitamin D level measured at ICU admit in ALL pts • Vitamin D <20: should receive 100,000 units of vitamin D_2 or D_3 for 5 d in first week and then 1–2× weekly (monitoring levels) for ICU stay	• Many vitamin D–deficient pts worldwide; vitamin D essential to immune function and muscle restoration and function • Data in ICU: significant relationship between vitamin D deficiency and adverse ICU outcomes • Recent large RCT in ICU: mortality benefit to repletion	58–63
Balanced TPN lipids (fish/olive oil)	• Recommend use of balanced lipid solutions containing fish oil and/or olive oil to minimize soy lipid content • Should not use pure soy lipid in sepsis or critical care setting for PN nutrition delivery	Soy lipids are • Immune suppressive • Associated with increased infections and LOS • Have elevated phytosterols, which increase cholestasis risk Meta-analysis data and recent RCTs: support use of balanced lipids with reduced infections and LOS	32,33,71,72
Antioxidants	Possible role for vitamin C in septic shock with thiamine and low-dose steroids (vitamin C: 1.5 g IV q 6 h for 4 d or until discharge from the ICU)	• Prevent organ failure/fluid leak • No clear benefit; for selenium or cocktail use possibly depends on dose and preillness deficiency status; more confirmatory literature needed for vitamin C	53–57

Trace element/ micronutrients	Routine administration of IV micronutrients/vitamins plus electrolyte replacement justified during acute phase of ICU until full enteral intake reached	• Many pts potentially deficient in trace element at ICU admit [22,48] • Depletion can lead to refeeding syndrome, with thiamine, Mg, K, and PO_4 deficiencies and potentially fatal complications (ie, cardiac failure, lactic acidosis, and respiratory failure)
Glutamine	Do not use early in shock, on vasopressors, or in renal failure (especially predialysis?) • Continued safety and use in TPN pts not in shock or renal failure at appropriate doses (<0.35 g/kg/d) supported by multiple meta-analyses	• Resupply conditional deficiency to improve outcomes [56,66–70] • Inconclusive and potentially harmful in higher doses (>0.5 g/kg/d EN/oral and >0.35 g/kg IV), early in shock or renal failure • Safety of EN/oral GLN and potential benefit indicated in ongoing trials in burn injury

B. Nutritional interventions in sepsis: chronic and recovery phase: (postresuscitation to hospital discharge)

EN	Protein: 1.2–2.0 g/kg/d Nonprotein kcal: 25–30 kcal/kg/d (ideally guided by indirect calorimetry) In recovery phase: greater kcal and protein delivery likely required	• Prevent ongoing LBM wasting, weakness, and infections to improve recovery [7,9,14–16,24,28] • Facilitate early mobility and physical therapy • Minnesota Starvation Study: >4000 kcal/d required for recovery
PN	• Well nourished: consider delay until d 3–7 if <60% EN protein/kcal goal • Malnourished pts: start at ICU admit goal: ~1.2 g/kg/d protein total kcal ~15–20 kcal/kg/d	• Prevent caloric deficit early to reduce LBM loss, enhance recovery, physical function, and QoL [2,5,9,15–18,22,24,25,29–31] • Signal of benefit in pts failing EN, EN contraindications, or pre-ICU malnutrition • No increased risk of infection over EN or other IV fluid delivery from TPN
Oral nutrition	Should not provide high protein oral nutrition supplements to all pts 2–3 × d when oral nutrition initiated	• Exceedingly poor oral intake in ICU pts [4,7,9,42–47] • Recent large RCT, large database observational data, and meta-analysis: reduced mortality, complications, LOS, and hospital costs • Minnesota Starvation Study: >4000 kcal/d required for recovery

(continued on next page)

Table 1
(continued)

Nutritional Intervention	Recommended Delivery/Dose	Rationale/Recent Evidence	References

Supplemental parenteral feeding	• Well nourished: consider delay until day 3–7 if <60% EN protein/kcal goal
	• Malnourished pts:
	  Start at ICU admit goal: ~1.2 g/kg/d protein total
	  kcal ~15–20 kcal/kg/d
	  Start at ICU admit in malnourished pts with NUTRIC >5 (w/o IL-6) and/or NRS ≥5
		• Prevent caloric deficit early to enhance recovery
		• No clear benefit of higher kcal dosages (>25 kcal/kg/d) in well-nourished ICU pts receiving dextrose-predominant, low-protein PN in first 3 d
		• Potential benefit in pts with contraindication to EN or failing EN, especially malnourished pts at ICU admit
			2,5,6,9,15–18,24,25,29–31

Vitamin D	• Vitamin D level measured at ICU admit in ALL pts • Vitamin D <20: should receive 100,000 units of vitamin D_2 or D_3 for 5 d in first week and then 1–2× weekly (monitoring levels) for ICU stay	• Many vitamin D- deficient pts worldwide, and vitamin D essential to immune function and muscle restoration and function • Data in ICU: significant relationship between vitamin D deficiency and adverse ICU outcomes • Mortality benefit to repletion shown in recent large RCT in ICU	58–63
Balanced TPN lipids (fish/olive oil)	• Recommend use of balanced lipid solutions containing fish oil and/or olive oil to minimize soy lipid content • Should not use pure soy lipid in sepsis or critical care setting for PN nutrition delivery	Soy lipids are • Immune suppressive • Associated with increased infections and LOS • Have elevated phytosterols, which increase cholestasis risk Use of balanced lipids with reduced infections and LOS supported by meta-analysis data and recent RCTs	32,33,71,72

Glutamine	Do not use early in shock, on vasopressors, or in renal failure (especially predialysis?) • Support from multiple meta-analyses for continued safety and use in TPN pts not in shock or renal failure at appropriate doses (<0.35 g/kg/d)	• Resupply conditional deficiency to improve outcomes • Inconclusive and potentially harmful in higher doses (>0.5 g/kg/d EN/oral and >0.35 g/kg/d IV), early in shock or renal failure • Safety of EN/oral GLN and potential benefit indicated in ongoing trials in burn injury	56,66–70

C. Nutritional interventions in sepsis: after hospital discharge

Oral nutrition	Should provide high-protein oral nutrition supplements to all pts 2–3 × d for 3 mo to 1 y after discharge Protein goal: 1.2–2.0 g/kg/d kcal goal: may be 4000–5000 kcal/d based on Minnesota Starvation Study	• Oral intake exceedingly poor in ICU pts • Recent large RCT, large database observational data, and meta-analysis: reduced mortality, complications, LOS, and hospital costs • Minnesota Starvation Study: >4000 kcal/d required for recovery • Potential for post-ICU hypermetabolism and catabolism to persist for months to years after ICU discharge	4,7,9,42–47
Vitamin D	• Measure vitamin D level at ICU admit in ALL pts • Vitamin D <20: receive 100,000 units of vitamin D_2 or D_3 for 5 d in first week and then 1–2× weekly (monitoring levels) for ICU stay and likely in post-hospital period	• Many vitamin D–deficient pts worldwide; vitamin D essential to immune function and muscle restoration and function • Data in ICU: significant relationship between vitamin D deficiency and adverse ICU outcomes • Recent large RCT in ICU: mortality benefit to repletion	58–63

Abbreviations: EN, enteral nutrition; GLN, glutamine; IL-6, interleukin 6; IV, intravenous; K, potassium; LBM, lean body mass; LOS, length of stay; Mg, magnesium; NRS, nutrition risk score; PN, parenteral nutrition; PO_4, phosphate; pts, patients; RCT, randomized controlled trial; TPN, total parenteral nutrition; w/o, without.

supplemental and full TPN support versus EN in the ICU setting demonstrated no increase in infection risk with TPN.[29–31] This finding is likely due to improvements in glucose control, central line infection control measures, and, potentially, improved (non–pure soy–based) balanced lipid formulations that reduce infection compared with pure soy lipid.[32,33] In support of early TPN use, the new SCCM/ASPEN guidelines indicate that for any patient at high nutrition risk (NRS 2002 ≥5 or NUTRIC score [without IL-6 score] ≥5) or found to be severely malnourished when EN is not feasible, *exclusive PN should be initiated as soon as possible following ICU admission.*[24]

Chronic and Recovery Phase of Sepsis: Significantly Increased Protein and Calorie Needs

Chronic phase: postresuscitation increase in nutrition delivery

As successful resuscitation of the acute phase of sepsis occurs and patients stabilize, an increasing amount of protein (1.2–2.0 g/kg/d) and calories (25–30 kcal/kg/d) needs to be delivered to reduce further loss of LBM, allow for early mobilization, and encourage functional recovery (see **Fig. 1**, **Table** 1B). The concept of adequate protein and calorie delivery improving QoL is well described in a recent study of ICU patients mechanically ventilated for greater than 8 days.[5] After adjustment for covariates, patients receiving inadequate nutrition over the first ICU week (<50% of predicted calorie/protein need) had an increased mortality compared with those patients receiving adequate nutrition delivery (>80% of calorie/protein needs). These data also demonstrate that for every 25% increase in calorie/protein delivery in the first ICU week, there was an improvement in 3-month post-ICU physical QoL scores (as measured by the 36-Item Short Form Health Survey [SF-36] score), with medical ICU patients showing significant improvements in both 3- and 6-month SF-36 scores.[5]

Recovery phase: continued increase in nutrition delivery needs: role of the Minnesota Starvation Study in intensive care unit recovery

As patients improve and enter the recovery phase, caloric intake likely needs to increase further, with implementation of aggressive rehabilitation and exercise interventions. The landmark Minnesota Starvation Study performed at the end of World War II[7,34] (a study all medical students and hospital practitioners should be taught or read for themselves) provides essential data on the nutritional needs required to recover from the fundamental severe LBM loss observed after sepsis. This seminal study demonstrates that a healthy 70-kg human, following significant weight loss, requires *an average of 5000 kcal/d for 6 months to 2 years to fully regain lost muscle mass and weight.*[7] As many ICU patients have similar marked weight/LBM loss, in addition to prolonged hypermetabolism and catabolism (which Minnesota subjects did not have as they were healthy volunteers), we must recognize that significant calorie/protein delivery will be required to restore this lost LBM and improve QoL. During the recovery phase of critical illness, the body experiences a massive increase in metabolic needs, with TEE increasing as much as approximately 1.7-fold greater than REE.[20] In the second week following sepsis, this increases to a TEE of approximately 3250 kcal/d or 47 kcal/kg/d, virtually identical to the World Health Organization's requirements for normal, healthy humans. In younger trauma patients (mean age: 34 years), Uehara and colleagues described an even greater increase in caloric need in the second week after injury to an *average of approximately 4120 kcal/d or 59 kcal/kg/d.* This amount is nearly identical to the 4000 kcal/d that Ancel Keys demonstrated was needed to recover from starvation in the young Minnesota subjects **(Table 2)**.

Table 2
Summary of caloric needs of critically ill and healthy individuals in the context of the Minnesota Starvation Study and actual current intensive care unit calories

	Mean REE (kcal/d)	TEE (kcal/d)	TEE/Weight (kcal/kg/d)
Uehara et al[20] ICU study			
Patients with sepsis (mean age: 67 y)			
Week 1	~1854	1927 ± 370	25 ± 5
Week 2	—	3257 ± 370	47 ± 6
Trauma patients (mean age: 34 y)			
Week 1	~2122	2380 ± 422	31 ± 6
Week 2	—	4123 ± 518	59 ± 7
WHO Calorie Requirements Healthy Subjects[a]			
Men	—	~3000	44 (Range: 35–53)
Women	—	~2500	36 (Range: 29–44)
Minnesota Starvation Study calorie delivery	—	Delivered energy (kcal/d)	Delivered energy/weight (kcal/kg/d)
Baseline period	—	3200	~50
Starvation period	—	~1800	23–30
Recovery period delivery (for recovery to occur)	—	~4000	~60

Actual average kcal/d: 1034 kcal/d.
Delivered in critically ill patients.
Over first 12 days of ICU stay.[15]
Abbreviations: REE, resting energy expenditure; TEE, total energy expenditure; WHO, World Health Organization.
[a] Data for healthy 7-kg person with intermediate physical activity (1.75 physical activity level factor) (Reference: Human energy requirements Report of a Joint FAO/WHO/UNU Expert Consultation - http://www.fao.org/docrep/007/y5686e/y5686e00.htm#Content. Accessed September 12, 2017).

Current Practice of Nutrition in Sepsis and Intensive Care Units Worldwide: Do We Already Hypocalorically Feed Our Patients Beyond the Acute Phase?

Extensive data for current international nutrition delivery in critical care are available from the International Nutrition Survey conducted regularly by the Canadian Critical Care Nutrition Group (www.criticalcarenutrition.com). These data reveal that *average calories delivered in ICU over the first 12 days is 1034 kcals and 47 g of protein* (see **Table 2**).[6] This period is far longer than the first 1 to 4 days of the acute phase whereby hypocaloric feeding (with moderated adequate protein) may make physiologic sense. More troubling is the fact that this total is far lower than the 1800 kcal/d calories and approximately 0.8 g/kg/d protein that led to severe starvation in the Minnesota Starvation Study. Thus, drawing comparison in nutrition delivery between ICUs worldwide and the landmark Starvation Study

Minnesota Starvation Study (Starvation Period)
    1800 kcal/d
    0.75 to 0.8 g/kg protein
ICU patients worldwide for first 12 days in ICU
    1034 kcal/d
    0.6 g/kg protein

These data confirm that ICU patients worldwide average far less energy and protein than healthy subjects in the legendary Minnesota Starvation Study. This study would likely never be repeated today because of the ethics of inducing potentially life-threatening starvation in healthy volunteers. We know that starvation in humans leads to slowing of metabolic rate and reduced protein catabolism over time. Unfortunately, after the first ICU week, critical illness leads to significant hypermetabolism and severe ongoing protein losses. Moreover, 30% to 50% of ICU patients are malnourished at hospital admission[35] (unlike the well-nourished men in Key's Minnesota Starvation study), thus, greatly increasing the risk of ongoing in-hospital starvation. We must critically examine and measure actual practice in our individual ICUs, as most already underfeed calories and protein well beyond the acute phase. Methods to improve EN, including prokinetic agents[36] and postpyloric feeding, have not been successful in addressing this global ICU iatrogenic malnutrition. New guidelines calling for the abandonment of checking gastric residual volumes (GRVs),[37] or changing GRV cutoffs to greater than 500 mL before feeding is stopped, may show promise to help improve EN delivery.[24] In a recent RCT, postpyloric feeding did not reliably prevent aspiration or increase EN delivery[38] so gastric feeding should be the primary route to deliver EN. Finally, could iatrogenic malnutrition in the ICU likely explain in part the increasing number of ICU survivors who ultimately become victims of PICS, never to walk again or return to a meaningful QoL after ICU discharge?[3,13,39,40]

These data demand that we ask whether our septic patients have been unable to recover their QoL after ICU for months to years because of our lack of understanding of their fundamental metabolic needs in different phases of their illness, especially following ICU and hospital discharge.

Intensive Care Unit/Hospital Discharge Nutrition Delivery to Optimize Recovery

Can patients discharged from critical care following sepsis consume adequate calories and protein to enable optimal recovery (see **Fig. 2**, **Table 1**C)? In the week following endotracheal extubation, an observational study demonstrated an average spontaneous calorie intake of 700 kcal/d; the entire population studied consumed less than 50% of calorie/protein needs for 7 days.[4] This study also emphasizes the importance of closely observing food intake in postoperative patients. In patients who have lost significant weight following surgery or illness, a considerable period of significantly increased calorie and protein delivery is required for recovery.[41] To address this, a large body of data demonstrates that oral nutrition supplements (ONS) must become a fundamental part of our post-ICU and hospital discharge care. A meta-analysis in a range of hospitalized patients demonstrates that ONS reduces mortality, reduces hospital complications, reduce hospital readmissions, shortens length of stay, and reduces hospital costs.[42–45] A large hospital database analysis of ONS use in 724,000 patients matched with controls not receiving ONS showed a 21% reduction in hospital LOS; for every $1 spent on ONS, $52.63 was saved in hospital costs.[46] Finally, a recent large RCT of 652 patients in 78 centers studied the effect of high-protein ONS (HP-ONS) with β-hydroxy-β-methyl butyrate (HP-HMB) versus placebo in elderly, malnourished (Subjective Global Assessment class B or C) hospitalized adults. HP-HMB reduced 90-day mortality by approximately 50% relative to placebo (4.8% vs 9.7%; relative risk 0.49, 95% confidence interval [CI]: 0.27–0.90; $P = .018$). The number needed to treat to prevent 1 death was 20.3 (95% CI: 10.9, 121.4).[47] As it is well known that ICU patients recovering from sepsis will not consume sufficient calories and protein to recover optimally, the use of HP-ONS will be essential. It is strongly recommended for all patients once oral intake is resumed for at least 3 months (and up to 1 year) following ICU discharge.

Correction of Vitamin/Micronutrient Deficiencies and Specific Nutrient Delivery

In addition to protein and calorie needs, a new and growing body of literature is identifying nutrients that should and should not be administered in the early acute phase of sepsis (see **Table 1**). These nutrients are discussed specifically later.

Micronutrients and electrolytes

Recent literature demonstrates a meaningful number of patients may be deficient in trace elements at ICU admissions or become deficient during their stay.[48] Refeeding syndrome is a real and present danger to malnourished ICU patients. This syndrome must be monitored via evaluation of electrolytes (phosphate, potassium, magnesium) and repletion when needed.[49,50] Casaer and van den Berghe[48] advocate for continuous infusion of trace elements: *"Routine administration of intravenous micronutrients and vitamins plus electrolyte replacement is justified during the acute phase of critical illness until full enteral intake is reached."*[48]

Thiamine

Thiamine is an essential vitamin for aerobic nutrient metabolism, playing a vital role in the Krebs' cycle and the pentose-phosphate shuttle.[51] New data indicate that thiamine deficiency occurs in up to 35% of patients with septic shock.[52] A recent double-blind RCT showed that administration of 200 mg thiamine to patients with septic shock did not improve lactate levels or other outcomes overall.[52] However, in thiamine-deficient patients, there was a statistically significant decrease in mortality over time, and a reduction in lactate at 24 hours, in those receiving thiamine ($P = .047$). These data have been supplemented by a recent retrospective before-after clinical study, showing significantly reduced mortality in patients with septic shock receiving thiamine, vitamin C, and low-dose steroids.[53] Hospital mortality was 8.5% (4 of 47) in the treatment group compared with 40.4% (19 of 47) in the earlier control group ($P<.001$). These trial data do, however, require confirmatory larger RCTs. As thiamine measurement is costly and not routinely performed, and thiamine itself is quite inexpensive and carries almost no risk, a recommendation for all patients with septic shock to receive 200 mg thiamine twice daily for 7 days after ICU admission seems reasonable to improve outcomes, though with the caveat that additional data are needed.

Vitamin C and antioxidants

As mentioned earlier, a potential benefit of vitamin C with thiamine and low-dose steroids has recently been described.[53] The doses of vitamin C used in this Marik trial are high, yet seemed to be safe and can be considered for use. Some concern for oxalate nephropathy should be considered, especially in patients with significant renal dysfunction, although the Marik group[53] has denied any incidence of this in their short-term vitamin C use. This practice has been seemingly safe in short-term use in the burn setting.[54] Consistent use of vitamin C at this level, as is often done in burn patients to reduce fluid leak and fluid requirements,[54] may challenge some ICU pharmacies to keep up with demand as this practice will be new to many centers. Routine use of selenium and other antioxidants has shown promise in meta-analysis[55]; however, recent large RCTs have not shown benefit.[56,57]

Vitamin D

A rapidly growing body of data demonstrates a significant proportion of the population of the United States and other industrialized nations is vitamin D deficient.[58] Data in ICU and surgical patients show that vitamin D deficiency has a significant association with postoperative complications and adverse ICU outcomes.[59–61] A key recent RCT found that ICU patients with vitamin D levels less than 12 ng/mL experienced a significant improvement in hospital survival with aggressive supplementation of vitamin D_3 given orally or via the nasogastric tube at a single dose of 540,000 IU followed by monthly maintenance doses of 90,000 IU for 5 months.[62] This dose will be difficult for many centers to administer if concentrated vitamin D solutions are not available. A recent double-blinded pilot RCT of 50,000 IU vitamin D_3 or 100,000 IU vitamin D_3 daily for 5 consecutive days enterally (total vitamin D_3 dose = 250,000 IU or 500,000 IU, respectively) reported a significant decrease in hospital length of stay in the 50,000 IU D_3 per day (25 ± 14 days) and 100,000 IU D_3 per day (18 ± 11 days) groups compared with the placebo group (36 ± 19 days; $P = .03$).[63] Vitamin D levels are, thus, recommended to be checked at ICU admission and once weekly thereafter in all patients with septic shock. For patients found to be deficient (<30 ng/mL), a repletion dose of 100,000 units of vitamin D_2 or D_3 for 5 days in the first week and 1 to 2 times per week thereafter (monitoring levels) for the duration of the ICU stay is reasonable. Larger trials on the role of vitamin D supplementation in sepsis and critical illness are currently underway.

Glutamine
Glutamine (GLN) is the most abundant nonessential free amino acid.[64] Low GLN levels have been associated with poor outcomes.[65] Thus, GLN has been labeled a conditionally essential amino acid during prolonged critical illness, leading to the hypothesis that GLN supplementation would improve outcomes.[64] However, signals showing a risk of harm have come from 2 large-scale multicenter trials evaluating mortality using a combination of high-dose intravenous/enteral GLN (the REDOXS (REducing Deaths due to OXidative Stress) study)[56] or a high-dose enteral mixture of different nutrients including GLN (the METAPLUS trial).[66] These new trials were both targeted to investigate GLN (and other nutrients) as primary pharmaconutrients and not as supplementation to PN. These data suggest that patients in the early phase of sepsis, on vasopressors, or in renal failure (especially without dialysis) should not get supplemental GLN. Two recent meta-analyses[67,68] have confirmed that traditional PN supplementation with intravenous GLN is safe, reduces mortality and LOS, and improves outcome. Based on 9 level 1 and 19 level 2 studies, the investigators concluded, *"When PN is prescribed to ICU patients, parenteral GLN supplementation should be considered."*[67] Patients in need of PN and those with burns, trauma, or malignancies may continue to benefit from supplemental GLN, administered either intravenously less than 0.35 g/kg/d or enterally less than 0.5 g/kg/d.[69,70] TPN routinely contains only 19 amino acids, so GLN must be supplemented, and not given pharmacologically, in a stable form to provide complete nutrition.

Lipids
Current use of pure soy lipid as part of PN should likely be abandoned, as it is immunosuppressive and proinflammatory.[71,72] This point is particularly true given the now worldwide availability of balanced lipid solutions containing various combinations of fish and/or olive oil. There are also data supporting a benefit of using fish oil containing balanced lipid formulations versus soy lipid alone in patients requiring TPN in the ICU or postoperative setting. These data include a recent meta-analysis of 23 RCTs, including 1502 surgical and ICU patients, which demonstrated that fish oil–containing lipids reduced length of stay and infectious complications versus traditional soy-only lipids.[32] A more recent meta-analysis of 10 RCTs demonstrated that fish oil–based intravenous lipids significantly reduced infections in critical illness.[33] It is, thus, recommended that when TPN is used, a modern, balanced lipid that reduces soy lipid content should be given.

SUMMARY

In conclusion, to optimize nutrition delivery, we need to consider basic metabolism and our historical understanding of data for recovery from severe LBM loss (starvation) to use targeted nutritional care in sepsis. If we are to optimize patient outcomes and start creating survivors and not victims following sepsis and intensive care, we must continue to evolve our delivery of personalized nutritional needs, which almost assuredly change over the course of illness. The presence of nutritional risk and metabolic reserve as defined by the NUTRIC score and CT scan- or ultrasound-guided LBM assessment should guide how we feed our patients, with high risk (NUTRIC ≥5 or patients with sarcopenia) getting aggressive early calorie and protein delivery via early EN and/or PN. Furthermore, we must all read and revel in the defining achievement that is the Minnesota Starvation Study[7] and learn from its landmark lessons. Most important among these is that even healthy subjects require significant calories (typically >4000 kcal/d) to recover from massive weight and LBM loss such as occurs following sepsis. How many of our care protocols, or our patients, acknowledge or achieve this well-described goal? Is it possible this lack of understanding of caloric and protein needs during recovery and, thus, suboptimal provision has led to the extremely poor long-term outcomes and QoL that follows ICU care? Only time and further research will tell for sure. This increase in calorie delivery should be targeted to when patients are recovering. Use of emerging metabolic cart technology[73] and, perhaps, even bedside C13 breath testing to target overfeeding/underfeeding and substrate delivery[74,75] will help guide this in the future. Finally, we must learn to target and incorporate nutritional therapies, such as vitamin D, probiotics, and anabolic/anticatabolic agents, to optimize our patients' chances of survival and to thrive against all evolutionary odds. We have long known Mother Nature does not want our ICU patients to win this war and become *survivors and not victims*. But to begin winning this war on long-term ICU outcomes and give our patients back the lives they came to us to restore, we must ensure we are giving the right nutrition, to the right patient, at the right time.

REFERENCES

1. Gillis C, Carli F. Promoting perioperative metabolic and nutritional care. Anesthesiology 2015;123(6):1455–72.
2. Preiser JC, van Zanten AR, Berger MM, et al. Metabolic and nutritional support of critically ill patients: consensus and controversies. Crit Care 2015;19:35.
3. Dinglas VD, Aronson Friedman L, Colantuoni E, et al. Muscle weakness and 5-year survival in acute respiratory distress syndrome survivors. Crit Care Med 2017;45(3):446–53.
4. Peterson SJ, Tsai AA, Scala CM, et al. Adequacy of oral intake in critically ill patients 1 week after extubation. J Am Diet Assoc 2010;110(3):427–33.
5. Wei X, Day AG, Ouellette-Kuntz H, et al. The association between nutritional adequacy and long-term outcomes in critically ill patients requiring prolonged mechanical ventilation: a multicenter cohort study. Crit Care Med 2015;43(8):1569–79.
6. Alberda C, Gramlich L, Jones N, et al. The relationship between nutritional intake and clinical outcomes in critically ill patients: results of an international multicenter observational study. Intensive Care Med 2009;35(10):1728–37.
7. Keys A, Brozek J, Henschel A, et al. The biology of human starvation, vols. I–II. Minneapolis (MN): University of Minnesota Press; 1950.

8. Stanojcic M, Finnerty CC, Jeschke MG. Anabolic and anticatabolic agents in critical care. Curr Opin Crit Care 2016;22(4):325–31.

9. Wischmeyer PE. Are we creating survivors…or victims in critical care? Delivering targeted nutrition to improve outcomes. Curr Opin Crit Care 2016;22(4):279–84.

10. Herridge MS, Cheung AM, Tansey CM, et al. One-year outcomes in survivors of the acute respiratory distress syndrome. N Engl J Med 2003;348(8):683–93.

11. Kaukonen KM, Bailey M, Suzuki S, et al. Mortality related to severe sepsis and septic shock among critically ill patients in Australia and New Zealand, 2000-2012. JAMA 2014;311(13):1308–16.

12. Weycker D, Akhras KS, Edelsberg J, et al. Long-term mortality and medical care charges in patients with severe sepsis. Crit Care Med 2003;31(9):2316–23.

13. Kamdar BB, Huang M, Dinglas VD, et al, National Heart, Lung, and Blood Institute Acute Respiratory Distress Syndrome Network. Joblessness and lost earnings after ARDS in a 1-year national multicenter study. Am J Respir Crit Care Med 2017. [Epub ahead of print].

14. Hoffer LJ, Bistrian BR. Appropriate protein provision in critical illness: a systematic and narrative review. Am J Clin Nutr 2012;96(3):591–600.

15. Hoffer LJ, Bistrian BR. What is the best nutritional support for critically ill patients? Hepatobiliary Surg Nutr 2014;3(4):172–4.

16. Oshima T, Deutz NE, Doig G, et al. Protein-energy nutrition in the ICU is the power couple: a hypothesis forming analysis. Clin Nutr 2016;35(4):968–74.

17. Rahman A, Hasan RM, Agarwala R, et al. Identifying critically-ill patients who will benefit most from nutritional therapy: further validation of the "modified NUTRIC" nutritional risk assessment tool. Clin Nutr 2016;35(1):158–62.

18. Heyland DK, Dhaliwal R, Jiang X, et al. Identifying critically ill patients who benefit the most from nutrition therapy: the development and initial validation of a novel risk assessment tool. Crit Care 2011;15(6):R268.

19. Looijaard WG, Dekker IM, Stapel SN, et al. Skeletal muscle quality as assessed by CT-derived skeletal muscle density is associated with 6-month mortality in mechanically ventilated critically ill patients. Crit Care 2016;20(1):386.

20. Uehara M, Plank LD, Hill GL. Components of energy expenditure in patients with severe sepsis and major trauma: a basis for clinical care. Crit Care Med 1999; 27(7):1295–302.

21. Kreymann G, Grosser S, Buggisch P, et al. Oxygen consumption and resting metabolic rate in sepsis, sepsis syndrome, and septic shock. Crit Care Med 1993;21(7):1012–9.

22. Casaer MP, Mesotten D, Hermans G, et al. Early versus late parenteral nutrition in critically ill adults. N Engl J Med 2011;365(6):506–17.

23. Fürst P. Protein and amino acid metabolism: composition of stressed and non-stressed states. In: Cresci G, editor. Nutrition support for the critically ill patient. Boca Raton (FL): Taylor & Francis (CRC); 2005. p. 29.

24. McClave SA, Taylor BE, Martindale RG, et al. Guidelines for the provision and assessment of nutrition support therapy in the adult critically ill patient: Society of Critical Care Medicine (SCCM) and American Society for Parenteral and Enteral Nutrition (A.S.P.E.N. JPEN J Parenter Enteral Nutr 2016;40(2):159–211.

25. Vanhorebeek I, Verbruggen S, Casaer MP, et al. Effect of early supplemental parenteral nutrition in the paediatric ICU: a preplanned observational study of post-randomisation treatments in the PEPaNIC trial. Lancet Respir Med 2017; 5(6):475–83.

26. National Heart, Lung, and Blood Institute Acute Respiratory Distress Syndrome Network, Rice TW, Wheeler AP, Thompson BT, et al. Initial trophic vs full enteral

feeding in patients with acute lung injury: the EDEN randomized trial. JAMA 2012; 307(8):795–803.

27. Arabi YM, Aldawood AS, Haddad SH, et al. Permissive underfeeding or standard enteral feeding in critically ill adults. N Engl J Med 2015;372(25):2398–408.

28. Hoffer LJ, Bistrian BR. Energy deficit is clinically relevant for critically ill patients: no. Intensive Care Med 2015;41(2):339–41.

29. Doig GS, Simpson F, Sweetman EA, et al. Early parenteral nutrition in critically ill patients with short-term relative contraindications to early enteral nutrition: a randomized controlled trial. JAMA 2013;309(20):2130–8.

30. Heidegger CP, Berger MM, Graf S, et al. Optimisation of energy provision with supplemental parenteral nutrition in critically ill patients: a randomised controlled clinical trial. Lancet 2013;381(9864):385–93.

31. Harvey SE, Parrott F, Harrison DA, et al. Trial of the route of early nutritional support in critically ill adults. N Engl J Med 2014;371(18):1673–84.

32. Pradelli L, Mayer K, Muscaritoli M, et al. n-3 fatty acid-enriched parenteral nutrition regimens in elective surgical and ICU patients: a meta-analysis. Crit Care 2012;16:R184.

33. Manzanares W, Langlois PL, Dhaliwal R, et al. Intravenous fish oil lipid emulsions in critically ill patients: an updated systematic review and meta-analysis. Crit Care 2015;19:167.

34. Kalm LM, Semba RD. They starved so that others be better fed: remembering Ancel Keys and the Minnesota experiment. J Nutr 2005;135(6):1347–52.

35. Norman K, Pichard C, Lochs H, et al. Prognostic impact of disease-related malnutrition. Clin Nutr 2008;27(1):5–15.

36. MacLaren R, Kiser TH, Fish DN, et al. Erythromycin vs metoclopramide for facilitating gastric emptying and tolerance to intragastric nutrition in critically ill patients. JPEN J Parenter Enteral Nutr 2008;32(4):412–9.

37. Reignier J, Mercier E, Le Gouge A, et al. Effect of not monitoring residual gastric volume on risk of ventilator-associated pneumonia in adults receiving mechanical ventilation and early enteral feeding: a randomized controlled trial. JAMA 2013; 309(3):249–56.

38. Davies AR, Morrison SS, Bailey MJ, et al. A multicenter, randomized controlled trial comparing early nasojejunal with nasogastric nutrition in critical illness. Crit Care Med 2012;40(8):2342–8.

39. Needham DM, Feldman DR, Kho ME. The functional costs of ICU survivorship. Collaborating to improve post-ICU disability. Am J Respir Crit Care Med 2011; 183(8):962–4.

40. Wischmeyer PE, San-Millan I. Winning the war against ICU-acquired weakness: new innovations in nutrition and exercise physiology. Crit Care 2015;19(Suppl 3):S6.

41. Puthucheary ZA, Wischmeyer P. Predicting critical illness mortality and personalizing therapy: moving to multi-dimensional data. Crit Care 2017;21(1):20.

42. Cawood AL, Elia M, Stratton RJ. Systematic review and meta-analysis of the effects of high protein oral nutritional supplements. Ageing Res Rev 2012;11(2): 278–96.

43. Elia M, Normand C, Norman K, et al. A systematic review of the cost and cost effectiveness of using standard oral nutritional supplements in the hospital setting. Clin Nutr 2016;35(2):370–80.

44. Stratton RJ, Hebuterne X, Elia M. A systematic review and meta-analysis of the impact of oral nutritional supplements on hospital readmissions. Ageing Res Rev 2013;12(4):884–97.

45. Stratton R, Green C, Elia M. Disease-related malnutrition: an evidence-based approach to treatment. Wallingford (United Kingdom): CABI Publishing; 2003.
46. Philipson TJ, Snider JT, Lakdawalla DN, et al. Impact of oral nutritional supplementation on hospital outcomes. Am J Manag Care 2013;19(2):121–8.
47. Deutz NE, Matheson EM, Matarese LE, et al, NOURISH Study Group. Readmission and mortality in malnourished, older, hospitalized adults treated with a specialized oral nutritional supplement: a randomized clinical trial. Clin Nutr 2016;35(1):18–26.
48. Casaer MP, Van den Berghe G. Nutrition in the acute phase of critical illness. N Engl J Med 2014;370(13):1227–36.
49. Stanga Z, Brunner A, Leuenberger M, et al. Nutrition in clinical practice-the refeeding syndrome: illustrative cases and guidelines for prevention and treatment. Eur J Clin Nutr 2008;62(6):687–94.
50. Doig GS, Simpson F, Heighes PT, et al, Refeeding Syndrome Trial Investigators Group. Restricted versus continued standard caloric intake during the management of refeeding syndrome in critically ill adults: a randomised, parallel-group, multicentre, single-blind controlled trial. Lancet Respir Med 2015;3(12):943–52.
51. Frank RA, Leeper FJ, Luisi BF. Structure, mechanism and catalytic duality of thiamine-dependent enzymes. Cell Mol Life Sci 2007;64(7–8):892–905.
52. Donnino MW, Andersen LW, Chase M, et al. Randomized, double-blind, placebo-controlled trial of thiamine as a metabolic resuscitator in septic shock: a pilot study. Crit Care Med 2016;44(2):360–7.
53. Marik PE, Khangoora V, Rivera R, et al. Hydrocortisone, vitamin C and thiamine for the treatment of severe sepsis and septic shock: a retrospective before-after study. Chest 2016;151(6):1229–38.
54. Tanaka H, Matsuda T, Miyagantani Y, et al. Reduction of resuscitation fluid volumes in severely burned patients using ascorbic acid administration: a randomized, prospective study. Arch Surg 2000;135(3):326–31.
55. Alhazzani W, Jacobi J, Sindi A, et al. The effect of selenium therapy on mortality in patients with sepsis syndrome: a systematic review and meta-analysis of randomized controlled trials. Crit Care Med 2013;41(6):1555–64.
56. Heyland D, Muscedere J, Wischmeyer PE, et al, Canadian Critical Care Trials Group. A randomized trial of glutamine and antioxidants in critically ill patients. N Engl J Med 2013;368(16):1489–97.
57. Bloos F, Trips E, Nierhaus A, et al. Effect of sodium selenite administration and procalcitonin-guided therapy on mortality in patients with severe sepsis or septic shock: a randomized clinical trial. JAMA Intern Med 2016;176(9):1266–76.
58. Holick MF. Vitamin D deficiency. N Engl J Med 2007;357(3):266–81.
59. Iglar PJ, Hogan KJ. Vitamin D status and surgical outcomes: a systematic review. Patient Saf Surg 2015;9:14.
60. Higgins DM, Wischmeyer PE, Queensland KM, et al. Relationship of vitamin D deficiency to clinical outcomes in critically ill patients. JPEN J Parenter Enteral Nutr 2012;36(6):713–20.
61. Moromizato T, Litonjua AA, Braun AB, et al. Association of low serum 25-hydroxyvitamin D levels and sepsis in the critically ill. Crit Care Med 2014;42(1):97–107.
62. Amrein K, Schnedl C, Holl A, et al. Effect of high-dose vitamin D3 on hospital length of stay in critically ill patients with vitamin D deficiency: the VITdAL-ICU randomized clinical trial. JAMA 2014;312(15):1520–30.
63. Han JE, Jones JL, Tangpricha V, et al. High dose vitamin D administration in ventilated intensive care unit patients: a pilot double blind randomized controlled trial. J Clin Transl Endocrinol 2016;4:59–65.

64. Bongers T, Griffiths RD, McArdle A. Exogenous glutamine: the clinical evidence. Crit Care Med 2007;35(9 Suppl):S545–52.

65. Rodas PC, Rooyackers O, Hebert C, et al. Glutamine and glutathione at ICU admission in relation to outcome. Clin Sci (Lond) 2012;122(12):591–7.

66. van Zanten AR, Sztark F, Kaisers UX, et al. High-protein enteral nutrition enriched with immune-modulating nutrients vs standard high-protein enteral nutrition and nosocomial infections in the ICU: a randomized clinical trial. JAMA 2014; 312(5):514–24.

67. Wischmeyer PE, Dhaliwal R, McCall M, et al. Parenteral glutamine supplementation in critical illness: a systematic review. Crit Care 2014;18(2):R76.

68. Bollhalder L, Pfeil AM, Tomonaga Y, et al. A systematic literature review and meta-analysis of randomized clinical trials of parenteral glutamine supplementation. Clin Nutr 2013;32(2):213–23.

69. Vanek VW, Matarese LE, Robinson M, et al. A.S.P.E.N. position paper: parenteral nutrition glutamine supplementation. Nutr Clin Pract 2011;26(4):479–94.

70. Wischmeyer P. Glutamine supplementation in parenteral nutrition and intensive care unit patients: are we throwing the baby out with the bathwater? JPEN J Parenter Enteral Nutr 2015;39(8):893–7.

71. Buenestado A, Cortijo J, Sanz MJ, et al. Olive oil-based lipid emulsion's neutral effects on neutrophil functions and leukocyte-endothelial cell interactions. JPEN J Parenter Enteral Nutr 2006;30(4):286–96.

72. Wischmeyer PE. Alternative lipid emulsions as a new standard of care for total parenteral nutrition: finally available in the United States? Crit Care Med 2015; 43(1):230–1.

73. De Waele E, Honore PM, Spapen HD. New generation indirect calorimeters for measuring energy expenditure in the critically ill: a rampant or reticent revolution? Crit Care 2016;20(1):138.

74. Butz DE, Weidmann D, Brownsword R, et al. Immediate biofeedback for energy balance via expired breath delta(13)CO2. Conf Proc IEEE Eng Med Biol Soc 2015;2015:8205–8.

75. Whigham LD, Butz DE, Johnson LK, et al. Breath carbon stable isotope ratios identify changes in energy balance and substrate utilization in humans. Int J Obes 2014;38(9):1248–50.

Common Sense Approach to Managing Sepsis

Anders Perner, MD, PhD*, Lars B. Holst, MD, PhD, Nicolai Haase, MD, PhD, Peter B. Hjortrup, MD, PhD, Morten H. Møller, MD, PhD

KEYWORDS

- Sepsis • Resuscitation • Hemodynamic monitoring • Antibiotics • Critical care
- Fluids

KEY POINTS

- Sepsis is frequent and deathly.
- The clinical management of patients with sepsis may be guided by applying the Surviving Sepsis Campaign guidelines together with common sense and flexibility based on patient-specific and setting-specific characteristics.
- Use 250-mL to 500-mL fluid boluses; continue only if there is clinical improvement.
- Use norepinephrine.
- Give broad-spectrum antibiotic early; de-escalate when the microbe is identified or the patient improves.

Sepsis is a syndrome, defined as life-threatening organ dysfunction caused by a dys-regulated host response to infection.[1] It is a global health challenge resulting in many deaths, prolonged suffering among survivors and relatives, and high use of resources both in developed and developing countries.[2,3]

Patients with sepsis may progress in disease severity from infection with a modest degree of organ dysfunction and in-hospital mortality of approximately 10% to severe circulatory impairment (ie, septic shock), to mortality rate above 40%.[4] This chain of progression represents a window of opportunity, in which correct identification of the patient and appropriate interventions and monitoring are likely to improve outcomes. Thus the recently updated clinical practice guidelines from the Surviving Sepsis Campaign (SSC) categorize sepsis and septic shock as medical emergencies for which treatment and resuscitation should begin immediately.[5] The diagnosis and care of patients with sepsis is complex because of the pathophysiologic involvement

---

Disclosure Statement: The Department of Intensive Care, Rigshospitalet receives funding for research from CSL Behring, Fresenius Kabi, and Ferring Pharmaceuticals.
Department of Intensive Care, Rigshospitalet, University of Copenhagen, Blegdamsvej 9, Copenhagen DK-2100, Denmark
* Corresponding author.
E-mail address: anders.perner@regionh.dk

Crit Care Clin 34 (2018) 127–138
http://dx.doi.org/10.1016/j.ccc.2017.08.009
criticalcare.theclinics.com

of several organ systems and many of the biological processes are far from understood.[6,7] Diagnosis and care are also complex because patients present with sepsis to different settings in the health care system (eg, prehospital, emergency department, operating room, ward, or intensive care unit [ICU]). The patients, therefore, have to be identified and cared for by different health care professionals.[7] Together this may lead to delayed diagnosis and less optimal treatment and care pathways for patients with sepsis.

The key items in the initial management of the patient with sepsis are microbiological culture and antibiotics, hemodynamic monitoring and interventions, source control, and supportive care, which for the severe cases most often occur in an ICU.

This narrative review discusses how to optimize the management of patients with sepsis by the application of the updated SSC guidelines and common sense.

THE SURVIVING SEPSIS CAMPAIGN GUIDELINES AND CARE BUNDLES

The 2016 SSC guidelines article represent the work of a consensus committee of 55 international experts representing 25 international organizations.[5] The guidelines are based on the best available evidence systematically synthesized and presented using the Grades of Recommendation Assessment, Development and Evaluation (GRADE) approach,[8] which was facilitated by methods experts. The 93 specific suggestions and recommendations are rarely supported by high-quality evidence. Only 7 are based on high-quality evidence, 28 on moderate evidence, and 58 on low-quality or very-low-quality evidence. Only 4 of the 26 statements on initial management, that is, screening, diagnosis, initial resuscitation, antibiotics, and source control, are based on moderate or high-quality evidence; the vast majority is based on low-level or very-low-level evidence. Also, there are 4 strong recommendations based on low-level evidence,[5] 1 of which is on initial fluid management, that is, the use of a fixed volume of 30 mL/kg for all patients with septic shock.

To operationalize the guidelines, SSC care bundles were developed together with the Institute for Healthcare Improvement. After the 2015 revision, the bundles now consist of 7 specific management goals to be completed before 3 hours or 6 hours within diagnostics (lactate measurement and blood culture), interventions (broad-spectrum antibiotics, fixed volume fluids, and vasopressors), and reassessment of the circulation in case of severe impairment (http://www.survivingsepsis.org/Bundles/Pages/default.aspx). In the 2016 guidelines, only 2 of the 7 items included in the revised bundles were graded as moderate quality of evidence (use of antibiotics and vasopressors); the remaining 5 were graded as low quality or very low quality of evidence.[5] Adherence in clinical practice to the items in the bundles has repeatedly been found to be low even with the use of focused implementation strategies.[9–11] The low compliance rates may indicate that the SSC guidelines are not standard of care in all settings.

HOW SHOULD THE SURVIVING SEPSIS CAMPAIGN GUIDELINES BE USED?

There has been vivid debate about how clinicians and heath care systems should use clinical practice guidelines, such as the SSC guidelines. On one hand, guidelines may be seen as a tool to provide the clinical application of the evidence base synthesized by experts through clear recommendation.[12] On the other hand, often guidelines are outdated, may contain few recommendations based on high-quality evidence, and may be used for legal or restrictive administrative purposes.[12] Guidelines may be colored by academic and fiscal conflicts of interest, and some investigators have argued that they cause regression toward the mean of care — poor performing centers improve while good performing ones get worse — and that guidelines hamper the conduct of clinical trials because uncertainties are rarely acknowledged in the guidelines.[13,14]

Some of the arguments from the guidelines pros and cons may be dampened by increasing emphasis on the World Health Organization definition of a clinical practice guideline (Version: 10 March 2003): "Guidelines are systematically developed evidence-based statements which assist providers, recipients and other stakeholders to make informed decisions about appropriate health interventions." Thus, clinical practice guidelines should assist and not mandate care; they are guidance to the clinicians. Applying this to the SSC, the 2016 guideline article is an extensive, fully updated document that may assist clinicians in delivering the best care to the patients with sepsis while adding flexibility based on patient-specific and setting-specific characteristics.

Where the SSC guidelines should advise clinicians, the SSC bundles may be another issue, because these quality-improvement tools may easily be used to mandate and measure care. Observational data suggest that adherence to the SSC guidelines and bundles is associated with improved outcome, despite low adherence to the items in bundles.[9–11] This challenges the outcome results, in particular because none of the bundles' items has been shown to improve outcomes in randomized trials, and observational data may overestimate the relative intervention effects by as much as 30%.[15,16] When coupled to outcome reports based on observational data with inherent high risk of bias,[9] then a self-fulfilling prophecy may be created. Interventions based on low-quality evidence recommendations may be mandated and further supported by low-quality evidence as is the case, for example, in fixed-volume fluid resuscitation in the SSC bundles and guidelines.[5] Forcing care based on lower-quality evidence may cause harm as suggested with certain antibiotics for pneumonia,[17] and the inclusion of tight blood sugar control in the original SSC bundle items.[18] It is, therefore, appropriate to raise concerns about mandating sepsis care items without high-quality evidence.[19]

HOW TO MANAGE THE PATIENT WITH SEPSIS?

What should clinicians managing patients with sepsis do when international standards are based on such uncertain evidence? With the Hippocratic Oath, they have promised to abstain from doing harm. For patients with septic shock, this is particularly difficult because of the uncertain risk-benefit ratio for interventions used in the initial management. In addition, the decision of whether or not to administer an intervention has to be balanced against the potential dire consequences of delaying interventions in these patients.[7] On the other hand, a constant theme in recent years is that less is often more in critical care. As many standard interventions and therapeutic targets in critical care are being challenged, simplifying care becomes increasingly rational both from patient, organizational, and financial perspectives.[7] How to use some of the specific items of the SSC guidelines together with a commonsense approach to aid clinical management of patients with sepsis while trying to balance the potential benefit and harm of the items is discussed.

IDENTIFICATION OF PATIENTS WITH SEPSIS

Although the updated definitions of sepsis and septic shock (Third International Consensus Definitions for Sepsis and Septic Shock [Sepsis-3])[1] should be applied in the broader context, the clinician standing in front of a sick patient should not rely solely on these or the previous syndrome criteria, because they were developed at a population level. Any patient with potential infection who seems very sick, that is, with new-onset warning signs or organ dysfunction (**Fig. 1**), will likely benefit from additional diagnostic work-up focusing on the circulation, markers of organ dysfunction, blood and other relevant cultures, and the most likely focus of infection. Importantly, the progression of sepsis is time dependent, so clinical reassessment should be planned within a short time frame and communicated to the entire clinical team.

INITIAL RESUSCITATION AND ONGOING CIRCULATORY MANAGEMENT

Because patients with septic shock have been consistently documented to have higher mortality than those with sepsis,[4] vigilant hemodynamic monitoring and intervention continue to be a central part of management of these patients and of the SSC guidelines. There is low-quality or very-low-quality evidence for 14 of the 20 statements in the guidelines on initial resuscitation, fluids, vasoactive drugs, and steroids. This is an obvious challenge, because some of the interventions used in these patients were shown ineffective or even harmful when a higher level of evidence was obtained from clinical trials and systematic reviews.[20–25]

Fluid Therapy

- For initial resuscitation, the SSC guidelines recommend at least 30 mL/kg of crystalloids be given to all patients with sepsis-induced hypoperfusion in the first 3 hours.[5] The physiologic rationale may be that all patients with sepsis-induced hypoperfusion are hypovolemic, but this may not be correct.[26] The evidence to support this recommendation is weak and comes from observational data and the notion that this volume was the average baseline fluid volume observed in the recent early goal-directed therapy (EGDT) trials (median 28 mL/kg given in the 3 trials combined),[27] in which overall low mortality was observed. Thus, more than half of the patients received less than the recommended 30 mL/kg, which may be in line with a large cohort study from a national US registry showing an average fluid volume of 4.4 L given on the first day in ICU.[28] Thus, the initial 30 mL/kg of fluids may not be current practice in many settings. More worrying, the only randomized trial done on fluid bolus versus no fluid bolus in sepsis-induced hypoperfusion indicated increased mortality with fluid bolusing.[29] This trial was done in children in sub-Saharan Africa, so the generalizability to adults with sepsis in more developed settings is unknown.
- For ongoing fluid therapy, the SSC recommends using fluid challenges as long as hemodynamic factors continue to improve. The physiologic rationale is likely that fluids given to maximize cardiac output are beneficial, which may have some support in the perioperative setting.[30] But the EDGT protocol, in which fluids, inotropes, and blood were given to optimize hemodynamic factors, was no better than usual care in patients with early septic shock in the recent large multicenter trials, neither overall nor in several subgroups based on disease or shock severity.[27] Furthermore, the recent CLASSIC trial showed that a protocol restricting fluid input after the initial resuscitation was feasible in ICU patients with septic shock and was associated with improved kidney function compared with a standard care protocol.[31] The hemodynamic parameters were identical in the 2 groups after randomization, indicating that additional fluid after the initial resuscitation did not result in improved circulation, at least not in terms of blood lactate level, vasopressor dose, or urine output.[32]
- A common-sense approach to fluid therapy in patients with sepsis-induced hypoperfusion is to give 250-mL to 500-mL boluses followed by regular

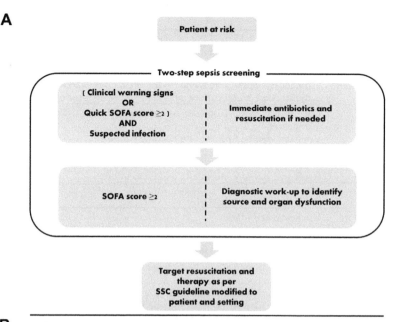

A

Patient at risk

Two-step sepsis screening

(Clinical warning signs
OR
Quick SOFA score ≥2)
AND
Suspected infection

Immediate antibiotics and
resuscitation if needed

SOFA score ≥2

Diagnostic work-up to identify
source and organ dysfunction

Target resuscitation and
therapy as per
SSC guideline modified to
patient and setting

B

Organ system	Clinical warning signs	Quick SOFA variables	SOFA variables
Central nervous system	Altered mental state	Altered mental state	Glasgow Coma Scale Score
Respiration	Dyspnea	Respiratory rate (>22 min⁻¹)	PaO₂/FiO₂-ratio
	High respiratory rate		
	Hypoxia		
	Expectoration of pus		
Cardiovascular	Cold extremities	Systolic blood pressure (<100 mm Hg)	Mean arterial pressure
	Mottling		Administration of vasopressors
	Tachycardia		(type and rate of infusion)
	Lactate above 2 mM		
	Delayed capillary refill		
Renal	Low urine output		S-creatinine
	High s-potassium		Urine output
	High s-creatinine		
	Metabolic acidosis		
Coagulation	Bleeding		Platelet count
	Suggillations		
	Petechiae		
Liver	Jaundice		S-bilirubin
Other	Fever		
	Chills		
	Shivering		
	Patient feeling severe acute sickness		

Fig. 1. Identifying sepsis among patients at risk being it in the ward, emergency department, operating room, or ICU. (*A*) Proposed flow chart for identifying sepsis in patients with clinical warning signs and suspected infection. Quick SOFA, SOFA variables, and suggested clinical warning signs are presented (*B*). SOFA, Sequential (Sepsis-related) Organ Failure Assessment. (*Modified from* Singer M, Deutschman CS, Seymour CW, et al. The Third International Consensus definitions for sepsis and septic shock (sepsis-3). JAMA 2016;315(8):801–10.)

reassessments of the circulation (**Table 1**). If a patient has had a documented fluid loss, then a fixed volume may be given to replace the documented loss. Although many patients improve their circulation with some fluid, those who do not should not receive any more because these patients may be at particular

Table 1	
A common sense approach to the initial management of patients with sepsis	
Identification of patients with sepsis	All patients with potential infection who seem very sick should have a diagnostic work-up focusing on the circulation, markers of organ dysfunction, blood culture, and the most likely focus of infection.
Fluid therapy	Use 250–500 mL fluid boluses; continue only if the circulation improves. Use fixed volume to substitute documented loss. Use crystalloid solutions (ie, isotonic saline and buffered solution) guided by repeated assessment of base excess and sodium in plasma. Avoid hydroxyethyl starch and gelatin solutions. Aim for fluid restriction and negative fluid balances as soon as the circulation has stabilized.
Vasopressor agents	Use norepinephrine. Early infusion of norepinephrine may be considered for severe hypotension, for example, MAP <50 mm Hg, and for those who have no documented loss of fluid. Peripheral infusion may be considered into a large vein proximal to the antecubital or popliteal fossae while waiting for central access or if a short infusion time is expected. Initially aim for MAP of 65 mm Hg; lower may be acceptable provided a patient is awake and adequately perfusing.
Inotropic agents	It is less likely that inotropic agents result in overall benefit, while the risk of adverse effects is high. Dobutamine may be tried in case of ongoing severe tissue hypoperfusion with signs of low cardiac output. In case of adverse effects, in particular tachycardia, the infusion should be decreased or stopped.
Blood transfusion	Transfuse at Hb threshold of 7 g/dL unless the patient has acute myocardial ischemia during which a higher Hb threshold may be considered.
Hemodynamic monitoring	Use repeated assessment of simple circulatory parameters, including blood pressure, heart rate, temperature gradients on the extremities, mottling, capillary refill time, and lactate.
Antibiotic therapy	Give an broad-spectrum antibiotic as soon as possible De-escalate when the microbe is identified or the patient is improving.

risk of being harmed by too much fluid. For ongoing fluid therapy, increasing evidence suggests a more restrictive approach should be used in preference to a more liberal strategy.[33]

- Crystalloid solutions can be used alone because the synthetic colloid solutions cause kidney and coagulation impairment[34–36] and have been shown to increase mortality with varying certainty (high certainty for hydroxyethyl starch and low for gelatin).[23,37] Albumin is likely safe in sepsis but has no obvious benefits and is an expensive and limited resource.[38] The SSC guidelines do suggest consideration of albumin use in patients expected to require large volumes of fluid.[5]

- As for the crystalloid solutions, both isotonic saline and buffered solutions may be used because they appear to cause no differences in outcome.[5,39] It may be rational to give patients with severe acidosis buffered solutions and isotonic saline to those at risk of severe hyponatremia.[40] Thus, ongoing fluid therapy may be guided by repeated assessment of plasma levels of base excess and sodium.

- Aiming at negative fluid balances may be of value for patients who have a positive fluid balance and are hemodynamically stable because such strategies may shorten the time of mechanical ventilation without increasing mortality.[33]

Vasopressors

- Norepinephrine is recommended as the first-line vasopressor in patients with septic shock in the SSC guidelines and in other clinical practice guidelines.[5,41] This choice should be uncontroversial because dopamine is associated with harm compared with norepinephrine,[21] and the overall benefit versus harm of other alternatives (eg, vasopressin analogs and phenylephrine) has been inadequately assessed.[41] The more challenging questions are when to start the norepinephrine infusion and what endpoints should be targeted where evidence from trials are limited.
- Early infusion of norepinephrine may be considered for sepsis patients with severe hypotension, for example, mean arterial pressure less than 50 mm Hg because very severe hypotension may pose a direct threat to a patient's life. In particular, patients with no documented fluid loss should be considered for early norepinephrine. In those who have a higher mean arterial pressure (MAP) and/or documented loss of fluid, IV fluid bolus(es) may be given before the initiation of norepinephrine, as described previously.
- A peripheral venous infusion may be considered to facilitate early initiation of norepinephrine while waiting for central access or if a short infusion time is expected. Taken together, the results of a cohort study and a systematic review of case series suggest that peripheral infusion of vasopressors may be safe if given into a large vein proximal to the antecubital or popliteal fossae for a few hours only, during which the infusion site should be monitored.[42,43] Such an approach has been suggested in the guidelines of the Canadian Association of Emergency Physicians.[44]
- Initially, aim for MAP of 65 mm Hg. To obtain this, patients should be allowed to have values of MAP both below and above 65 mm Hg; if not, patients will likely have time-averaged means of MAP well above the target as has been observed in recent MAP target trials.[45,46] The overshoot observed in these trials hampers interpretation of their results. Thus, there is no good evidence to support any particular level of MAP, but increasing doses of norepinephrine seem to result in increased rates of adverse effects (eg, atrial fibrillation).[45,46] Therefore, the lowest possible MAP target should be accepted as long as the patient is awake and makers of perfusion and kidney function remains unaltered. With this approach, some patients can be handled with MAP target below 65 mm Hg, whereas other patients (eg, those with chronic hypertension) may need a higher target.[45]

Inotropes

- The use of inotropes in patients with septic shock should be carefully considered because there are no placebo-controlled trials showing their efficacy, and safety. Recent trials in patients with septic shock and in patients with impaired heart function prior to or after cardiac surgery indicated no beneficial effects from levosimendan and even harm in those with septic shock.[47–49] Based on a physiologic rationale, the SSC guidelines suggest using dobutamine in patients with evidence of persistent tissue hypoperfusion despite adequate fluid loading and the use of vasopressor agents.[5] One strategy of applying this concept was extensively accessed in the EGDT trials; however, outcomes were not improved by the use of dobutamine in patents in the EGDT groups who had a persistently low central venous oxygen saturation (ScvO$_2$) compared with patients in the usual-care groups.[27] Judging the effects of dobutamine based on the EGDT trial is not straightforward; however, the results of a recent propensity-adjusted cohort study suggested increased mortality with the use of dobutamine in patients with septic shock.[50] Taken together, it is less likely that the use of inotropes (ie, dobutamine, levosimendan, and milrinone) improves patient-important outcomes yet the risk of harm is imminent.

Blood Transfusion

- Transfusion with red blood cells should be performed at a hemoglobin (Hb) level of 7.0 g/dL.[5,24,25,51] There is limited evidence that extenuating circumstances should alter this threshold level except for ongoing myocardial ischemia, during which a higher Hb threshold for transfusion may be considered.[52] There is limited evidence for the use of alternative triggers of transfusion other than Hb.

Hemodynamic Monitoring

- The repeated assessment of circulatory parameters is likely to be important in guiding therapy; this may be done using simple markers of perfusion including lactate (see **Table 1**). Urine output may be used, but it may result in overtreatment, because oliguria may be due to causes other than a low renal blood flow in sepsis.[26]
- On the other hand, it is less likely that more advanced hemodynamic monitoring improves outcomes of patients with septic shock. No hemodynamic target used to guide therapy has been shown to improve outcomes of patients with sepsis. Guidance by ScvO$_2$ monitoring, at least as part of the EGDT protocol,[27] and guidance using cardiac output, at least in general ICU patients and those with early shock,[53,54] does not lead to improved outcomes. The use of alternative strategies, such as echocardiography, has not been tested in trials of sepsis resuscitation. Furthermore, the validity of some of the measures obtained by echocardiography may be questioned.[55,56] The use of markers predictive of fluid responsiveness has shown proof-of-concept,[57,58] but it is still unknown if outcomes are improved by applying these in the management of patients with sepsis.

ANTIMICROBIAL THERAPY

- Broad-spectrum antibiotic therapy should be given as soon as possible to patients with septic shock because this, together with source control, is the only specific intervention against sepsis.[5] The choice of antimicrobial cover should be made according to the likely focus of infection and knowledge about the local antibiogram, in particular the likelihood of infections with multiresistant bacteria. If needed, more than 1 antibiotic may be given to broaden the cover, but there is limited evidence supporting the use of combination therapy with the specific aim of covering the suspected microbe with more than 1 antibiotic.[59]
- Antibiotic cover should be narrowed as soon as the pathogenic microbe has been identified or the patient has improved.[5] If repeated sampling of procalcitonin is used, there is evidence to suggest that antibiotics may be stopped when procalcitonin is normal or has decreased below 80% of the peak value.[60,61] This protocol will likely reduce the use of antibiotics without adverse effects on patient outcomes.

PERSPECTIVE

The clinical management of patients with sepsis and septic shock may be guided by applying the SSC guidelines together with common sense and flexibility based on patient-specific and setting-specific characteristics. A balanced approach is particularly important in areas of uncertainty of which there are still many, as exemplified by the low number of recommendations in the guidelines supported by high-quality evidence.[5] These areas of uncertainty should be broadly acknowledged for clinicians, clinical researchers, and policy makers to act cautiously and together point to the interventions needed to be tested in trials. The aim should be to assess as many current and novel interventions for sepsis as possible in large, multicenter, randomized trials with the lowest possible risk of bias. The results of such trials should improve clinical practice guidelines and patient care and outcomes.

REFERENCES

1. Singer M, Deutschman CS, Seymour CW, et al. The Third International Consensus definitions for sepsis and septic shock (sepsis-3). JAMA 2016;315:801–10.
2. GBD 2013 Mortality and Causes of Death Collaborators. Global, regional, and national age-sex specific all-cause and cause-specific mortality for 240 causes of death, 1990-2013: a systematic analysis for the Global Burden of Disease Study 2013. Lancet 2015;385:117–71.
3. Prescott HC, Langa KM, Liu V, et al. Increased 1-year healthcare use in survivors of severe sepsis. Am J Respir Crit Care Med 2014;190:62–9.
4. Shankar-Hari M, Phillips GS, Levy ML, et al. Developing a new definition and assessing new clinical criteria for septic shock: for the Third International Consensus definitions for sepsis and septic shock (sepsis-3). JAMA 2016;315: 775–87.
5. Rhodes A, Evans LE, Alhazzani W, et al. Surviving sepsis campaign: international guidelines for management of sepsis and septic shock: 2016. Intensive Care Med 2017;43:304–77.
6. Perner A, Gordon AC, De Backer D, et al. Sepsis: frontiers in diagnosis, resuscitation and antibiotic therapy. Intensive Care Med 2016;42:1958–69.
7. Perner A, Rhodes A, Venkatesh B, et al. Sepsis: frontiers in supportive care, organisation and research. Intensive Care Med 2017;43:496–508.
8. Balshem H, Helfand M, Schunemann HJ, et al. GRADE guidelines: 3. Rating the quality of evidence. J Clin Epidemiol 2011;64:401–6.
9. Levy MM, Rhodes A, Phillips GS, et al. Surviving Sepsis Campaign: association between performance metrics and outcomes in a 7.5-year study. Intensive Care Med 2014;40:1623–33.
10. Noritomi DT, Ranzani OT, Monteiro MB, et al. Implementation of a multifaceted sepsis education program in an emerging country setting: clinical outcomes and cost-effectiveness in a long-term follow-up study. Intensive Care Med 2014;40:182–91.
11. Rhodes A, Phillips G, Beale R, et al. The surviving sepsis campaign bundles and outcome: results from the international multicentre prevalence study on sepsis (the IMPreSS study). Intensive Care Med 2015;41:1620–8.
12. Shekelle P, Aronson MD, Melin JA. Overview of clinical practice guidelines. UpToDate 2017. 9-5-2017. Ref Type: Online Source.
13. Girbes AR, Robert R, Marik PE. Protocols: help for improvement but beware of regression to the mean and mediocrity. Intensive Care Med 2015;41:2218–20.

14. Bonten MJ. Dangers and opportunities of guidelines in the data-free zone. Lancet Respir Med 2015;3:670–2.
15. Hemkens LG, Contopoulos-Ioannidis DG, Ioannidis JP. Agreement of treatment effects for mortality from routinely collected data and subsequent randomized trials: meta-epidemiological survey. BMJ 2016;352:i493.
16. Ziff OJ, Lane DA, Samra M, et al. Safety and efficacy of digoxin: systematic review and meta-analysis of observational and controlled trial data. BMJ 2015; 351:h4451.
17. Kett DH, Cano E, Quartin AA, et al. Implementation of guidelines for management of possible multidrug-resistant pneumonia in intensive care: an observational, multicentre cohort study. Lancet Infect Dis 2011;11:181–9.
18. Finfer S, Chittock DR, Su SY, et al. Intensive versus conventional glucose control in critically ill patients. N Engl J Med 2009;360:1283–97.
19. Rhee C, Gohil S, Klompas M. Regulatory mandates for sepsis care–reasons for caution. N Engl J Med 2014;370:1673–6.
20. Angus DC, Barnato AE, Bell D, et al. A systematic review and meta-analysis of early goal-directed therapy for septic shock: the ARISE, ProCESS and ProMISe Investigators. Intensive Care Med 2015;41:1549–60.
21. De Backer D, Biston P, Devriendt J, et al. Comparison of dopamine and norepinephrine in the treatment of shock. N Engl J Med 2010;362:779–89.
22. Perner A, Haase N, Guttormsen AB, et al. Hydroxyethyl starch 130/0.42 versus Ringer's acetate in severe sepsis. N Engl J Med 2012;367:124–34.
23. Haase N, Perner A, Hennings LI, et al. Hydroxyethyl starch 130/0.38-0.45 versus crystalloid or albumin in patients with sepsis: systematic review with meta-analysis and trial sequential analysis. BMJ 2013;346:f839.
24. Holst LB, Haase N, Wetterslev J, et al. Lower versus higher hemoglobin threshold for transfusion in septic shock. N Engl J Med 2014;371:1381–91.
25. Holst LB, Petersen MW, Haase N, et al. Restrictive versus liberal transfusion strategy for red blood cell transfusion: systematic review of randomised trials with meta-analysis and trial sequential analysis. BMJ 2015;350:h1354.
26. Perner A, Prowle J, Joannidis M, et al. Fluid management in acute kidney injury. Intensive Care Med 2017;43(6):807–15.
27. The Prism Investigators, Rowan KM, Angus DC, Bailey M, et al. Early, goal-directed therapy for septic shock - a patient-level meta-analysis. N Engl J Med 2017;376(23):2223–34.
28. Marik PE, Linde-Zwirble WT, Bittner EA, et al. Fluid administration in severe sepsis and septic shock, patterns and outcomes: an analysis of a large national database. Intensive Care Med 2017;43:625–32.
29. Maitland K, Kiguli S, Opoka RO, et al. Mortality after fluid bolus in African children with severe infection. N Engl J Med 2011;364:2483–95.
30. Pearse RM, Harrison DA, MacDonald N, et al. Effect of a perioperative, cardiac output-guided hemodynamic therapy algorithm on outcomes following major gastrointestinal surgery: a randomized clinical trial and systematic review. JAMA 2014;311:2181–90.
31. Hjortrup PB, Haase N, Bundgaard H, et al. Restricting volumes of resuscitation fluid in adults with septic shock after initial management: the CLASSIC randomised, parallel-group, multicentre feasibility trial. Intensive Care Med 2016;42: 1695–705.
32. Hjortrup PB, Haase N, Wetterslev J, et al. Effects of fluid restriction on measures of circulatory efficacy in adults with septic shock. Acta Anaesthesiol Scand 2017; 61:390–8.

33. Silversides JA, Major E, Ferguson AJ, et al. Conservative fluid management or deresuscitation for patients with sepsis or acute respiratory distress syndrome following the resuscitation phase of critical illness: a systematic review and meta-analysis. Intensive Care Med 2017;43:155–70.

34. Rochwerg B, Alhazzani W, Gibson A, et al. Fluid type and the use of renal replacement therapy in sepsis: a systematic review and network meta-analysis. Intensive Care Med 2015;41:1561–71.

35. Haase N, Ostrowski SR, Wetterslev J, et al. Thromboelastography in patients with severe sepsis: a prospective cohort study. Intensive Care Med 2015;41:77–85.

36. Mittermayr M, Streif W, Haas T, et al. Hemostatic changes after crystalloid or colloid fluid administration during major orthopedic surgery: the role of fibrinogen administration. Anesth Analg 2007;105:905–17, table.

37. Moeller C, Fleischmann C, Thomas-Rueddel D, et al. How safe is gelatin? A systematic review and meta-analysis of gelatin-containing plasma expanders vs crystalloids and albumin. J Crit Care 2016;35:75–83.

38. Perner A, Junttila E, Haney M, et al. Scandinavian clinical practice guideline on choice of fluid in resuscitation of critically ill patients with acute circulatory failure. Acta Anaesthesiol Scand 2014;59:274–85.

39. Young P, Bailey M, Beasley R, et al. Effect of a buffered crystalloid solution vs saline on acute kidney injury among patients in the intensive care unit: the SPLIT randomized clinical trial. JAMA 2015;314:1701–10.

40. Burdett E, Dushianthan A, Bennett-Guerrero E, et al. Perioperative buffered versus non-buffered fluid administration for surgery in adults. Cochrane Database Syst Rev 2012;(12):CD004089.

41. Moller MH, Claudius C, Junttila E, et al. Scandinavian SSAI clinical practice guideline on choice of first-line vasopressor for patients with acute circulatory failure. Acta Anaesthesiol Scand 2016;60:1347–66.

42. Cardenas-Garcia J, Schaub KF, Belchikov YG, et al. Safety of peripheral intravenous administration of vasoactive medication. J Hosp Med 2015;10:581–5.

43. Loubani OM, Green RS. A systematic review of extravasation and local tissue injury from administration of vasopressors through peripheral intravenous catheters and central venous catheters. J Crit Care 2015;30:653.e9-17.

44. Djogovic D, MacDonald S, Wensel A, et al. Vasopressor and inotrope use in Canadian emergency departments: evidence based consensus guidelines. CJEM 2015;17(Suppl 1):1–16.

45. Asfar P, Meziani F, Hamel JF, et al. High versus low blood-pressure target in patients with septic shock. N Engl J Med 2014;370:1583–93.

46. Lamontagne F, Meade MO, Hebert PC, et al. Higher versus lower blood pressure targets for vasopressor therapy in shock: a multicentre pilot randomized controlled trial. Intensive Care Med 2016;42:542–50.

47. Gordon AC, Perkins GD, Singer M, et al. Levosimendan for the prevention of acute organ dysfunction in sepsis. N Engl J Med 2016;375:1638–48.

48. Landoni G, Lomivorotov VV, Alvaro G, et al. Levosimendan for hemodynamic support after cardiac surgery. N Engl J Med 2017;376(21):2021–31.

49. Mehta RH, Leimberger JD, van DS, et al. Levosimendan in patients with left ventricular dysfunction undergoing cardiac surgery. N Engl J Med 2017;376(21):2032–42.

50. Wilkman E, Kaukonen KM, Pettila V, et al. Association between inotrope treatment and 90-day mortality in patients with septic shock. Acta Anaesthesiol Scand 2013;57:431–42.

51. Yealy DM, Kellum JA, Huang DT, et al. A randomized trial of protocol-based care for early septic shock. N Engl J Med 2014;370:1683–93.

52. Carson JL, Stanworth SJ, Roubinian N, et al. Transfusion thresholds and other strategies for guiding allogeneic red blood cell transfusion. Cochrane Database Syst Rev 2016;(10):CD002042.

53. Rajaram SS, Desai NK, Kalra A, et al. Pulmonary artery catheters for adult patients in intensive care. Cochrane Database Syst Rev 2013;(2):CD003408.

54. Takala J, Ruokonen E, Tenhunen JJ, et al. Early non-invasive cardiac output monitoring in hemodynamically unstable intensive care patients: a multi-center randomized controlled trial. Crit Care 2011;15:R148.

55. Wetterslev M, Moller-Sorensen H, Johansen RR, et al. Systematic review of cardiac output measurements by echocardiography vs. thermodilution: the techniques are not interchangeable. Intensive Care Med 2016;42:1223–33.

56. Wetterslev M, Haase N, Johansen RR, et al. Predicting fluid responsiveness with transthoracic echocardiography is not yet evidence based. Acta Anaesthesiol Scand 2013;57:692–7.

57. Marik PE, Cavallazzi R, Vasu T, et al. Dynamic changes in arterial waveform derived variables and fluid responsiveness in mechanically ventilated patients: a systematic review of the literature. Crit Care Med 2009;37:2642–7.

58. Monnet X, Marik P, Teboul JL. Passive leg raising for predicting fluid responsiveness: a systematic review and meta-analysis. Intensive Care Med 2016;42: 1935–47.

59. Sjovall F, Perner A, Hylander MM. Empirical mono- versus combination antibiotic therapy in adult intensive care patients with severe sepsis - a systematic review with meta-analysis and trial sequential analysis. J Infect 2017;74:331–44.

60. Bouadma L, Luyt CE, Tubach F, et al. Use of procalcitonin to reduce patients' exposure to antibiotics in intensive care units (PRORATA trial): a multicentre randomised controlled trial. Lancet 2010;375:463–74.

61. De Jong E, van Oers JA, Beishuizen A, et al. Efficacy and safety of procalcitonin guidance in reducing the duration of antibiotic treatment in critically ill patients: a randomised, controlled, open-label trial. Lancet Infect Dis 2016;16:819–27.

Biomarkers in Sepsis

Tjitske S.R. van Engelen, MD[a],*, Willem Joost Wiersinga, MD[a,b],
Brendon P. Scicluna, PhD[a,c], Tom van der Poll, MD[a,b]

KEYWORDS

- Sepsis • Biomarkers • Procalcitonin • Omics technologies • Transcriptomics
- Diagnosis • Prognosis

KEY POINTS

- A biomarker is a characteristic by which a pathophysiologic process can be identified.
- In the clinical setting, a biomarker needs to quickly assist physicians confronted with an ill patient in their decision on the best possible treatment.
- Biomarkers can be of diagnostic value, prognostic value, and in the future may be of theranostic value.
- The omics field of systems biology provides a promising tool for the discovery of novel biomarkers.
- Biomarkers, measured in simply obtainable samples with limited hands-on time or need for specialized laboratories, may be the key to personalized targeted treatment in the future clinical management of sepsis.

INTRODUCTION

Sepsis is characterized by complex pathophysiology and heterogeneous phenotypes of affected patients regarding their symptoms, response to treatment, and outcomes. At present there is no gold standard to diagnose sepsis; no tool to select, evaluate, and de-escalate treatment; and no reliable way to assign risk profiles or predict outcome.[1] Biomarkers can be the key to personalized medicine in sepsis whereby patients receive tailored treatment based on their unique characteristics.[2,3]

Biomarkers are naturally occurring molecules, genes, or other characteristics by which particular physiologic or pathologic processes can be identified. In the clinical setting a biomarker is useful once it can aid decision making. The ideal biomarker has

Disclosure: The authors have nothing to disclose.
[a] Division of Laboratory Specialties, Center for Experimental Molecular Medicine, Academic Medical Center, University of Amsterdam, Meibergdreef 9, Room G2-130, Amsterdam 1105AZ, The Netherlands; [b] Division of Infectious Diseases, Academic Medical Center, University of Amsterdam, Meibergdreef 9, Room G2-130, Amsterdam 1105AZ, The Netherlands; [c] Department of Clinical Epidemiology, Biostatistics and Bioinformatics, Academic Medical Center, University of Amsterdam, Meibergdreef 9, Room G2-130, Amsterdam 1105AZ, The Netherlands
* Corresponding author.
E-mail address: t.s.vanengelen@amc.uva.nl

fast kinetics, high sensitivity and specificity, can be identified by fully automated technology, has a short turnaround time, and is available as a point-of-care test with low production costs.[1] A biomarker therefore needs to quickly assist physicians confronted with an ill patient in their decision on the best possible treatment. Current clinical biomarkers can be roughly divided into 2 types: diagnostic and prognostic markers (**Fig. 1**). Biomarkers that can discriminate sepsis from noninfectious critical illness or can differentiate between causative organisms in sepsis can be regarded as diagnostic biomarkers. A diagnostic biomarker can diminish improper use of antibiotics and could be used for antibiotic stewardship. Although pathogen detection remains the gold standard in establishing the cause of infection, blood cultures are only positive in 30% to 40% of the sepsis cases and in one-third of (clinically defined) sepsis cases all cultures are sterile.[4,5] In addition, the presence of a pathogen does not prove the presence of disease and infections can be caused by multiple pathogens, further showing the need for biomarkers that indicate infection. Prognostic biomarkers can help predict outcomes in patients with sepsis by assigning risk profiles. In addition, biomarkers can aid in stratifying patients in subgroups based on specific pathophysiologic features, thereby paving the way to personalized therapy with biomarker-guided follow-up of response to treatment.[6] The approach to using biomarker tests to select and evaluate specific therapies is known as theranostics and is seen as a main tool in the future management of many diseases.[7] Such biomarker tests should be applicable on easily obtained samples such as urine or blood. Rapid testing should identify subgroups of patients that would benefit from certain targeted therapies. The biomarker test could further be of use by evaluating the effect of the therapy on its target.

Biomarkers have been implemented in clinical practice in various fields of medicine, including cardiology (eg, troponin T in myocardial infarction), vascular medicine (eg, D-dimer in patients suspected of pulmonary embolism), and in particular oncology

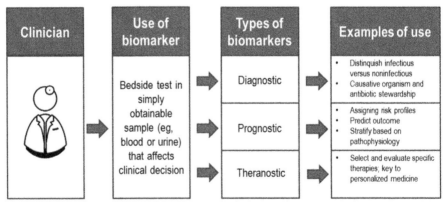

Fig. 1. What is a biomarker? Biomarkers are host characteristics, such as molecules or genes, by which particular physiologic or pathologic processes can be identified. When developing and validating novel biomarkers their potential clinical use is of utmost importance. Biomarkers can be used to distinguish sepsis from noninfectious critical illness or to determine causative pathogens to initiate the best possible treatment, thereby contributing to antibiotic stewardship. Furthermore, biomarkers can help stratify patients based on risk profiles, and predict outcome or identify pathophysiologic pathways that can be the target for personalized therapy. Biomarker tests that select and monitor specific therapies are known as theranostics and are seen as a future aid for a targeted personalized approach in patients with sepsis.

(numerous examples). In contrast, in sepsis management the use of biomarkers is still at its beginning. In a comprehensive systematic review, conducted nearly a decade ago, 178 biomarkers were evaluated in the context of sepsis.[8] A crude search in the PubMed database shows that biomarkers in sepsis is a trending topic (**Fig. 2**). In the last 10 years almost 5000 articles on biomarkers in sepsis have been published, whereas before 2007 the total number of published articles was less than 3000. Roughly 100 clinical trials are currently enrolling patients to study biomarkers in sepsis.[9] Even though numerous biomarkers for sepsis have been identified,[8,10] the recently updated guidelines of the Surviving Sepsis Campaign only see a minor role for 1 biomarker in clinical practice; that is, procalcitonin (PCT).[11] This guideline underlines the current status of biomarkers in sepsis. So far, no biomarker has been found reliable enough to diagnose sepsis or predict prognosis; only PCT is used in some medical centers to guide antibiotic treatment in critically ill patients.[12] This limitation is largely attributed to the complex pathophysiology of sepsis, and it seems unlikely that a single biomarker can provide accurate information about the main drivers of the disturbed host response in individual patients with sepsis. A panel of biomarkers may deliver unique sepsis signatures that are informative for specific pathophysiologic derailments and/or prognosis, which is very much desired for the development of targeted therapies.[3,13–15] New developments such as omics technologies and the human genome project are promising aids in the search for new useful biomarkers in sepsis. This article reviews current and novel biomarkers in sepsis and their potential use at the bedside to guide clinical decision making.

TRADITIONAL (PROTEIN) BIOMARKERS

Many protein biomarkers have been evaluated for their ability to discriminate between sepsis and noninfectious conditions. In critical care, antibiotic therapy is almost invariably initiated on (even modest) suspicion of infection. However, the infection diagnosis in critically ill patients is likely overestimated. A recent study involving more than 2500 patients treated for sepsis on the intensive care unit (ICU) reported that 13% had a post-hoc infection likelihood of none, and an additional 30% of only possible, as determined by well-defined criteria and making use of all clinical, radiological, and microbiological information.[16] Remarkably, patients who were initially treated for sepsis but were post hoc determined to have noninfectious disease had higher mortality,[16] thereby underlining the necessity for a diagnostic biomarker to correctly diagnose sepsis.

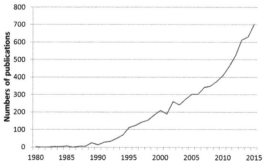

Fig. 2. Articles published on biomarkers in sepsis. An exploratory search in the PubMed database regarding "sepsis AND biomarkers" shows an increase in number of publications from 1980 to 2015.

By far the most studied biomarker, and the only biomarker that is currently implemented in clinical sepsis guidelines, is PCT. PCT levels increase in response to a proinflammatory stimulus. Because of the short time between stimulus and induction of PCT (detectable after 4 hours, peak at 6 hours)[17,18] and its long half-life of 25 to 30 hours,[19] it is a widely investigated biomarker in sepsis. A recent meta-analysis showed a pooled sensitivity of 0.77 (95% confidence interval [CI] 0.72–0.81) and a pooled specificity of 0.79 (95% CI, 0.74–0.84) of PCT to distinguish between sepsis and a systemic inflammatory response syndrome of noninfectious origin.[20] Levels of PCT between 0.1 and 0.5 ng/mL suggest the presence of bacterial infection for which antimicrobial therapy is required,[21] but no consensus has been reached about the correct cutoff value for PCT in this decision making.[20] Furthermore, PCT levels associate with severity of illness in patients with severe pneumonia,[22] and decreasing PCT levels associate with improved survival rates.[23] Likewise, in a prospective observational study conducted in 858 patients with sepsis, inability to decrease PCT level by greater than 80% from baseline to day 4 and day 28 was an independent predictor of mortality.[24] Although the use of PCT as a biomarker for the diagnosis of sepsis is limited because PCT levels also increase in noninfectious diseases, it differentiates better between infectious and noninfectious causes of critical illness than C-reactive protein (CRP), lipopolysaccharide binding protein (LBP), and interleukin (IL)-6.[25]

Different PCT algorithms have been developed to help decision making regarding the start and duration of antibiotic treatment. In patients with acute respiratory infections the use of PCT algorithms reduces the initiation of antibiotic treatment (mostly in primary care settings) and duration of antibiotic treatment (mostly in emergency departments [EDs] and ICU settings) without affecting mortality.[26] Similarly, a randomized controlled trial found a decrease of 4.5% in use of antibiotics without differences in mortality, diagnostic procedures, or therapeutic procedures in patients with severe sepsis or septic shock.[27] In a prospective, multicenter, randomized controlled, open-label intervention trial in 15 hospitals in the Netherlands involving 1575 patients, PCT guidance of antibiotic therapy, consisting of a nonbinding advice to discontinue antibiotics if PCT concentration decreased by 80% or PCT levels were less than 0.5 ng/mL, was associated with a reduced consumption of antibiotics and a diminished mortality at 28 days (20% vs 27% in the standard-of-care group).[12] This finding suggests that PCT concentrations might assist in identifying bacterial infections, which may result in more adequate diagnosis and treatment.[12] Another randomized controlled trial in critically ill patients, using a PCT algorithm wherein a 0.1-ng/mL cutoff determined antibiotic cessation, found no reduction in duration of antibiotic treatment.[28] A recent investigation determined the use of PCT and associated outcomes in the real-world clinical setting of ICUs in the United States.[29] Among more than 20,000 critically ill patients in 107 hospitals with PCT testing available, 18% of patients had PCT levels checked; in this population the use of PCT was not associated with improved antibiotic use or other clinical outcomes.[29] Hence, current data on the use of PCT for antibiotic stewardship in critically ill patients with sepsis are not consistent.

Examples of other well-studied protein biomarkers are CRP,[30] LBP,[31] IL-6,[31] soluble triggering receptor expressed on myeloid cells-1 (sTREM-1),[32,33] and soluble urokinase plasminogen activator receptor (suPAR),[34] all with a lower sensitivity and specificity as a biomarker for sepsis compared with PCT. The biggest potential of PCT so far seems to be to help reduce exposure to antibiotics in patients with acute respiratory infections and perhaps as a stimulant to physicians to safely reduce the duration of antibiotic treatment in critically ill patients with presumed bacterial infection. Nonetheless, PCT cannot be used as a single diagnostic test for sepsis, because false-negative results could lead to mortality. Considering the weak evidence for the use of PCT in clinical settings, the Surviving Sepsis Campaign guidelines stress the point that a clinical decision to initiate, alter, or stop antimicrobial treatment should never be based solely on changes in any current biomarker, including PCT.[11]

NEW BIOMARKERS DERIVED FROM OMICS RESEARCH

Considering the huge potential of biomarkers for personalized medicine in sepsis, the search for biomarkers has shifted focus from traditional protein and cytokine markers to systems-based approaches. The omics field of systems biology seeks to characterize and quantify molecules that translate in the structure, function, and dynamics of an organism. Omics encompasses genomics, epigenetics, transcriptomics, proteomics, and metabolomics (**Fig. 3**). Omics-based methodologies have developed into more feasible and less costly tools[35] and are increasingly used to study host-pathogen interactions,[36] the host response, and biomarkers in sepsis.[37] Traditional biomarkers or sets of biomarkers measure the concentration of circulating proteins, but the rapidly growing field of systems biology integrates and analyses complex data sets of various aspects of host signaling and response pathways. In this respect, transcriptomics has been studied most. The use of RNA molecules as biomarkers has the advantage that these can be incorporated in polymerase chain reaction–based bedside tests with limited or no hands-on time, making them attractive for implementation in clinical practice. Such tests could measure a set of RNA biomarkers concurrently, which is likely to improve sensitivity and specificity. Several publications on traditional protein biomarkers have indicated that sets of host proteins are superior to single biomarkers to diagnose sepsis.[13,15]

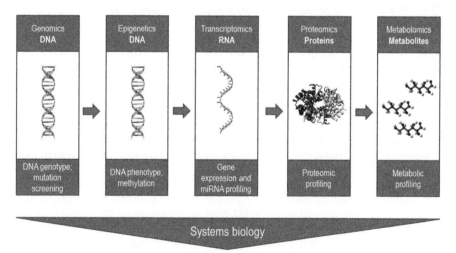

Fig. 3. Omics technologies. Omics is the characterization and quantification of molecules that translate into the structure, function, and dynamics of an organism. (Epi)genomics studies methylation of DNA and screens for single nucleotide polymorphisms. Transcriptomics studies messenger RNA and microRNA (miRNA) expression. Proteomics and metabolomics comprise the study of, respectively, protein and metabolic profiling. Systems biology integrates these fields by analyzing complex data sets of various aspects of host signaling and response pathways in sepsis.

RNA Biomarkers

The genomic response to sepsis shows alterations in the transcriptome of peripheral white blood cells with significant differences of their RNA transcripts compared with healthy individuals.[7] Several investigations have reported on the ability of host transcriptome analyses to discriminate between infection and noninfectious acute disease, and even between different causative pathogens[38] (**Fig. 4**). Among these diagnostic RNA biomarkers the molecular host response classifier SeptiCyte LAB was recently approved by the US Food and Drug Administration as an aid in differentiating infection-positive (sepsis) from infection-negative systemic inflammation in critically ill patients on their first day of ICU admission.[39] This 4-gene classifier combines *CEACAM4*, *LAMP1*, *PLA2G7*, and *PLAC8* to produce a summary area under the receiver operating characteristic (ROC) curve (AUC) of 0.89 (95% CI, 0.85–0.93) to differentiate sepsis from noninfectious systemic inflammatory response syndrome.[40] This rapid molecular assay is the first RNA-based clinical diagnostic tool derived from whole blood approved as a diagnostic test in critically ill patients.[40] Another investigation, performed in a large number of independent cohorts, reported an 11-gene biomarker, named the Sepsis MetaScore, that could reliably distinguish patients with sepsis from patients with sterile inflammation[41] with an AUC of 0.87 (range, 0.70–0.98). Furthermore, a recent study, using genome-wide messenger RNA (mRNA) expression profiles, identified a set panel of markers composed of 3 upregulated transcripts (Toll-like receptor 5, protectin, and clusterin) and 4 downregulated transcripts (fibrinogenlike 2, IL-7 receptor, major histocompatibility complex class II, carboxypeptidase, and vitellogeniclike) that best described the extent of immune alterations.[42] A gene expression score was created that was greater in patients with definite as well as with possible/probable infection than in those without infection.[42] Our group focused on the development of context-specific molecular biomarkers; that is, in patients with a particular clinical presentation, such as suspected community-acquired pneumonia (CAP).[43] We compared whole-genome mRNA profiles in blood leukocytes of patients treated for suspected CAP on ICU admission, who were designated CAP (cases) and no-CAP patients (control subjects) by post-hoc assessment. A 78-gene signature was defined for the diagnosis of CAP, from which a *FAIM3:PLAC8* gene expression ratio was derived that outperformed plasma PCT in discriminating between CAP and no-CAP patients.[43] Moreover, other groups have evaluated the *FAIM3:PLAC8* score in the context of all-cause adult, pediatric, and neonatal sepsis with favorable ROC AUCs.[44,45] This finding indicates that, although the *FAIM3:PLAC8* score was derived as a context-specific biomarker (ie, CAP diagnosis), its applicability may be broadened. These studies have shown that transcriptomics coupled with sophisticated machine learning and statistical tests may provide an invaluable tool to identify diagnostic biomarkers of sepsis.

Several studies have indicated that host gene expression signatures can assist in discriminating between causative pathogens in infected patients. In an observational cohort study in adults presenting to the ED, host gene expression profiling was used to classify the cause of suspected community-acquired acute respiratory tract infections (ARIs) into bacterial, viral, or noninfectious origin. The overall accuracy of gene expression classifiers was 87%, which was significantly better than the use of procalcitonin, which could assign patients as having bacterial ARI or nonbacterial ARI with 78% accuracy.[46] Furthermore, transcriptional profiling of blood leukocytes from hospitalized patients with lower respiratory tract infections was superior in differentiating bacterial from viral causes compared with the use of PCT.[47] Transcriptome analyses of blood leukocytes of adult ICU patients with influenza A pneumonia, bacterial pneumonia,

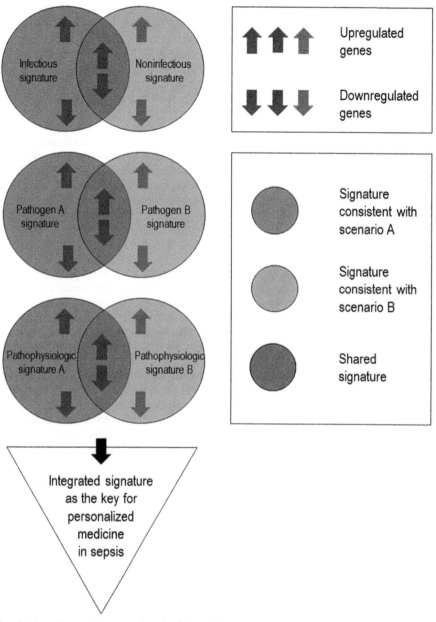

Fig. 4. Host signatures as molecular biomarkers using omics technologies. Using omics-based methodologies, various host signatures can be determined in an integrated systems biology approach aiding the development of targeted therapies. This article describes several molecular biomarkers with diagnostic value (eg, discriminating infectious from noninfectious critically ill patients or distinguishing between causative pathogens) and prognostic value (eg, stratifying patients in risk groups correlating with outcome measures such as mortality). The key is to identify omic biomarkers unique for a certain scenario. An ideal biomarker can quickly assist physicians confronted with an ill patient in the decision on the best possible treatment.

and noninfectious respiratory compromise delineated a 29-gene classifier of viral infection that discriminated viral from bacterial infection and noninfectious disease; this classifier could not distinguish bacterial infection and noninfectious disease.[48] A set of 7 genes was derived from a multicohort analysis that could discriminate bacterial from viral infections.[49] This gene classifier was validated in 30 independent cohorts and integrated together with the 11-gene Sepsis MetaScore in an antibiotics decision model, which had a sensitivity and specificity for bacterial infections of 94.0% and 59.8%, respectively.[49] Several investigations examined the value of transcriptomics to build host response classifiers that can assist in the discrimination between viral and bacterial causes of acute infections in children.[50,51] A 35-gene set was able to divide infections based on broad groups of causative pathogens in pediatric patients, with distinct gene signatures for infections caused by influenza A virus, *Escherichia coli*, or *Streptococcus pneumoniae*.[50] Discrimination within viral pathogens (respiratory syncytial virus, human rhinovirus, and influenza) was achieved with 95% accuracy using a 70-gene classifier in children.[52] In febrile children presenting to the hospital, a 38-transcript signature distinguishing bacterial from viral infection was discovered, which was reduced to a 2-transcript signature (*FAM89A* and *IFI44L*) by removing highly correlated mRNA levels.[53]

Transcriptomics has also been used to develop biomarkers that potentially can provide insight into the prognosis of patients with sepsis. In a prospective cohort study of ICU patients with sepsis caused by CAP, transcriptomics of peripheral blood leukocytes defined 2 sepsis response signatures (named SRS1 and SRS2), wherein SRS1 had a immunosuppressive phenotype with a higher 14-day mortality than the SRS2.[54] These signatures not only provide insight into the main pathophysiology of individual patients but could be the start of targeted therapy and better outcome prediction. In pediatric sepsis, the Pediatric Sepsis Biomarker Risk Model (PERSEVERE) was developed to estimate baseline mortality risk in children with septic shock, consisting of serum proteins selected based on gene expression profiles.[55,56] PERSEVERE has recently been adapted for adults with septic shock.[57] Notably, biomarkers associated with mortality were in part different between adult and pediatric patients; that is, although in children with septic shock granzyme B, heat shock protein 70 kDa 1B, C-C chemokine ligand (CCL) 3, IL-8, and matrix metalloproteinase 8 (MMP8) contributed to the predictive capacity of the model, in adult patients, granzyme B, heat shock protein 70 kDa 1B, CCL3, IL-8, IL-1α, and CCL4 contributed to its prognostic capability.[57] Considering that the initial approach to selecting the PERSEVERE protein biomarkers left 68 genes unconsidered, in a subsequent study this group of investigators determined whether these previously not incorporated genes could advance the performance of PERSEVERE.[58] A network containing 18 mortality risk assessment genes related to tumor protein 53 (TP53) was revealed and combined with PERSEVERE into the so-called PERSEVERE-XP, which was superior to PERSEVERE in differentiating between survivors and nonsurvivors.[58]

Note that all these studies on host gene expression have led to the publication of multiple gene expression data sets with only partially overlapping classifier genes, underlining the necessity to critically determine the study population when developing or validating these host gene expression signatures. Along the same lines, direct comparison of different gene signatures should be done with caution, especially when evaluated outside the context in which they were discovered and validated.[45,59]

Proteomics and Metabolomics

The developments of mass spectrometry have paved the way to the study of changes in proteomics and metabolomics during sepsis.[60] Initial enthusiasm about the application of proteomics to discovering protein biomarkers was reduced because of technical difficulties and low reproducibility. Nonetheless, several studies have reported using proteomics to discover biomarkers for infection diagnosis and sepsis prognosis. A recent proteomics study screened 600 proteins in 765 patients presenting to the ED with fever and identified a 3-protein signature that could discriminate bacterial, viral, and noninfectious disease accurately.[61] The plasma concentrations of tumor necrosis factor–related apoptosis-inducing ligand 1, chemokine (C-X-C motif) ligand 10 (CXCL10) and CRP distinguished bacterial from viral, and infectious (bacterial and viral) from noninfectious disease with an AUC of 0.94 (95% CI, 0.92–0.96). The 3-protein signature was strongest in differentiating bacterial from viral causes in lower respiratory tract infections and fever of no known source.[61] Notably, although this study suggests that proteomics can be useful for the discovery of biomarkers of infection, this population is different from patients with sepsis, and similar studies in sepsis are warranted to evaluate protein signatures as biomarkers in this context. A limitation of conventional proteomic techniques, such as two-dimensional gel electrophoresis, is that the abundant plasma proteins, such as albumin, limit identification and measurement of changes in low-abundance plasma proteins (or peptides). A pilot study conducted in 20 patients with sepsis sought to circumvent this technical issue by making use of the fact that albumin is not glycosylated, and used a plasma glycoproteomic evaluation for analysis of low-abundance plasma proteins.[62] N-linked plasma glycopeptides were quantified by solid-phase extraction coupled with mass spectrometry, after which protein differences between sepsis survivors and nonsurvivors were validated by immunoblotting.[62] A total of 501 glycopeptides corresponding with 234 proteins were identified, of which 66 glycopeptides (54 proteins) were unique to survivors, 60 glycopeptides (43 proteins) were unique to nonsurvivors, and 375 glycopeptides (137 proteins) were common between groups. Nonsurvivors showed increased total kininogen, and decreased total cathepsin-L1, vascular cell adhesion molecule, periostin, neutrophil gelatinase–associated lipocalin, and glycosylated clusterin levels.[62]

Several recent studies have focused on investigating plasma metabolomic profiles as predictive signatures of ICU mortality in adult patients.[63–67] An investigation that sought to identify metabolic biomarkers for differentiation of sepsis and noninfectious acute disease analyzed 186 metabolites comprising 6 analyte classes (acylcarnitines, amino acids, biogenic amines, glycerophospholipids, sphingolipids, and carbohydrates) to reveal 2 markers (acylcarnitine C10:1 and glycerophospholipid PCaaC32:0) that had higher concentrations in sepsis, suggesting that they may be helpful for differentiation of infectious from noninfectious systemic inflammation.[63] Carnitine, the product of acylcarnitine, is used to transport fatty acids into the mitochondria, whereas glycerophosphatidylcholines are major constituents of cell membranes and play a role in cell signaling. A metabolomics approach was also adopted to identify markers that distinguish between sepsis and noninfectious causes of critical illness.[67] Serum concentrations of most acylcarnitines, glycerophospholipids, and sphingolipids were altered in sepsis compared with noninfectious critical illness, and a regression model combining the sphingolipid sphingomyelin (SM) C22:3 and the glycerophospholipid lysoPCaC24:0 was discovered for sepsis diagnosis with a sensitivity of 0.84 and specificity of 0.86. Furthermore, specific metabolites could be used for the discrimination of different types of infection. Patients with sepsis with bloodstream infection could be discriminated by a decrease of acetylornithine level. Putrescine, lysoPCaC18:0, and SM C16:1 were associated with unfavorable outcome in patients with sepsis caused by CAP, intra-abdominal infections, and bloodstream infections, respectively.[67] Sphingolipids are involved in signal transmission and cell recognition, whereas putrescine mediates the complex interplay between bacterial infection and the host immune response. Another investigation tested variable metabolites for association with 28-day mortality in patients with sepsis and found 31 metabolites that differed among ICU survivors versus those who died. In those who died, the levels of 25 metabolites were increased and 6 were decreased (all of which were lipids). The investigators developed a metabolomic network of 7 metabolites associated with death [gamma-glutamylphenylalanine, gamma-glutamyltyrosine, 1-arachidonoylGPC(20;4), taurochenodeoxycholate, 3-(4-hydroxyphenyl) lactate, sucrose, kynurenine].[64] In a retrospective analysis conducted in 20 patients with septic shock, changes in the levels of circulating metabolites were studied in relation to mortality using a targeted mass spectrometry–based quantitative metabolomic approach.[68] Low levels of unsaturated long-chain phosphatidylcholines and lysophosphatidylcholine species (among which are glycerophospholipid lysoPCaC24:0 and lysoPCaC18:0) were associated with 90-day survival together with low levels of circulating kynurenine, which is relevant for tryptophan catabolism.[68]

In a comprehensive proteomic-metabolomic analysis on patients with community-acquired sepsis, patients at higher risk of death were found to be deficient in fatty acid transport and beta-oxidation, gluconeogenesis, and the citric acid cycle.[66] Alterations in the metabolome were correlated with changes in the proteome and a 7-metabolite panel could predict sepsis mortality at the time of presentation to the ED.[66] In an approach that integrated human genetics, patient metabolite and cytokine measurements, and testing in a mouse model, the methionine salvage pathway was revealed as a regulator of sepsis pathophysiology that can predict prognosis in patients.[69] Increased plasma levels of the pathway's substrate methylthioadenosine were associated with mortality in 2 cohorts of patients with sepsis and correlated with levels of proinflammatory cytokines, indicating that increased methylthioadenosine level marks a subgroup of patients with excessive inflammation. A machine-learning model combining methylthioadenosine and other variables produced 80% accuracy in predicting death.[69] These studies show differences in altered metabolites (eg, glycerophospholipid PCaaC32:0 in one study and glycerophospholipid lysoPCaC24:0 in another) and similarities (eg, higher levels of circulating kynurenine, putrescine, lysoPCaC18:0, and lysoPCaC24:0) associated with unfavorable outcome. This finding could be the result of well-known pathophysiologic lipid induction by bacterial components as part of the metabolic changes in patients with sepsis, as well as altered pathogen-host interactions.

FUTURE PERSPECTIVES

The clinical use of biomarkers in sepsis is still at its infancy, especially compared with other fields such as vascular medicine and oncology. Thus far, biomarker research in sepsis has primarily focused on discrimination between infectious and noninfectious causes of critical illness, and sepsis prognosis. Biomarkers can likely also be used to stratify patients with sepsis according to biochemical and/or immunologic profiles, which can provide insight into the main pathophysiologic mechanisms in individual patients and in pathways that can potentially be targeted. New omics technologies can be of great help, associating expression at RNA, protein, and metabolite levels with specific complications and outcomes. The challenge will be to develop biomarker sets that can be measured in simply obtainable samples such as blood and urine but that mirror pathophysiologic events at different body sites. Such biomarker sets could guide the inclusion of patients who might benefit from a targeted therapy and monitor the effect of the therapeutic on its target using an approach that has been named theranostics. The authors foresee a future for sepsis management in which therapies are guided by repeated measurements of biomarker sets reflecting aberrations in host response pathways that can be specifically modified by targeted therapeutics, using rapid bedside tests with limited hands-on time and no need for specialized laboratories. In this personalized medicine approach, individualized therapies would be provided in a pathology-specific way, and not purely based on clinical presentation.

REFERENCES

1. Cohen J, Vincent JL, Adhikari NK, et al. Sepsis: a roadmap for future research. Lancet Infect Dis 2015;15(5):581–614.
2. Singer M. Biomarkers in sepsis. Curr Opin Pulm Med 2013;19(3):305–9.
3. Perner A, Rhodes A, Venkatesh B, et al. Sepsis: frontiers in supportive care, organisation and research. Intensive Care Med 2017;43(4):496–508.
4. Bochud PY, Glauser MP, Calandra T. Antibiotics in sepsis. Intensive Care Med 2001;27(Suppl 1):S33–48.
5. Bochud PY, Bonten M, Marchetti O, et al. Antimicrobial therapy for patients with severe sepsis and septic shock: an evidence-based review. Crit Care Med 2004; 32(11 Suppl):S495–512.
6. Sims CR, Nguyen TC, Mayeux PR. Could biomarkers direct therapy for the septic patient? J Pharmacol Exp Ther 2016;357(2):228–39.
7. van der Poll T, van de Veerdonk FL, Scicluna BP, et al. The immunopathology of sepsis and potential therapeutic targets. Nat Rev Immunol 2017;17:407–20.
8. Pierrakos C, Vincent JL. Sepsis biomarkers: a review. Crit Care 2010;14(1):R15.
9. Clinical Trials. List of open studies regarding "sepsis" AND "biomarkers" 2017. Available at: https://www.clinicaltrials.gov/ct2/results?term=sepsis+AND+biomarkers&recr=Open. Accessed August 24, 2017.
10. Bloos F, Reinhart K. Rapid diagnosis of sepsis. Virulence 2014;5(1):154–60.
11. Rhodes A, Evans LE, Alhazzani W, et al. Surviving Sepsis Campaign: international guidelines for management of sepsis and septic shock: 2016. Intensive Care Med 2017;43(3):304–77.
12. de Jong E, van Oers JA, Beishuizen A, et al. Efficacy and safety of procalcitonin guidance in reducing the duration of antibiotic treatment in critically ill patients: a randomised, controlled, open-label trial. Lancet Infect Dis 2016;16(7):819–27.
13. Gibot S, Bene MC, Noel R, et al. Combination biomarkers to diagnose sepsis in the critically ill patient. Am J Respir Crit Care Med 2012;186(1):65–71.
14. Casserly B, Read R, Levy MM. Multimarker panels in sepsis. Crit Care Clin 2011; 27(2):391–405.
15. Kofoed K, Andersen O, Kronborg G, et al. Use of plasma C-reactive protein, procalcitonin, neutrophils, macrophage migration inhibitory factor, soluble urokinase-type plasminogen activator receptor, and soluble triggering receptor expressed on myeloid cells-1 in combination to diagnose infections: a prospective study. Crit Care 2007;11(2):R38.
16. Klein Klouwenberg PM, Cremer OL, van Vught LA, et al. Likelihood of infection in patients with presumed sepsis at the time of intensive care unit admission: a cohort study. Crit Care 2015;19:319.
17. Dandona P, Nix D, Wilson MF, et al. Procalcitonin increase after endotoxin injection in normal subjects. J Clin Endocrinol Metab 1994;79(6):1605–8.
18. Brunkhorst FM, Heinz U, Forycki ZF. Kinetics of procalcitonin in iatrogenic sepsis. Intensive Care Med 1998;24(8):888–9.

19. Meisner M, Lohs T, Huettemann E, et al. The plasma elimination rate and urinary secretion of procalcitonin in patients with normal and impaired renal function. Eur J anaesthesiology 2001;18(2):79–87.

20. Wacker C, Prkno A, Brunkhorst FM, et al. Procalcitonin as a diagnostic marker for sepsis: a systematic review and meta-analysis. Lancet Infect Dis 2013;13(5): 426–35.

21. Schuetz P, Briel M, Christ-Crain M, et al. Procalcitonin to guide initiation and duration of antibiotic treatment in acute respiratory infections: an individual patient data meta-analysis. Clin Infect Dis 2012;55(5):651–62.

22. Bloos F, Marshall JC, Dellinger RP, et al. Multinational, observational study of procalcitonin in ICU patients with pneumonia requiring mechanical ventilation: a multicenter observational study. Crit Care 2011;15(2):R88.

23. Schuetz P, Maurer P, Punjabi V, et al. Procalcitonin decrease over 72 hours in US critical care units predicts fatal outcome in sepsis patients. Crit Care 2013; 17(3):R115.

24. Schuetz P, Birkhahn R, Sherwin R, et al. Serial procalcitonin predicts mortality in severe sepsis patients: results from the Multicenter Procalcitonin Monitoring Sepsis (MOSES) study. Crit Care Med 2017;45(5):781–9.

25. Reinhart K, Meisner M. Biomarkers in the critically ill patient: procalcitonin. Crit Care Clin 2011;27(2):253–63.

26. Schuetz P, Muller B, Christ-Crain M, et al. Procalcitonin to initiate or discontinue antibiotics in acute respiratory tract infections. Cochrane Database Syst Rev 2012;(9):CD007498.

27. Bloos F, Trips E, Nierhaus A, et al. Effect of sodium selenite administration and procalcitonin-guided therapy on mortality in patients with severe sepsis or septic shock: a randomized clinical trial. JAMA Intern Med 2016;176(9):1266–76.

28. Shehabi Y, Sterba M, Garrett PM, et al. Procalcitonin algorithm in critically ill adults with undifferentiated infection or suspected sepsis. A randomized controlled trial. Am J Respir Crit Care Med 2014;190(10):1102–10.

29. Chu DC, Mehta AB, Walkey AJ. Practice patterns and outcomes associated with procalcitonin use in critically ill patients with sepsis. Clin Infect Dis 2017;64(11): 1509–15.

30. Simon L, Gauvin F, Amre DK, et al. Serum procalcitonin and C-reactive protein levels as markers of bacterial infection: a systematic review and meta-analysis. Clin Infect Dis 2004;39(2):206–17.

31. Sakr Y, Burgett U, Nacul FE, et al. Lipopolysaccharide binding protein in a surgical intensive care unit: a marker of sepsis? Crit Care Med 2008;36(7):2014–22.

32. Bouchon A, Facchetti F, Weigand MA, et al. TREM-1 amplifies inflammation and is a crucial mediator of septic shock. Nature 2001;410(6832):1103–7.

33. Wu Y, Wang F, Fan X, et al. Accuracy of plasma sTREM-1 for sepsis diagnosis in systemic inflammatory patients: a systematic review and meta-analysis. Crit Care 2012;16(6):R229.

34. Backes Y, van der Sluijs KF, Mackie DP, et al. Usefulness of suPAR as a biological marker in patients with systemic inflammation or infection: a systematic review. Intensive Care Med 2012;38(9):1418–28.

35. Skibsted S, Bhasin MK, Aird WC, et al. Bench-to-bedside review: future novel diagnostics for sepsis - a systems biology approach. Crit Care 2013;17(5):231.

36. Goh C, Knight JC. Enhanced understanding of the host-pathogen interaction in sepsis: new opportunities for omic approaches. Lancet Respir Med 2017;5(3): 212–23.

37. Reinhart K, Bauer M, Riedemann NC, et al. New approaches to sepsis: molecular diagnostics and biomarkers. Clin Microbiol Rev 2012;25(4):609–34.

38. Holcomb ZE, Tsalik EL, Woods CW, et al. Host-based peripheral blood gene expression analysis for diagnosis of infectious diseases. J Clin Microbiol 2017; 55(2):360–8.

39. PR newswire. News releases: revolutionary diagnostic septiCyte™ LAB cleared by FDA for suspected sepsis patients. 2017. Available at: http://www.prnewswire. com/news-releases/revolutionary-diagnostic-septicyte-lab-cleared-by-fda-for-suspected-sepsis-patients-300411470.html. Accessed April 19, 2017.

40. McHugh L, Seldon TA, Brandon RA, et al. A molecular host response assay to discriminate between sepsis and infection-negative systemic inflammation in critically ill patients: discovery and validation in independent cohorts. PLoS Med 2015;12(12):e1001916.

41. Sweeney TE, Shidham A, Wong HR, et al. A comprehensive time-course-based multicohort analysis of sepsis and sterile inflammation reveals a robust diagnostic gene set. Sci translational Med 2015;7(287):287ra71.

42. Bauer M, Giamarellos-Bourboulis EJ, Kortgen A, et al. A transcriptomic biomarker to quantify systemic inflammation in sepsis - a prospective multicenter phase II diagnostic study. EBioMedicine 2016;6:114–25.

43. Scicluna BP, Klein Klouwenberg PM, van Vught LA, et al. A molecular biomarker to diagnose community-acquired pneumonia on intensive care unit admission. Am J Respir Crit Care Med 2015;192(7):826–35.

44. Sweeney TE, Khatri P. Comprehensive validation of the FAIM3:PLAC8 ratio in time-matched public gene expression data. Am J Respir Crit Care Med 2015; 192(10):1260–1.

45. Sweeney TE, Khatri P. Benchmarking sepsis gene expression diagnostics using public data. Crit Care Med 2017;45(1):1–10.

46. Tsalik EL, Henao R, Nichols M, et al. Host gene expression classifiers diagnose acute respiratory illness etiology. Sci translational Med 2016;8(322):322ra11.

47. Suarez NM, Bunsow E, Falsey AR, et al. Superiority of transcriptional profiling over procalcitonin for distinguishing bacterial from viral lower respiratory tract infections in hospitalized adults. J Infect Dis 2015;212(2):213–22.

48. Parnell GP, McLean AS, Booth DR, et al. A distinct influenza infection signature in the blood transcriptome of patients with severe community-acquired pneumonia. Crit Care 2012;16(4):R157.

49. Sweeney TE, Wong HR, Khatri P. Robust classification of bacterial and viral infections via integrated host gene expression diagnostics. Sci translational Med 2016;8(346):346ra91.

50. Ramilo O, Allman W, Chung W, et al. Gene expression patterns in blood leukocytes discriminate patients with acute infections. Blood 2007;109(5):2066–77.

51. Hu X, Yu J, Crosby SD, et al. Gene expression profiles in febrile children with defined viral and bacterial infection. Proc Natl Acad Sci U S A 2013;110(31): 12792–7.

52. Mejias A, Dimo B, Suarez NM, et al. Whole blood gene expression profiles to assess pathogenesis and disease severity in infants with respiratory syncytial virus infection. PLoS Med 2013;10(11):e1001549.

53. Herberg JA, Kaforou M, Wright VJ, et al. Diagnostic test accuracy of a 2-transcript host RNA signature for discriminating bacterial vs viral infection in febrile children. JAMA 2016;316(8):835–45.

54. Davenport EE, Burnham KL, Radhakrishnan J, et al. Genomic landscape of the individual host response and outcomes in sepsis: a prospective cohort study. Lancet Respir Med 2016;4(4):259–71.

55. Wong HR, Salisbury S, Xiao Q, et al. The pediatric sepsis biomarker risk model. Crit Care 2012;16(5):R174.

56. Wong HR. Genome-wide expression profiling in pediatric septic shock. Pediatr Res 2013;73(4 Pt 2):564–9.

57. Wong HR, Lindsell CJ, Pettila V, et al. A multibiomarker-based outcome risk stratification model for adult septic shock*. Crit Care Med 2014;42(4):781–9.

58. Wong HR, Cvijanovich NZ, Anas N, et al. Improved risk stratification in pediatric septic shock using both protein and mRNA Biomarkers: PERSEVERE-XP. Am J Respir Crit Care Med 2017;196:494–501.

59. Scicluna BP, van der Poll T. Turning a new page in sepsis molecular diagnostics necessitates context-specific biomarkers. Crit Care Med 2017;45(4):e457.

60. Ludwig KR, Hummon AB. Mass spectrometry for the discovery of biomarkers of sepsis. Mol Biosystems 2017;13:648–64.

61. Oved K, Cohen A, Boico O, et al. A novel host-proteome signature for distinguishing between acute bacterial and viral infections. PLoS One 2015;10(3):e0120012.

62. DeCoux A, Tian Y, DeLeon-Pennell KY, et al. Plasma glycoproteomics reveals sepsis outcomes linked to distinct proteins in common pathways. Crit Care Med 2015;43(10):2049–58.

63. Schmerler D, Neugebauer S, Ludewig K, et al. Targeted metabolomics for discrimination of systemic inflammatory disorders in critically ill patients. J Lipid Res 2012;53(7):1369–75.

64. Rogers AJ, McGeachie M, Baron RM, et al. Metabolomic derangements are associated with mortality in critically ill adult patients. PLoS One 2014;9(1):e87538.

65. Mickiewicz B, Duggan GE, Winston BW, et al. Metabolic profiling of serum samples by 1H nuclear magnetic resonance spectroscopy as a potential diagnostic approach for septic shock. Crit Care Med 2014;42(5):1140–9.

66. Langley RJ, Tsalik EL, van Velkinburgh JC, et al. An integrated clinico-metabolomic model improves prediction of death in sepsis. Sci translational Med 2013;5(195):195ra95.

67. Neugebauer S, Giamarellos-Bourboulis EJ, Pelekanou A, et al. Metabolite profiles in sepsis: developing prognostic tools based on the type of infection. Crit Care Med 2016;44(9):1649–62.

68. Ferrario M, Cambiaghi A, Brunelli L, et al. Mortality prediction in patients with severe septic shock: a pilot study using a target metabolomics approach. Scientific Rep 2016;6:20391.

69. Wang L, Ko ER, Gilchrist JJ, et al. Human genetic and metabolite variation reveals that methylthioadenosine is a prognostic biomarker and an inflammatory regulator in sepsis. Sci Adv 2017;3(3):e1602096.

Personalizing Sepsis Care

Mervyn Singer, MB BS, MD, FRCP(Lon), FRCP(Edin), FFICM

KEYWORDS

- Sepsis • Personalized medicine • Precision medicine • Biomarker • Theranostic

KEY POINTS

- Although sepsis represents a syndrome of organ dysfunction related to a dysregulated host response to infection, it covers a wide range of causative microorganisms and sites of infection in heterogenous patient populations with differing comorbidities, clinical features, illness severity, and outcomes.
- A 1-size-fits-all approach, adopting a rigid, homogenized treatment approach, is unlikely to offer optimal care to individual patients.
- Biological signatures are increasingly being unraveled that can identify subsets of septic patients who may either respond positively or negatively to therapeutic interventions.
- Rapid access to such biomarker information will allow identification of suitable patients and titration of therapy to optimal effect

PROTOCOLS, GUIDELINES, AND PROCESS OF CARE

The term, *evidence-based guidelines*, first appeared in press in a series of articles in *JAMA* in 1990.[1] These articles differentiated between guidelines based on consensus, evidence, outcomes, and preference and proposed that evidence based should take precedence over the other forms. Sackett and colleagues[2] later described evidence-based medicine as "the conscientious, explicit, and judicious use of current best evidence in making decisions about the care of individual patients." Crucially, they continued, "Good doctors use both individual clinical expertise and the best available external evidence, and neither alone is enough. Without clinical expertise, practice risks becoming tyrannised by evidence, for even excellent external evidence may be inapplicable to or inappropriate for an individual patient. Without current best evidence, practice risks becoming rapidly out of date, to the detriment of patients."[2]

Eddy[3] promoted this personalized, educational, bedside-based philosophy, coining the description of "Evidence-based individual decision-making (EBID)." He contended that EBID should be undertaken "by individual physicians, using implicit and personal methods, to make decisions about individual patients and directly determine their care." He distinguished EBID from evidence-based guidelines, where generic

Division of Medicine, Bloomsbury Institute of Intensive Care Medicine, University College London, Gower Street, London WC1E 6BT, UK
E-mail address: m.singer@ucl.ac.uk

Crit Care Clin 34 (2018) 153–160
http://dx.doi.org/10.1016/j.ccc.2017.08.011
0749-0704/18/© 2017 Elsevier Inc. All rights reserved.

guidelines and other policies address the needs of institutions and groups of people and thus affect individual patients indirectly. He argued, "guidelines need to be tailored to individual cases, and EBID improves physicians' ability to do this. Many problems fall through the cracks of guidelines, and EBID is the only way to get evidence-based medicine to them. Physicians work on guideline teams, and the educational approach of EBID enables them to be better participants. EBID also helps physicians understand the rationale for evidence-based guidelines, which greatly improves their acceptance, especially when the evidence contradicts a time-honored practice."[3]

Evidence-based guidelines have been incorporated into clinical practice within critical care, in particular, the management of sepsis and septic shock within the Surviving Sepsis Campaign guidelines.[4–7] These guidelines perhaps have not taken sufficient note of Sackett and colleagues' and Eddy's strictures that individual expertise be brought to bear to guide management of individual patients. Didactic recommendations suit populations but may not be best suited to individuals. Although aiming to raise mediocre or poor practice and offering a framework for management, especially among practitioners who may be inexperienced in dealing with critically ill patients, there is a significant risk that strict adherence to guidelines may, in some cases, detract from best care. This is particularly pertinent when the bulk of recommendations is based on a poor evidence base and, often, a weak strength of recommendation because full consensus could not be achieved among the guidelines committee members. Strict blood pressure targets, fluid resuscitation volumes, and duration of antibiotic therapy are examples of rigid directives applied to patients and situations where a more tailored approach is likely preferable.

Guidelines should perhaps be differentiated from protocols. Although protocols may be viewed as mandatory, guidelines can be perceived as advisory. A protocolized approach can be reasonably applied to processes of care that should happen automatically. This includes, for example, a daily methodical clinical examination, daily review of drug chart and fluid balance, good infection control practices, and an individualized management plan reviewed at least daily. On the other hand, advisory guidelines should incorporate Eddy's EBID dictum, as described previously. This allows clinicians to be aware of the wider evidence base and follow appropriate general recommendations. Yet it still permits a more flexible management approach that varies according to a patient's age, comorbidities, condition (cause of sepsis and affected organs), and initial response to treatment.

INDIVIDUALIZED PHYSIOLOGIC ENDPOINTS

As with any critically ill patient, septic or otherwise, one size does not — should not —fit all. Didactic treatment endpoints and management strategies serve a general population but not necessarily individuals. Thus, a hypertensive patient may benefit from a higher targeted blood pressure in sepsis.[8,9] In other patients, however, a lower-than-recommended mean blood pressure (eg, 55–60 mm Hg) may still be compatible with adequacy of tissue perfusion, thereby avoiding unnecessary and potentially deleterious vasopressor therapy (or high dosing). Avoidance of a rigid mindset and a stepwise evaluation of the adequacy of tissue perfusion at different pressures are key to a likely more beneficial individualized approach. Similarly, fluid resuscitation should not involve fixed-volume administration because patients vary markedly in requirements.[10] Some patients may require much less than 30 mL/kg over the first few hours of sepsis presentation, especially in the presence of significant sepsis-induced myocardial depression because this may be compromised further by unnecessary fluid. Some patients may require very little fluid resuscitation if the pathophysiology relates more to loss of vascular tone rather than hypovolemia. Careful, titrated fluid administration, assessing incrementally the impact of smaller fluid boluses on tissue perfusion, is a more physiologically appropriate strategy that should avoid fluid overload.

Key to a personalized approach is adequate monitoring of circulatory, respiratory, and metabolic variables. This enables optimization of the circulation, gas exchange, fluid status, and metabolic status to suit patients and their baseline physiologic status; however, this should not be a short-term strategy delivered at the expense of long-term detriment. For example, increasing minute ventilation generally improves oxyhemoglobin levels and carbon dioxide clearance, but this should not be at the cost of a significantly increased risk of barotrauma. Current technology is still, however, limited in terms of the ability to gauge cellular distress accurately at the bedside. Plasma lactate levels are frequently used but lack both sensitivity and specificity as markers of organ hypoperfusion.[11] An important factor is that the plasma level represents the balance between production and utilization. Excess production may be counterbalanced by large-scale use of lactate as an important fuel source for varied organs, such as brain, heart, liver, and kidney; lactate levels may thus remain within the normal range despite significant organ compromise. Septic, fluid-resuscitated, normotensive patients in multiorgan failure had similar mortality rates irrespective of their lactate level.[12]

SEPSIS — AN UMBRELLA SYNDROME

Sepsis requires a definition that captures the essence of the condition and embraces both the pathophysiologic basis and the clinical manifestation. In addition, there needs to be accompanying clinical criteria that allow operationalization of the definition to enable consistency for the purpose of improved epidemiology, research, and coding. The new version of the international sepsis definitions — the Third International Consensus Definitions for Sepsis and Septic Shock [Sepsis-3] — was published in 2016.[13] This updates the current concept of sepsis as a dysregulated host response to infection that leads to life-threatening organ dysfunction. As a failing of previous definitions, strict descriptors of organ dysfunction were never rigidly applied, allowing marked variations in reported incidence and mortality.[12] Sepsis-3 offers a change in Sequential Organ Failure Assessment (SOFA) score greater than or equal to 2 points as a more precise means of characterizing new organ dysfunction over and above a patient's baseline. Although the SOFA score is not perfect, it is nevertheless well established, has widespread familiarity within critical care, and has a well-validated relationship to mortality risk.[14]

Sepsis-3 also offered a similar rebranding of septic shock. Previously, myriad permutations of thresholds of blood pressure and/or lactate and/or base deficit and/or fluid resuscitation volumes and/or organ dysfunction and/or use/dose of vasoactive agents resulted in a 10-fold variation in incidence and 4-fold variation in mortality.[12] Septic shock is now defined by Sepsis-3 as "a subset of sepsis in which particularly profound circulatory, cellular, and metabolic abnormalities are associated with a greater risk of mortality than with sepsis alone."[13] This is operationalized clinically by a vasopressor requirement to maintain a mean arterial pressure greater than or equal to 65 mm Hg and serum lactate greater than 2 mmol/L despite adequate volume resuscitation.

These syndromic descriptions necessarily cover a wide range of microbiological causes and sites of infection, affecting a broad spectrum of patients varying by age, gender, underlying health status, medications, and coexisting acute conditions, such as surgery and trauma. All these factors have an impact, to greater or lesser degrees, on patient outcome. An *Escherichia coli* sepsis arising from the urinary tract carries a far lower mortality rate than an *E coli* bacteremia consequent to abdominal sepsis.[15] A previously healthy 18-year-old patient with toxic shock syndrome has different clinical, biological, and outcome responses compared with a 40-year-old neutropenic patient undergoing chemotherapy for leukemia who develops a pneumonia or an 83-year-old patient with chronic obstructive airways disease, diabetes, chronic renal failure, and fecal peritonitis from a perforated diverticulum. Yet these patients are lumped together as septic into clinical trials simply by fulfilling physiologic criteria, such as fluid-refractory hypotension.

SEPSIS — A SERIES OF BIOLOGICAL PHENOTYPES WITH DIFFERING OUTCOMES

It is also becoming increasingly apparent that a disparity often exists between the clinical manifestations of sepsis and underlying biological phenotypes, which vary both between individuals and in the same individual over time. Sepsis triggers a dysregulated host response that includes an exaggerated but highly variable degree of systemic inflammation and, at the same time, an exaggerated but highly variable anti-inflammatory response. The GENIMS (Genetic and Inflammatory Markers of Sepsis) study examined 1886 patients hospitalized with community acquired pneumonia in 28 US hospitals.[16] Approximately a third developed sepsis, and a third of this more severe subset died. Elevated levels of both the proinflammatory cytokine, interleukin (IL)-6, and the anti-inflammatory cytokine, IL-10, measured in plasma sampled in the emergency department gave a 20-fold increase in risk of death at 90 days compared with low levels of both. Unbalanced (high/low) cytokine patterns had intermediate outcomes.

This disparity between eventual survivors and nonsurvivors extends beyond inflammation into many other pathways. Davenport and colleagues[17] performed a transcriptomic analysis in blood leukocytes taken from ICU patients admitted with sepsis secondary to community-acquired pneumonia and characterized two endotypes; 41% had a more immunosuppressed phenotype that included features of endotoxin tolerance, T-cell exhaustion, and down-regulation of HLA class II. Such patients had a higher mortality compared with the remainder not showing these features (hazard ratio 2.4–2.8 in 2 separate cohorts). A recent follow-up article[18] compared the 2 types of sepsis response signature in these pneumonia patients against a separate cohort of patients with fecal peritonitis. The transcriptomic response was largely independent of the source of infection and included signatures that reflected the immune response state and prognosis in both conditions. Similarly, Langley and colleagues[19] measured the plasma metabolome and proteome in patients with and without community-acquired sepsis from different causes on arrival in an emergency department and at 24 hours later. Differences in plasma metabolites and proteins (predominantly involved in fatty acid transport and ß-oxidation, gluconeogenesis, and the Krebs cycle) were able to discriminate between eventual survivors and nonsurvivors on admission. This prognostic differentiation was more pronounced 24 hours later. The metabolome/proteome were similar in survivors, regardless of severity.

Multiple other biomarkers measured either in emergency departments or within 24 hours of ICU admission have also shown prognostic utility. These range from simple physiologic measures, such as heart rate[20]; point-of-care tests, such as troponin[21] and lactate[22]; and formal laboratory tests, such as thyroid function,[23] coagulation markers,[24] and high-density lipoprotein cholesterol[25] to more esoteric tests ranging from plasma DNA[26] to autonomic dysfunction[27] to fecal pH.[28]

SEPSIS — OUTCOMES DIFFER BY INTERVENTION ACCORDING TO BIOLOGICAL PHENOTYPE

Two retrospective analyses have arisen from the Acute Respiratory Distress Syndrome Clinical Trials Network interrogating laboratory and clinical data taken from patients enrolled in acute respiratory distress syndrome intervention studies.[29,30] Calfee and colleagues[29] applied latent class modeling to split the patients into 2 subphenotypes. A quarter of patients had a hyperinflammatory subphenotype (characterized by higher plasma levels of inflammatory biomarkers, more acidosis, vasopressor use, and sepsis) and the remainder had a less inflammatory subphenotype where these markers were not so prevalent. The group with the hyperinflammatory subphenotype had higher mortality, morbidity, ventilator requirement, and length of stay. This subset responded positively in terms of outcome improvement (90-day mortality, ventilator-free days, and organ failure-free days) to an increase in positive end-expiratory pressure (PEEP) (in the ALVEOLI trial) whereas detriment was seen in the less inflamed subset. Famous and colleagues[30] confirmed a similar subphenotype picture and distribution in another of the Acute Respiratory Distress Syndrome Clinical Trials Network studies (the Fluid and Catheter Treatment Trial fluid management study) and found a different outcome response to fluid management. The hyperinflammatory subphenotype had 90-day mortality rates of 40% with a fluid-conservative strategy versus 50% in those managed with a more liberal approach. The less inflamed subphenotype showed an opposite effect (26% mortality with fluid-conservative and 18% with fluid-liberal). They reported that a 3-variable model of IL-8, bicarbonate, and tumor necrosis factor receptor 1 accurately discriminated between these subphenotypes, with sensitivity and specificity of 87% and 93%, respectively. This was superior to a model reliant only on clinical variables (bicarbonate, vasopressor use, creatinine, minute ventilation, heart rate, primary acute respiratory distress syndrome risk factor, and systolic blood pressure), which was still good at prognostication (sensitivity and specificity both 84%).

On similar lines, 2 further studies based on retrospective analyses of data also reveal interesting outcome differences in response to therapeutic interventions. Russell and colleagues[31] reanalyzed the database of the VASST comparing vasopressin against norepinephrine on the basis of the new Sepsis-3 septic shock criteria. Only half of the enrolled patients would have fulfilled the new criteria (mean arterial pressure $\geq$65 mm Hg and lactate >2 mmol/L after adequate volume resuscitation) and with an absolute 12% increase in 90-day mortality rate. Mortality in the subset of hypotensive patients with a lactate less than 2 mmol/L was significantly lower in the vasopressin-treated limb, but no difference was seen in those with a lactate greater than 2 mmol/L, in whom circulating cytokine levels were markedly higher. This implies benefit was only seen from vasopressin in the less inflamed subset of patients, who likely also had less cellular/metabolic abnormalities. On the other hand, Wong and colleagues[32] conducted a secondary analysis of 288 pediatric septic shock patients and divided them into 2 endotypes based on a 100-gene transcript signature focusing on adaptive immunity and glucocorticoid receptor signaling pathways.[33] In the endotype with increased expression of glucocorticoid receptor signaling genes, corticosteroids were independently associated with a 10-fold reduction in the risk of persisting organ failure at day 7.

TRIAL DESIGN

The studies described previously — albeit all retrospective — suggest that patient groups differentiated by a biological signature respond positively or negatively to standard ICU interventions, such as fluid, choice of vasopressor, and level of PEEP. The same principle should also be applied to trials of novel therapies or management strategies. For example, immunosuppression is increasingly recognized in critically ill patients and often present on ICU admission.[33] In a study of postoperative cardiac surgical patients, HLA-DR expression was significantly decreased in all patients on ICU admission.[34] It is rational, therefore, to avoid immunosuppressive therapies in such patients, for instance, corticosteroids or antibodies directed against proinflammatory cytokines. Conversely, the use of immune stimulating agents could be considered in such patients to reduce the risk of secondary infections but avoided in those patients with preexisting excessive activation. The challenge in such trials is to find a reliable, rapidly available (ideally point-of-care) theranostic that can both indicate the suitability of a patient for entry and then allow titration of the drug or other intervention accordingly for optimal effect. Thus, use of an immunostimulant therapy could be guided by several possible indicators, including lymphopenia,[34] monocyte HLA-DR level,[35] or other markers, including ex vivo stimulation testing.[36,37] This does, however, create a chicken-and-egg dilemma in that the worth of a theranostic will only be realized once the trial is concluded, so a leap of faith is necessary that the purported biomarker will appropriately guide the intervention and is not simply an epiphenomenon.

REFERENCES

1. Eddy DM. Practice policies: where do they come from? JAMA 1990;263:1265–75.
2. Sackett DL, Rosenberg WM, Gray JA, et al. Evidence based medicine: what it is and what it isn't. BMJ 1996;312:71–2.
3. Eddy DM. Evidence-based medicine: a unified approach. Health Aff (Millwood) 2005;24:9–17.
4. Levy MM, Fink MP, Marshall JC, et al. 2001 SCCM/ESICM/ACCP/ATS/SIS International Sepsis Definitions Conference. Crit Care Med 2003;31:1250–6.
5. Dellinger RP, Levy MM, Carlet JM, et al. Surviving Sepsis Campaign: international guidelines for management of severe sepsis and septic shock. Crit Care Med 2008;2008(36):296–327.
6. Dellinger RP, Levy MM, Rhodes A, et al. Surviving Sepsis Campaign: International Guidelines for Management of severe sepsis and septic shock. Intensive Care Med 2012;2013(39):165–228.
7. Rhodes A, Evans LE, Alhazzani W, et al. Surviving sepsis Campaign: International Guidelines for Management of sepsis and septic shock. Intensive Care Med 2016;2017(43):304–77.
8. Asfar P, Meziani F, Hamel JF, et al. High versus low blood-pressure target in patients with septic shock. N Engl J Med 2014;370:1583–93.
9. Lamontagne F, Meade MO, Hébert PC, et al. Higher versus lower blood pressure targets for vasopressor therapy in shock: a multicentre pilot randomized controlled trial. Intensive Care Med 2016;42:542–50.
10. Perner A, Singer M. Fixed minimum fluid volume for resuscitation: con. Intensive Care Med 2016. http://dx.doi.org/10.1007/s00134-016-4581-3.
11. Garcia-Alvarez M, Marik P, Bellomo R. Sepsis-associated hyperlactatemia. Crit Care 2014;18:503.
12. Shankar-Hari M, Phillips GS, Levy ML, et al. Developing a new definition and assessing new clinical criteria for septic shock: for the Third International Consensus Definitions for Sepsis and Septic Shock (Sepsis-3). JAMA 2016; 315:775–87.

13. Singer M, Deutschman CS, Seymour CW, et al. The Third International Consensus Definitions for Sepsis and Septic Shock (Sepsis-3). JAMA 2016;315:801–10.
14. Raith EP, Udy AA, Bailey M, et al. Prognostic accuracy of the SOFA score, SIRS criteria, and qSOFA score for in-hospital mortality among adults with suspected infection admitted to the intensive care unit. JAMA 2017;317:290–300.
15. Jauréguy F, Carbonnelle E, Bonacorsi S, et al. Host and bacterial determinants of initial severity and outcome of Escherichia coli sepsis. Clin Microbiol Infect 2007; 13:854–62.
16. Kellum JA, Kong L, Fink MP, et al. Understanding the inflammatory cytokine response in pneumonia and sepsis: results of the genetic and inflammatory markers of sepsis (GenIMS) study. Arch Intern Med 2007;167:1655–63.
17. Davenport EE, Burnham KL, Radhakrishnan J, et al. Genomic landscape of the individual host response andoutcomes in sepsis: a prospective cohort study. Lancet Respir Med 2016;4:259–71.
18. Burnham KL, Davenport EE, Radhakrishnan J, et al. Shared and distinct aspects of the sepsis transcriptomic response to fecal peritonitis and pneumonia. Am J Respir Crit Care Med 2017;196(3):328–39.
19. Langley RJ, Tsalik EL, Velkinburgh JCV, et al. An integrated clinico-metabolomic model improves prediction of death in sepsis. Sci Transl Med 2013;5:195ra95.
20. Beesley SJ, Wilson EL, Lanspa MJ, et al. Relative bradycardia in patients with septic shock requiring vasopressor therapy. Crit Care Med 2017;45:225–33.
21. de Groot B, Verdoorn RC, Lameijer J, et al. High-sensitivity cardiac troponin T is an independent predictor of inhospital mortality in emergency department patients with suspected infection: a prospective observational derivation study. Emerg Med J 2014;31:882–8.
22. Houwink API, Rijkenberg S, Bosman RJ, et al. The association between lactate, mean arterial pressure, central venous oxygen saturation and peripheral temperature and mortality in severe sepsis: a retrospective cohort analysis. Crit Care 2016;20:56.
23. Wang F, Pan W, Wang H, et al. Relationship between thyroid function and ICU mortality: a prospective observation study. Crit Care 2012;16:R11.
24. McClintock D, Zhuo H, Wickersham N, et al. Biomarkers of inflammation, coagulation and fibrinolysis predict mortality in acute lung injury. Crit Care 2008;12:R41.
25. Cirstea M, Walley KR, Russell JA, et al. Decreased high-density lipoprotein cholesterol level is an early prognostic marker for organ dysfunction and death in patients with suspected sepsis. J Crit Care 2017;38:289–94.
26. Kung C-T, Hsiao S-Y, Tsai T-C, et al. Plasma nuclear and mitochondrial DNA levels as predictors of outcome in severe sepsis patients in the emergency room. J Transl Med 2012;10:130.
27. Schmidt H, Müller-Werdan U, Hoffmann T, et al. Autonomic dysfunction predicts mortality in patients with multiple organ dysfunction syndrome of different age groups. Crit Care Med 2005;33:1994–2002.
28. Osuka A, Shimizu K, Ogura H, et al. Prognostic impact of fecal pH in critically ill patients. Crit Care 2012;16:R119.
29. Calfee CS, Delucchi K, Parsons PE, et al. Subphenotypes in acute respiratory distress syndrome: latent class analysis of data from two randomised controlled trials. Lancet Respir Med 2014;2:611–20.
30. Famous KR, Delucchi K, Ware LB, et al. Acute respiratory distress syndrome subphenotypes respond differently to randomized fluid management strategy. Am J Respir Crit Care Med 2017;195:331–8.

31. Russell JA, Lee T, Singer J, et al, Vasopressin and Septic Shock Trial (VASST) Group. The septic shock 3.0 definition and trials: a vasopressin and septic shock trial experience. Crit Care Med 2017;45(6):940–8.
32. Wong HR, Atkinson SJ, Cvijanovich NZ, et al. Combining prognostic and predictive enrichment strategies to identify children with septic shock responsive to corticosteroids. Crit Care Med 2016;44:e1000–3.
33. Lukaszewicz AC, Grienay M, Resche-Rigon M, et al. Monocytic HLA-DR expression in intensive care patients: interest for prognosis and secondary infection prediction. Crit Care Med 2009;37:2746–52.
34. Oczenski W, Krenn H, Jilch R, et al. HLA-DR as a marker for increased risk for systemic inflammation and septic complications after cardiac surgery. Intensive Care Med 2003;29:1253–7.
35. Drewry AM, Samra N, Skrupky LP, et al. Persistent lymphopenia after diagnosis of sepsis predicts mortality. Shock 2014;42:383–91.
36. Meisel C, Schefold JC, Pschowski R, et al. Granulocyte-macrophage colony-stimulating factor to reverse sepsis-associated immunosuppression: a double-blind, randomized, placebo-controlled multicenter trial. Am J Respir Crit Care Med 2009;180:640–8.
37. Bermejo-Martin JF, Andaluz-Ojeda D, Almansa R, et al. Defining immunological dysfunction in sepsis: a requisite tool for precision medicine. J Infect 2016;72: 525–36.

Novel Interventions
What's New and the Future

Jean-Louis Vincent, MD, PhD*, David Grimaldi, MD, PhD

KEYWORDS

- Septic shock • Microcirculation • Interferon • Thrombomodulin
- Immunosuppression • Personalization • Biomarkers • Organ dysfunction

KEY POINTS

- Rather than testing new interventions in poorly characterized patient populations, the current trend is to study interventions in well-defined patient populations characterized by a special feature or a particular biomarker.
- The current focus is on immunomodulation in a broader sense rather than on only antiinflammatory strategies or strategies designed to improve the host response.
- Improving endothelial cell function, blood purification and immunostimulation are important areas of current research in sepsis therapeutics.

INTRODUCTION

Despite several decades of sepsis research, no specific therapies for sepsis have emerged and current management still relies on source control, antibiotics, and organ support. One of the reasons for the many failed trials of potential new interventions has been the lack of clear patient inclusion criteria, resulting in heterogeneous populations unlikely to all respond positively to the intervention in question. As the understanding of sepsis pathophysiology continues to improve and new techniques are developed to help better characterize patients with sepsis, particularly in terms of their immune status, clinical trials are beginning to better target new interventions at those patients most likely to respond, rather than at the poorly characterized heterogeneous groups of patients widely used in the past. Biomarkers are also being used to identify groups of patients most likely to respond to specific therapies.

Given the complexity of sepsis, there are almost limitless potential avenues for novel therapeutic agents, but this article concentrates on 3 of the most important current trends that show promise:

- Decreasing harmful capillary leak and edema formation by protecting or restoring endothelial cell function

Conflicts of Interest: The authors have no conflicts of interest to declare.
Department of Intensive Care, Erasme Hospital, Université libre de Bruxelles, Route de Lennik 808, Brussels 1070, Belgium
* Corresponding author. Department of Intensive Care, Erasme University Hospital, Route de Lennik 808, Brussels 1070, Belgium.
E-mail address: jlvincent@intensive.org

Crit Care Clin 34 (2018) 161–173
http://dx.doi.org/10.1016/j.ccc.2017.08.012
0749-0704/18/© 2017 Elsevier Inc. All rights reserved.

criticalcare.theclinics.com

- Reversing sepsis-induced immunosuppression by immunostimulation
- Removal of harmful mediators from the blood using extracorporeal techniques

PHARMACOLOGIC TREATMENT OPTIONS
Endothelial Cell Protection

Disturbed endothelial function plays a key role in the development of sepsis and associated organ dysfunction, partly as a result of altered endothelial permeability leading to edema formation. Several potential therapies have been developed that have endothelial cell protective functions, including vasopressin, interferon (IFN)-beta, and thrombomodulin.

Vasopressin

Patients with septic shock are said to have a relative deficiency of vasopressin,[1] hence the rationale for using exogenous arginine vasopressin (AVP) as an adjunct therapy in these patients. Several studies using AVP in conjunction with catecholamines have shown that AVP administration enables doses of catecholamines to be reduced.[2] This finding is not surprising. The question is whether the use of vasopressin is associated with better outcomes, and this has not been shown.[3,4] Therefore the latest Surviving Sepsis Campaign guidelines do not make any specific recommendation about the use of vasopressin in septic shock.

Vasopressin acts via 3 specific receptors: in addition to its V1A receptor–mediated vasopressor actions, its actions on other receptors, including V2 and oxytocin receptors, may aggravate sepsis-induced vasodilation and promote fluid accumulation. Therefore, AVP analogues that are highly specific for the V1A receptor and may thus avoid the potentially negative effects of AVP mediated via other receptors have been developed. Selepressin is one of these substances, and its use was shown to reduce vascular leak in an ovine model of pneumonia-induced sepsis.[5] In an ovine model of peritonitis-induced septic shock, selepressin use was associated with better hemodynamic stabilization, preserved lung and renal function, reduced cumulative fluid balance, and prolonged survival, particularly when given early in the course of shock.[6] In a small randomized controlled trial, 50 patients with septic shock were randomized to receive selepressin 1.25 ng/kg/min, selepressin 2.5 ng/kg/min, or placebo. The results suggested a dose-dependent reduction in norepinephrine requirements, reduced need for mechanical ventilation, and shorter time to shock resolution.[7] In view of these encouraging data, a larger clinical trial, targeting 1800 patients, is now ongoing (Selepressin Evaluation Program for Sepsis-Induced Shock - Adaptive Clinical Trial [SEPSIS-ACT]; ClinicalTrials.gov identifier, NCT02508649) in which patients with vasopressor-dependent septic shock are randomized to receive 1 of 4 doses of selepressin or placebo. This study will use an adaptive clinical trial design, which will enable enrollment in nonpromising treatment arms to be stopped during the course of the study, so improving the study efficiency. The primary end point is a composite of 30-day vasopressor-free and mechanical ventilator–free days.

Interferon-beta

Adenosine is an extracellular signaling molecule that regulates multiple immunologic processes and is thought to play an important role in regulating the host response to sepsis.[8] Inhibition of adenosine deaminase was associated with reduced vascular leakage and improved survival in septic mice.[9] Cluster of differentiation 73 (CD73) is a cell surface enzyme that catalyzes the dephosphorylation of soluble AMP into adenosine, and is upregulated by IFN-β.[10,11] IFN-β may, therefore, help restore endothelial integrity by increasing local adenosine levels. IFN-β may also upregulate silent information regulator transcript-1 (SIRT1), a protein thought to be involved in regulating the inflammatory response.[12] Treatment with IFN-β was shown to prevent vascular leakage in a mouse model of acute lung injury (ALI).[11] Recombinant human IFN-β1a was assessed for the treatment of ALI and acute respiratory distress syndrome (ARDS) in a phase I/II study in 37 patients.[10] Patients treated with IFN-β had increased survival compared with control patients (8% vs 32%; odds ratio, 0.19 [95% confidence interval, 0.03–0.72]; $P = .01$). There were no safety concerns during the study period. Following this successful study, a phase III double-blind, randomized, parallel-group trial, the INTEREST study, is currently ongoing (European Union Clinical Trials Register no. 2014-005260-15). The study is intended to include 300 patients and has a composite primary end point of any cause of death at 28 days plus days free of mechanical ventilation within 28 days among survivors; more than 200 patients have been enrolled so far.

Thrombomodulin

Sepsis is known to be associated with coagulopathy,[13,14] and this is linked to endothelial damage.[15] These observations formed part of the rationale behind investigating natural anticoagulants, such as activated protein C, in the treatment of sepsis. Clinicians are aware of the so-called rise and demise of activated protein C (APC) for the treatment of sepsis.[16] APC may be effective in some patients, but it is too difficult to define which patients will benefit. Thrombomodulin is another natural anticoagulant but with a different mode of action from that of APC. Thrombomodulin, a cell surface protein expressed by endothelial cells, binds thrombin and enhances activation of protein C.[17,18] Thrombomodulin also inhibits complement and neutralizes high mobility group box 1 protein (HMGB1), a proinflammatory protein that has been associated with vascular endothelial integrity.[19] In a phase 2b, multicenter, randomized controlled trial in 750 patients with sepsis and suspected disseminated intravascular coagulopathy, patients who received recombinant thrombomodulin in addition to standard care seemed to have a lower 28-day mortality compared with patients who received placebo (17.8% vs 21.6%; 2-sided P value of 0.273, suggestive of efficacy of thrombomodulin).[20] In subgroup analyses, patients with at least 1 organ system dysfunction and an International Normalized Ratio (INR) greater than 1.4 at baseline seemed to benefit most from the thrombomodulin. As a result of these findings, a large phase 3 study (NCT01598831) is now ongoing targeting this specific population. An estimated 800 patients with infection, organ dysfunction (respiratory or cardiovascular), and an INR greater than 1.40 will be enrolled and randomized to receive recombinant thrombomodulin or placebo for 6 days in addition to standard care. The study is now about 75% complete.

Other experimental agents

As more is learned about the importance of the endothelial barrier in the pathogenesis of sepsis, other potential targets will no doubt come to light. One such target is FX06 (peptide Bβ15-42), a natural product of fibrin that interacts with VE-cadherin, one of the key molecules involved in endothelial integrity and the opening and closing of cell junctions.[21] FX06 was shown to reduce vascular leak and mortality in a mouse model of dengue shock and in rats injected with lipopolysaccharide.[21] In a mouse model of polymicrobial sepsis, FX06 administration was associated with reduced inflammation, which the investigators attributed to sustained vascular integrity.[22] In a case report published in *The Lancet*, Wolf and colleagues[23] used FX06 as compassionate treatment of a patient with severe Ebola virus disease, respiratory failure, and vascular leak syndrome. The vascular leak improved with treatment.

Other potential targets for endothelial cell protection include angiopoietin,[24] sphingosine-1 phosphate receptors,[25] and the Slit-ROBO pathway.[26]

Immunostimulation

As the pathogenesis of sepsis began to be unraveled, the role of proinflammatory mediators came to the fore and the search for therapeutic agents focused on reducing the inflammatory response. However, it has become increasingly obvious that, after the initial proinflammatory phase, patients then develop immunosuppression that increases the risk of intensive care unit (ICU)–acquired infections despite cure of the initial infection.[27] Each patient's immune status thus varies during the course of the disease, and the precise response also differs among patients. Some patients may, therefore, benefit more from an immune-stimulating than an immunosuppressive agent, depending on their particular immune profile at the time of treatment.[28] The originality of this strategy is that it moves away from the idea of just fighting the initial infection and toward preventing subsequent sepsis-induced morbidity. Several agents have been investigated for this purpose.

Granulocyte-colony stimulating factor and granulocyte-macrophage colony stimulating factor

Some of the first immunostimulating agents to be investigated were granulocyte-colony stimulating factor (G-CSF) and granulocyte-macrophage colony stimulating factor (GM-CSF), which are involved in the regulation of neutrophil production and function. GM-CSF can also induce monocyte differentiation into dendritic cells (DCs) and promote maturation and activation of these cells and is therefore an interesting molecule to reverse sepsis-induced monocyte and DC deactivation. Despite promising early experimental data, clinical trials with these agents showed no beneficial effects on mortalities in heterogeneous groups of patients.[29] However, in a small study by Meisel and colleagues,[30] in which only patients with proven immunosuppression (as determined by low human leukocyte antigen, antigen D related [HLA-DR] levels) were included, patients treated with GM-CSF had increased mHLA-DR levels and Toll-like receptor–induced cytokine production, and reduced duration of mechanical ventilation. Following these promising results, a multicenter phase III trial is now ongoing to assess the effects of GM-CSF versus placebo in ICU patients with sepsis or septic shock and reduced HLA-DR levels (NCT02361528).

Interferon-gamma

IFN-γ is a cytokine secreted predominantly by T-helper cells and natural killer cells and plays a key role in mounting an efficient immune response against invading pathogens. IFN-γ secretion by T cells is reduced in sepsis and this impairment was correlated with death or development of secondary infections.[31] In healthy volunteers given endotoxin, injection of IFN-γ reduced the endotoxin-induced inflammatory response and increased monocyte HLA-DR expression compared with placebo injection.[32] In addition, in a series of patients with invasive fungal infections, adjunctive IFN-γ therapy restored immune function.[33] However, in old trials using IFN-γ in unselected patients with trauma there was no reduction in secondary infections.[34] A clinical trial is planned to further determine the effects of IFN-γ on sepsis-induced immunoparalysis (NCT01649921).

Interleukin-7 and interleukin-15

Other cytokines, such as interleukin (IL)-7 and IL-15, which promote lymphocyte proliferation, have also been proposed as potential therapies to reverse sepsis-induced apoptosis and stimulate the immune system. IL-15 activates T cells, natural killer cells, and DCs, and increases IFN-γ production.[35,36] In patients with severe lymphopenia as a result of sepsis, IL-15 levels were significantly higher than in patients with sepsis without lymphopenia, but these patients still had downregulated B-cell lymphoma 2 messenger RNA expression in peripheral blood mononuclear cells, suggesting that the IL-15 levels were inadequate to maintain lymphocyte homeostasis.[37] In one cecal ligation and puncture mouse model of sepsis, IL-15 administration improved survival.[35] However, in another study, IL-15 knockout mice had improved survival after sepsis induction, and exogenous IL-15 administration exacerbated the severity of sepsis.[38] These apparently conflicting results may be related to different models and different dosing regimens but they highlight the difficulties in trying to influence an isolated mediator of the sepsis response. In clinical trials in patients with cancer, IL-15 administration was associated with increased release of multiple inflammatory cytokines, hypotension, thrombocytopenia, and liver damage,[39] again raising concerns regarding any potential therapeutic role in patients with sepsis.

IL-7 has similar actions to those of IL-15 and has been shown to improve T-cell proliferation and enhance IFN-γ production.[40-42] In animal models of sepsis, IL-7 administration increased survival.[42-44] IL-7 seemed to be well tolerated in phase 2 trials in patients infected with human immunodeficiency virus.[45] Phase 2 clinical trials assessing the ability of recombinant IL-7 treatment to restore absolute lymphocyte counts in patients with sepsis with reduced levels of circulating lymphocytes are currently ongoing (NCT02797431) or have recently been completed (NCT02640807).

Programmed cell death 1 and programmed death ligand 1

Programmed cell death 1 (PD-1), a negative costimulatory molecule, and its ligand, programmed death ligand 1 (PD-L1), are another potential target because they negatively regulate the immune response. Patients with septic shock had increased PD-1 and PD-L1 monocyte and T-lymphocyte expression compared with patients with trauma and healthy volunteers and the increased levels were associated with reduced survival and a greater incidence of secondary nosocomial infections.[46] In patients 3 to 4 days after onset of sepsis symptoms, monocyte PD-L1 expression was an independent predictor of 28-day mortality.[47] Anti–PD-1 and anti–PD-L1 antibodies have been shown to improve immune function and survival in mouse models of sepsis,[48-50] even when given some time after sepsis induction.[48,50] In a mouse model of sepsis, IL-7 and anti–PD-L1 antibody had additive effects on lymphocyte proliferation and splenic secretion of IFN-γ, suggesting a possible benefit of combined therapy.[41] Anti–PD-1 and anti–PD-L1 antibodies were shown to reverse sepsis-induced so-called immune exhaustion in peripheral blood monocytes from patients with sepsis, supporting a potential role in patients with sepsis-induced immunosuppression.[51] Anti–PD-1 and anti–PD-L1 antibodies have been shown to be effective in patients with various cancers, with tolerable adverse effect profiles.[52,53] Although concerns have been raised regarding the development of autoimmune conditions with anti–PD-1 and anti–PD-L1 antibodies,[54] because of the immune checkpoint nature of PD-1 and PD-L1, the shorter-term use in patients with sepsis compared with those with cancer may make such events less likely in these patients.[55] In a recent case report of a patient with fungal sepsis and documented immunosuppression who was unresponsive to conventional therapy, combined treatment with IFN-γ and an anti–PD-1 antibody restored immune function.[56] Phase 1 and 2 multicenter, randomized clinical trials of anti–PD-L1 and anti–PD-1 antibodies in patients with sepsis are currently underway using an adaptive enrichment design in which enrollment criteria will be adjusted according to response in different biomarker-identified subgroups (NCT02576457 and NCT02960854).

NONPHARMACOLOGIC EXPERIMENTAL TREATMENT OPTIONS
Blood Purification

Renal replacement therapy is designed to remove uremic toxins, but since the late 1980s it has been suggested that it could also be used to remove circulating mediators of sepsis[57,58] and, by so doing, attenuate the sepsis response and potentially improve outcomes. However, this was not supported by the evidence. In a small pilot study of 24 patients with early septic shock, Cole and colleagues[59] were unable to show any change in cytokine levels or organ dysfunction in patients treated with continuous venovenous hemofiltration (CVVH) at 2 L/h compared with those who received no hemofiltration. In addition, a randomized controlled study in 80 patients with early sepsis was discontinued early because of a greater occurrence of organ failures in the CVVH (25 mL/kg/h) group; there were again no difference in cytokine levels between groups.[60]

Because of the lack of benefit with conventional-dose hemofiltration, it was suggested that higher-volume hemofiltration may be more effective at removing cytokines and several small studies suggested improved hemodynamics and outcomes with this approach.[61–63] However, a multicenter trial comparing high-volume hemofiltration (70 mL/kg/h) and standard-volume hemofiltration (35 mL/kg/h) in patients with catecholamine-dependent septic shock showed no differences in organ dysfunction or mortality between groups, although it was stopped prematurely because of slow recruitment. Similarly, Park and colleagues[64] reported no differences in 28-day mortality or 28-day kidney survival in patients with septic acute kidney injury randomized to receive high-volume (80 mL/kg/h) or conventional (40 mL/kg/h) continuous venovenous hemodiafiltration, despite significantly greater reduction in measured cytokine levels in the high-volume group. High-volume hemofiltration may result in the excessive removal of many substances, including antimicrobial agents, thus reducing its potential for benefit.

Hemoperfusion using specific sorbents has also been suggested in an attempt to improve mediator removal. CytoSorb is one such device, composed of porous polymer beads. When placed in the hemodialysis circuit, this device removes molecules in the range of 5 to 60 kDa, which includes most cytokines and inflammatory mediators. Case series have shown promising results on hemodynamic stabilization[65] and several clinical trials are currently ongoing.

Another sorbent that has been investigated widely in this context, particularly in Japan, is polymyxin-B, which binds and neutralizes endotoxin. In a pilot study of patients with sepsis secondary to intra-abdominal infection, treatment with the polymyxin cartridge seemed to be associated with improved hemodynamics and reduced need for continuous renal replacement therapy (CRRT) compared with standard treatment.[66] In the multicenter EUPHAS (Early Use of Polymyxin B Hemoperfusion in Abdominal Sepsis) study, patients with sepsis secondary to intra-abdominal infection who underwent polymyxin hemoperfusion had improved hemodynamics and organ function compared with those managed without hemoperfusion.[67] It may even reduce 28-day mortality, although the study was unblinded and the differences were not statistically significant.[68] In a larger study in patients with septic shock secondary to peritonitis, there were no significant differences in organ dysfunction or mortality between patients who received hemoperfusion and those who did not.[69] More recently, the EUPHRATES (Evaluating the Use of Polymyxin B Hemoperfusion in a Randomized Controlled Trial of

Adults Treated for Endotoxemia and Septic Shock) trial, a well-conducted double-blinded trial in 446 patients with septic shock and high endotoxin activity assay values,[70] failed to show a survival benefit with polymyxin hemoperfusion in the whole population.

Other blood purification techniques have been suggested for the treatment of sepsis, including plasma exchange and coupled plasma filtration adsorption (CPFA) (**Fig. 1**). A recent meta-analysis of 4 randomized trials reported that plasma exchange was associated with reduced mortality in adult patients, but noted that the trial hetero-geneity was moderate and all trials were at unclear or high risk of bias.[71] A randomized clinical trial in patients with early septic shock and high catecholamine doses is ongoing to assess the potential role of this approach in addition to standard sepsis management (NCT03065751). A multicenter randomized trial of CPFA in 192 patients with septic shock was stopped early for futility; there were no overall differences be-tween groups in terms of mortality, ICU-free days, or new organ failures.[72] However, subgroup analyses suggested reduced mortality in patients who had larger volumes of plasma treated per day ($\geq$0.18 L/kg/d) and 2 studies are currently ongoing to confirm these findings in patients with septic shock using CPFA at doses of greater than 0.20 L/kg/d (NCT01639664[73]). These blood purification strategies do not act specif-ically against the pathogen, although this may be achieved with the development of opsonin-coated blood purification devices,[74] which still require human evaluation.

In summary, although no recommendations can currently be given regarding blood purification techniques in patients with sepsis because of the poor quality and con-flicting evidence available,[75] some systems may be effective in some patients and the results of the ongoing studies should help identify who can benefit from this approach.

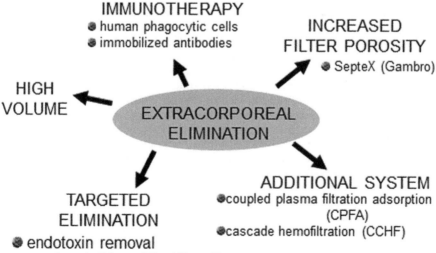

Fig. 1. Some of the blood purification systems under investigation for the management of sepsis.

CHALLENGES

Despite decades of ongoing research into therapies for sepsis, no specific antisepsis interventions have been consistently shown to improve outcomes. However, the years of research and unsuccessful trials have not been in vain.

1. Much has been learned about sepsis pathogenesis, providing multiple new potential targets for antisepsis interventions. This article focuses on interventions that may protect the endothelium or enhance the immune response, two important trends in current clinical research, but there are many other potential avenues of study.

2. Clinicians have increasingly realized that not all patients with sepsis are the same and no single intervention will work in all patients with sepsis. Therapies needs to be adapted to individual patients, depending on their immune status and associated organ dysfunction at the time of intervention. There has been a principal focus on blocking the proinflammatory response, but many patients with sepsis become rapidly immunosuppressed and may benefit from immunostimulation rather than antiinflammatory interventions. The principal shortcoming of an individualized approach is that circulating cells may not reflect the immune status of noncirculating cells.

3. Clinicians have begun to understand that their focus on mortality as the primary study end point, although easy to measure, may not provide an adequate indication of efficacy. Mortality can be influenced by many factors, including the primary disease, comorbidities, non–sepsis-related events, and patient preferences. Moreover, the effects of the intervention may not be strong enough to influence survival (especially now, when outcomes are already optimized by high-quality standard of care in many centers). End points of morbidity, including organ dysfunction, should therefore be used more often and several ongoing studies have incorporated such end points into their design; for example, the study on IFN-β in patients with ARDS mentioned earlier (European Union Clinical Trials register no. 2014-005260-15) is using a composite end point of 28-day mortality plus days free of mechanical ventilation, and an ongoing study assessing alkaline phosphatase in patients with sepsis-associated acute kidney injury has the area under the time-corrected endogenous creatinine clearance curve from day 1 to day 7 as the primary end point.[76] The sequential organ failure assessment (SOFA) score[77] is widely used to assess outcomes and is increasingly used as an outcome (albeit often a secondary end point) in clinical trials. Changes in SOFA score over time have been shown to be associated with mortality in randomized clinical trials.[78] Obviously, mortality should not be totally discarded as an end point, but it should not be the only outcome measure.

4. Clinicians have learned that clinical trials in heterogeneous groups of patients with sepsis do not provide positive results.[79] Studies need to be conducted in groups of patients who are most likely to benefit from the intervention in question and new studies are increasingly including this approach in their design. Several studies have used sophisticated techniques to better characterize patients with sepsis, which could be used to more appropriately target interventions. For example, Davenport and colleagues[80] identified 2 subphenotypes of patients with community-acquired pneumonia: patients with a type 1 sepsis response signature (SRS) profile had an immunosuppressed phenotype and higher 14-day mortality than patients with the type 2 SRS profile. In pediatric patients, Wong and colleagues[81] identified 2 subphenotypes of septic shock and reported different mortalities in the 2 groups when they were prescribed corticosteroids. Clinicians are

some way from being able to incorporate these high-technology approaches into clinical trial inclusion criteria, but biomarkers can already help identify patients who are more likely to respond to specific therapies and follow their response.[82,83] This biomarker-driven approach to clinical trials is already well established in oncology, but less so in sepsis. In the ongoing study of thrombomodulin mentioned earlier (NCT01598831), the inclusion criteria have been developed based on the results from earlier studies that identified patients with coagulopathy as being most likely to respond. In the ongoing study of an anti–PD-L1 antibody (NCT02576457), biomarkers will be used to adapt enrollment criteria according to response. As another example, studies assessing the effects of recombinant gelsolin in patients with community-acquired pneumonia will only enroll patients with low gelsolin levels; this is a known biomarker associated with higher mortalities in patients with sepsis.[84]

SUMMARY

Advances in sepsis therapeutics continue to be made on a regular basis and important avenues of current research include improving endothelial cell function to protect the endothelium and limit edema formation, blood purification techniques to help restore immune homeostasis, and immunostimulatory therapies for patients with immune exhaustion. The key challenge at present is how best to identify those patients who are most likely to respond to any particular therapy so that inclusion criteria can be selected accordingly.

REFERENCES

1. Landry DW, Levin HR, Gallant EM, et al. Vasopressin deficiency contributes to the vasodilation of septic shock. Circulation 1997;95:1122–5.
2. Dunser MW, Mayr AJ, Ulmer H, et al. Arginine vasopressin in advanced vasodilatory shock: a prospective, randomized, controlled study. Circulation 2003;107:2313–9.
3. Russell JA, Walley KR, Singer J, et al. Vasopressin versus norepinephrine infusion in patients with septic shock. N Engl J Med 2008;358:877–87.
4. Gordon AC, Mason AJ, Thirunavukkarasu N, et al. Effect of early vasopressin vs norepinephrine on kidney failure in patients with septic shock: the VANISH randomized clinical trial. JAMA 2016;316:509–18.
5. Maybauer MO, Maybauer DM, Enkhbaatar P, et al. The selective vasopressin type 1a receptor agonist selepressin (FE 202158) blocks vascular leak in ovine severe sepsis. Crit Care Med 2014;42:e525–33.
6. He X, Su F, Taccone FS, et al. A selective V1A receptor agonist, selepressin, is superior to arginine vasopressin and to norepinephrine in ovine septic shock. Crit Care Med 2016;44:23–31.
7. Russell JA, Vincent JL, Kjolbye AL, et al. Selepressin, a novel selective vasopressin V1A receptor agonist, reduces norepinephrine requirements and shortens duration of organ dysfunction in septic shock patients [abstract]. Crit Care Med 2012;40(Suppl 1):62.
8. Hasko G, Csoka B, Koscso B, et al. Ecto-5'-nucleotidase (CD73) decreases mortality and organ injury in sepsis. J Immunol 2011;187:4256–67.
9. Cohen ES, Law WR, Easington CR, et al. Adenosine deaminase inhibition attenuates microvascular dysfunction and improves survival in sepsis. Am J Respir Crit Care Med 2002;166:16–20.

10. Bellingan G, Maksimow M, Howell DC, et al. The effect of intravenous interferon-beta-1a (FP-1201) on lung CD73 expression and on acute respiratory distress syndrome mortality: an open-label study. Lancet Respir Med 2014;2:98–107.
11. Kiss J, Yegutkin GG, Koskinen K, et al. IFN-beta protects from vascular leakage via up-regulation of CD73. Eur J Immunol 2007;37:3334–8.
12. Yoo CH, Yeom JH, Heo JJ, et al. Interferon beta protects against lethal endotoxic and septic shock through SIRT1 upregulation. Sci Rep 2014;4:4220.
13. Angus DC, van der Poll T. Severe sepsis and septic shock. N Engl J Med 2013; 369:840–51.
14. Johansson P, Stensballe J, Ostrowski S. Shock induced endotheliopathy (SHINE) in acute critical illness - a unifying pathophysiologic mechanism. Crit Care 2017; 21:25.
15. Ostrowski SR, Haase N, Muller RB, et al. Association between biomarkers of endothelial injury and hypocoagulability in patients with severe sepsis: a prospective study. Crit Care 2015;19:191.
16. Vincent JL. The rise and fall of drotrecogin alfa (activated). Lancet Infect Dis 2012;12:649–51.
17. Davis RP, Miller-Dorey S, Jenne CN. Platelets and coagulation in infection. Clin Transl Immunol 2016;5:e89.
18. Ito T, Maruyama I. Thrombomodulin: protectorate God of the vasculature in thrombosis and inflammation. J Thromb Haemost 2011;9(Suppl 1):168–73.
19. Zheng YJ, Xu WP, Ding G, et al. Expression of HMGB1 in septic serum induces vascular endothelial hyperpermeability. Mol Med Rep 2016;13:513–21.
20. Vincent JL, Ramesh MK, Ernest D, et al. A randomized, double-blind, placebo-controlled, phase 2b study to evaluate the safety and efficacy of recombinant human soluble thrombomodulin, ART-123, in patients with sepsis and suspected disseminated intravascular coagulation. Crit Care Med 2013;41:2069–79.
21. Groger M, Pasteiner W, Ignatyev G, et al. Peptide $B\beta_{15-42}$ preserves endothelial barrier function in shock. PLoS One 2009;4:e5391.
22. Jennewein C, Mehring M, Tran N, et al. The fibrinopeptide bβ15-42 reduces inflammation in mice subjected to polymicrobial sepsis. Shock 2012;38:275–80.
23. Wolf T, Kann G, Becker S, et al. Severe Ebola virus disease with vascular leakage and multiorgan failure: treatment of a patient in intensive care. Lancet 2015;385: 1428–35.
24. Alfieri A, Watson JJ, Kammerer RA, et al. Angiopoietin-1 variant reduces LPS-induced microvascular dysfunction in a murine model of sepsis. Crit Care 2012;16:R182.
25. Zhang G, Yang L, Kim GS, et al. Critical role of sphingosine-1-phosphate receptor 2 (S1PR2) in acute vascular inflammation. Blood 2013;122:443–55.
26. Zhao H, Anand AR, Ganju RK. Slit2-Robo4 pathway modulates lipopolysaccharide-induced endothelial inflammation and its expression is dysregulated during endotoxemia. J Immunol 2014;192:385–93.
27. Hotchkiss RS, Monneret G, Payen D. Sepsis-induced immunosuppression: from cellular dysfunctions to immunotherapy. Nat Rev Immunol 2013;13:862–74.
28. Leentjens J, Kox M, van der Hoeven JG, et al. Immunotherapy for the adjunctive treatment of sepsis: from immunosuppression to immunostimulation. Time for a paradigm change? Am J Respir Crit Care Med 2013;187:1287–93.
29. Bo L, Wang F, Zhu J, et al. Granulocyte-colony stimulating factor (G-CSF) and granulocyte-macrophage colony stimulating factor (GM-CSF) for sepsis: a meta-analysis. Crit Care 2011;15:R58.

30. Meisel C, Schefold JC, Pschowski R, et al. Granulocyte-macrophage colony-stimulating factor to reverse sepsis-associated immunosuppression: a double-blind, randomized, placebo-controlled multicenter trial. Am J Respir Crit Care Med 2009;180:640–8.

31. Boomer JS, Shuherk-Shaffer J, Hotchkiss RS, et al. A prospective analysis of lymphocyte phenotype and function over the course of acute sepsis. Crit Care 2012;16:R112.

32. Leentjens J, Kox M, Koch RM, et al. Reversal of immunoparalysis in humans in vivo: a double-blind, placebo-controlled, randomized pilot study. Am J Respir Crit Care Med 2012;186:838–45.

33. Delsing CE, Gresnigt MS, Leentjens J, et al. Interferon-gamma as adjunctive immunotherapy for invasive fungal infections: a case series. BMC Infect Dis 2014;14:166.

34. Mock CN, Dries DJ, Jurkovich GJ, et al. Assessment of two clinical trials: interferon-gamma therapy in severe injury. Shock 1996;5:235–40.

35. Inoue S, Unsinger J, Davis CG, et al. IL-15 prevents apoptosis, reverses innate and adaptive immune dysfunction, and improves survival in sepsis. J Immunol 2010;184:1401–9.

36. Ward PA. The curiosity of IL-15. Nat Med 2007;13:903–4.

37. Chung KP, Chang HT, Lo SC, et al. Severe lymphopenia is associated with elevated plasma interleukin-15 levels and increased mortality during severe sepsis. Shock 2015;43:569–75.

38. Guo Y, Luan L, Patil NK, et al. IL-15 enables septic shock by maintaining NK cell integrity and function. J Immunol 2017;198:1320–33.

39. Conlon KC, Lugli E, Welles HC, et al. Redistribution, hyperproliferation, activation of natural killer cells and CD8 T cells, and cytokine production during first-in-human clinical trial of recombinant human interleukin-15 in patients with cancer. J Clin Oncol 2015;33:74–82.

40. Venet F, Foray AP, Villars-Mechin A, et al. IL-7 restores lymphocyte functions in septic patients. J Immunol 2012;189:5073–81.

41. Shindo Y, Unsinger J, Burnham CA, et al. Interleukin-7 and anti-programmed cell death 1 antibody have differing effects to reverse sepsis-induced immunosuppression. Shock 2015;43:334–43.

42. Shindo Y, Fuchs AG, Davis CG, et al. Interleukin 7 immunotherapy improves host immunity and survival in a two-hit model of Pseudomonas aeruginosa pneumonia. J Leukoc Biol 2017;101:543–54.

43. Unsinger J, McGlynn M, Kasten KR, et al. IL-7 promotes T cell viability, trafficking, and functionality and improves survival in sepsis. J Immunol 2010;184:3768–79.

44. Unsinger J, Burnham CA, McDonough J, et al. Interleukin-7 ameliorates immune dysfunction and improves survival in a 2-hit model of fungal sepsis. J Infect Dis 2012;206:606–16.

45. Thiebaut R, Jarne A, Routy JP, et al. Repeated cycles of recombinant human interleukin 7 in HIV-infected patients with low CD4 T-cell reconstitution on antiretroviral therapy: results of 2 phase II multicenter studies. Clin Infect Dis 2016;62:1178–85.

46. Guignant C, Lepape A, Huang X, et al. Programmed death-1 levels correlate with increased mortality, nosocomial infection and immune dysfunctions in septic shock patients. Crit Care 2011;15:R99.

47. Shao R, Fang Y, Yu H, et al. Monocyte programmed death ligand-1 expression after 3-4 days of sepsis is associated with risk stratification and mortality in septic patients: a prospective cohort study. Crit Care 2016;20:124.

48. Brahmamdam P, Inoue S, Unsinger J, et al. Delayed administration of anti-PD-1 antibody reverses immune dysfunction and improves survival during sepsis. J Leukoc Biol 2010;88:233–40.

49. Zhang Y, Zhou Y, Lou J, et al. PD-L1 blockade improves survival in experimental sepsis by inhibiting lymphocyte apoptosis and reversing monocyte dysfunction. Crit Care 2010;14:R220.

50. Shindo Y, McDonough JS, Chang KC, et al. Anti-PD-L1 peptide improves survival in sepsis. J Surg Res 2017;208:33–9.

51. Chang K, Svabek C, Vazquez-Guillamet C, et al. Targeting the programmed cell death 1: programmed cell death ligand 1 pathway reverses T cell exhaustion in patients with sepsis. Crit Care 2014;18:R3.

52. Ott PA, Piha-Paul SA, Munster P, et al. Safety and antitumor activity of the anti-PD-1 antibody pembrolizumab in patients with recurrent carcinoma of the anal canal. Ann Oncol 2017;28:1036–41.

53. Ott PA, Bang YJ, Berton-Rigaud D, et al. Safety and antitumor activity of pembrolizumab in advanced programmed death ligand 1-positive endometrial cancer: results from the KEYNOTE-028 study. J Clin Oncol 2017;35(22):2535–41.

54. Michot JM, Bigenwald C, Champiat S, et al. Immune-related adverse events with immune checkpoint blockade: a comprehensive review. Eur J Cancer 2016;54:139–48.

55. Monneret G, Gossez M, Venet F. Sepsis in PD-1 light. Crit Care 2016;20:186.

56. Grimaldi D, Pradier O, Hotchkiss RS, et al. Nivolumab plus interferon-gamma in the treatment of intractable mucormycosis. Lancet Infect Dis 2017;17:18.

57. Gotloib L, Barzilay E, Shustak A, et al. Hemofiltration in septic ARDS. The artificial kidney as an artificial endocrine lung. Resuscitation 1986;13:123–32.

58. Bellomo R, Tipping P, Boyce N. Continuous veno-venous hemofiltration with dialysis removes cytokines from the circulation of septic patients. Crit Care Med 1993;21:522–6.

59. Cole L, Bellomo R, Hart G, et al. A phase II randomized, controlled trial of continuous hemofiltration in sepsis. Crit Care Med 2002;30:100–6.

60. Payen D, Mateo J, Cavaillon JM, et al. Impact of continuous venovenous hemofiltration on organ failure during the early phase of severe sepsis: a randomized controlled trial. Crit Care Med 2009;37:803–10.

61. Honore PM, Jamez J, Wauthier M, et al. Prospective evaluation of short-term, high-volume isovolemic hemofiltration on the hemodynamic course and outcome in patients with intractable circulatory failure resulting from septic shock. Crit Care Med 2000;28:3581–7.

62. Cornejo R, Downey P, Castro R, et al. High-volume hemofiltration as salvage therapy in severe hyperdynamic septic shock. Intensive Care Med 2006;32:713–22.

63. Joannes-Boyau O, Rapaport S, Bazin R, et al. Impact of high volume hemofiltration on hemodynamic disturbance and outcome during septic shock. ASAIO J 2004;50:102–9.

64. Park JT, Lee H, Kee YK, et al. High-dose versus conventional-dose continuous venovenous hemodiafiltration and patient and kidney survival and cytokine removal in sepsis-associated acute kidney injury: a randomized controlled trial. Am J Kidney Dis 2016;68:599–608.

65. Kogelmann K, Jarczak D, Scheller M, et al. Hemoadsorption by CytoSorb in septic patients: a case series. Crit Care 2017;21:74.

66. Vincent JL, Laterre PF, Cohen J, et al. A pilot-controlled study of a polymyxin B-immobilized hemoperfusion cartridge in patients with severe sepsis secondary to intra-abdominal infection. Shock 2005;23:400–5.

67. Cruz DN, Antonelli M, Fumagalli R, et al. Early use of polymyxin B hemoperfusion in abdominal septic shock: the EUPHAS randomized controlled trial. JAMA 2009; 301:2445–52.

68. Vincent JL. Sepsis: clearing the blood in sepsis. Nat Rev Nephrol 2009;5:559–60.

69. Payen DM, Guilhot J, Launey Y, et al. Early use of polymyxin B hemoperfusion in patients with septic shock due to peritonitis: a multicenter randomized control trial. Intensive Care Med 2015;41:975–84.

70. Klein DJ, Foster D, Schorr CA, et al. The EUPHRATES trial (Evaluating the Use of Polymyxin B Hemoperfusion in a Randomized controlled trial of Adults Treated for Endotoxemia and Septic shock): study protocol for a randomized controlled trial. Trials 2014;15:218.

71. Rimmer E, Houston BL, Kumar A, et al. The efficacy and safety of plasma exchange in patients with sepsis and septic shock: a systematic review and meta-analysis. Crit Care 2014;18:699.

72. Livigni S, Bertolini G, Rossi C, et al. Efficacy of coupled plasma filtration adsorption (CPFA) in patients with septic shock: a multicenter randomised controlled clinical trial. BMJ Open 2014;4:e003536.

73. Colomina-Climent F, Gimenez-Esparza C, Portillo-Requena C, et al. Mortality reduction in septic shock by plasma adsorption (ROMPA): a protocol for a randomised clinical trial. BMJ Open 2016;6:e011856.

74. Kang JH, Super M, Yung CW, et al. An extracorporeal blood-cleansing device for sepsis therapy. Nat Med 2014;20:1211–6.

75. Rhodes A, Evans LE, Alhazzani W, et al. Surviving sepsis campaign: international guidelines for management of sepsis and septic shock: 2016. Crit Care Med 2017;45:486–552.

76. Peters E, Mehta RL, Murray PT, et al. Study protocol for a multicentre randomised controlled trial: safety, tolerability, efficacy and quality of life of a human recombinant alkaline phosphatase in patients with sepsis-associated acute kidney injury (STOP-AKI). BMJ Open 2016;6:e012371.

77. Vincent JL, Moreno R, Takala J, et al. The SOFA (sepsis-related organ failure assessment) score to describe organ dysfunction/failure. On behalf of the Working Group on Sepsis-related Problems of the European Society of Intensive Care Medicine. Intensive Care Med 1996;22:707–10.

78. de Grooth HJ, Geenen IL, Girbes AR, et al. SOFA and mortality endpoints in randomized controlled trials: a systematic review and meta-regression analysis. Crit Care 2017;21:38.

79. Vincent JL. Improved survival in critically ill patients: are large RCTs more useful than personalized medicine? No. Intensive Care Med 2016;42:1778–80.

80. Davenport EE, Burnham KL, Radhakrishnan J, et al. Genomic landscape of the individual host response and outcomes in severe sepsis. Lancet Respir Med 2016;4:259–71.

81. Wong HR, Cvijanovich NZ, Anas N, et al. Developing a clinically feasible personalized medicine approach to pediatric septic shock. Am J Respir Crit Care Med 2015;191:309–15.

82. Sims CR, Nguyen TC, Mayeux PR. Could biomarkers direct therapy for the septic patient? J Pharmacol Exp Ther 2016;357:228–39.

83. Vincent JL. The clinical challenge of sepsis identification and monitoring. PLoS Med 2016;13:e1002022.

84. Lee PS, Patel SR, Christiani DC, et al. Plasma gelsolin depletion and circulating actin in sepsis—a pilot study. PLoS One 2008;3(11):e3712.

Improving Long-Term Outcomes After Sepsis

Hallie C. Prescott, MD, MSc[a],*, Deena Kelly Costa, PhD, RN[b]

KEYWORDS

- Cognitive impairment • Physical disability • Re-hospitalization • Anxiety
- Depression • Stress

KEY POINTS

- Acute survival from sepsis has improved dramatically in recent years, resulting in a large population of sepsis survivors.
- Many sepsis survivors experience long-term sequelae of sepsis, including weakness, cognitive impairment, frequent hospital readmission, and increased risk for death.
- In-hospital care should focus on treatment of sepsis; minimizing exposure to delirium, distress, and immobility; and preparing patients and families both emotionally and physically for hospital discharge.
- Posthospital care should focus on validating a patient's experience, referral to appropriate therapies (eg, physical or speech therapy), and actively screening for and preventing medical deterioration.

INTRODUCTION

Short-term survival from sepsis has improved dramatically in recent years.[1,2] As a result, there is a growing population of sepsis survivors.[3] These patients frequently experience new symptoms, long-term disability,[4] worsening of chronic health conditions, and increased risk for death following sepsis hospitalization.[5] In light of these poor outcomes, the Society for Critical Care Medicine has defined "post–intensive care syndrome" as new or worsening cognitive, physical, and mental health impairments that persist beyond acute hospitalization.[6] Sepsis survivors are at particularly high risk for this syndrome.

Funding: This work was supported by grants K08 GM115859 [HCP] from the National Institute of General Medical Sciences of the National Institutes of Health and K08 HS024552 [DKC] from the Agency for Healthcare Research and Quality.
Disclosures: This work does not represent the position or policy of the US government of the Department of Veterans Affairs. The authors have no financial conflicts of interest.
[a] Department of Internal Medicine, University of Michigan, VA Center for Clinical Management Research, HSR&D Center of Innovation, North Campus Research Center, 2800 Plymouth Road, Building 16, 341E, Ann Arbor, MI 48109-2800, USA; [b] Department of Systems, Populations & Leadership, School of Nursing, University of Michigan, 400 North Ingalls Street #4351, Ann Arbor, MI 48109-5482, USA
* Corresponding author.
E-mail address: hprescot@med.umich.edu

Elderly sepsis survivors experience a 10% absolute increase in moderate-to-severe cognitive impairment relative to their own presepsis rates,[4] and middle-aged adult patients fare similarly.[7] Elderly patients also develop an average 1 to 2 new limitations of activities of daily living (eg, dressing, bathing) and instrumental activities of daily living (eg, taking medications, managing money) around the time of sepsis hospitalization.[4] Rates of anxiety, depression, and posttraumatic stress disorder are higher than population norms.[8–10] For these reasons, sepsis hospitalization often represents a pivotal downturn in patients' ability to function independently.[11]

These new disabilities after sepsis represent a significant public health burden, with an estimated 500,000 older sepsis survivors with functional impairments in the United States and 100,00 with moderate-severe cognitive impairment.[12] More than 1 in 4 older survivors is discharged to a post-acute care facility.[13] Approximately 40% are readmitted to the hospital at least once in the next 90 days.[14] One in 5 survivors has a late death that is not explained by presepsis health status.[5]

Not all sepsis survivors experience poor long-term outcomes. Of patients surviving hospitalization, approximately one-third die during the following year,[13,15] one-sixth experience severe persistent impairments, and one-half have a good recovery. The severity of impairments immediately after hospitalization do not correlate well with later outcomes[16] because patients have different trajectories (eg, progressive decline vs recovery) after sepsis.[17] Although there are no routinely used tools to predict long-term disability after sepsis, several factors have been associated with worse outcomes (**Box 1**).

Although the long-term burdens of sepsis survivorship are increasingly recognized, the best in–intensive care unit (ICU), in-hospital, and postdischarge practices for improving long-term outcomes after sepsis are still evolving. In this article, we review the available evidence on management strategies to improve long-term outcomes after sepsis hospitalization.

MANAGEMENT GOALS
In the Intensive Care Unit

Delirium,[18] acute distress,[19] and immobility have each been identified as a key in-ICU factor that is associated with long-term cognitive impairment and physical

---

Box 1
Risk factors associated with poor long-term functional outcomes

- Burden of chronic health conditions[81]
- Duration of delirium during hospitalization[82]
- Hearing impairment[83]
- Immobility
- Frailty[84]
- No spouse[81]
- Older age
- Premorbid disability[85]
- Prior nursing home care
- Severity of acute illness[81]
- Vision impairment[83]

disability.[20,21] Thus, in addition to rapid treatment of infection and support for vital organs, the ICU treatment of septic patients should focus on limiting exposure to these risk factors. One evidence-based approach is the "ABCDEF" bundle.[22] This is a collection of multidisciplinary practices for mechanically ventilated patients (**Table 1**) that is designed to improve long-term outcomes by minimizing exposure to delirium, distress, and immobility. Aspects of the ABCDEF bundle, in its entirety or paired bundled components, have been shown to double the odds of walking and halving the odds of delirium, without a subsequent increased risk for self-extubation or reintubation.[23,24] Newer evidence further suggests the ABCDEF bundle as newly conceptualized,[22] when implemented effectively, is associated with more days alive, and free of delirium and coma for patients cared for in 7 community hospitals in California.[25]

In the Hospital

Patients' risk for poor long-term outcomes does not end on ICU discharge. Medical care on the ward should focus on increasing mobility, preparing patients and

Table 1
ABCDEF bundle and selected evidence in support of each bundle element

Bundle Element	Evidence
A Assess, Prevent, and Manage Pain	Pain is a common memory of intensive care unit (ICU) survivors[85,86] and increases risk for posttraumatic stress disorder.[18,19] When pain is routinely assess using a validated pain scale and controlled with intravenous narcotics, sedation often can be avoided.[39,86,87]
B Both Spontaneous Awakening and Spontaneous Breathing Trials	Spontaneous awakening and breathing trials are associated with shorter duration of mechanical ventilation, better psychological outcomes, and significantly improved 1-y mortality.[65–67]
C Choice of Analgesia and Sedation	Nonbenzodiazepine sedatives are associated with less delirium,[87,88] particularly in septic patients. In general, patients do better with less sedation.[88,89] Less sedation may be achieved by spontaneous awakening trials, bolus vs continuous sedation, and targeting a lighter depth of sedation.[88,89]
D Delirium Monitoring and Management	Delirium is associated with greater mortality and cognitive impairment.[18,89,90] Screening for delirium with tools such as the Confusion Assessment Method for the ICU (CAM-ICU) can increase recognition of delirium,[90,91] prompting clinicians to address driving factors such as medications, environment and medical conditions.
E Early Mobility and Exercise	Skeletal muscle wasting begins within 24 h of critical illness.[55,56] Early mobility, including walking patients during invasive mechanical ventilation, has been shown to be safe and effective at reducing short-term physical disability associated with critical illness, as well as at reducing delirium.[52–54]
F Family Engagement and Empowerment	Families are important supports for patients' recovery, also experience poor outcomes related to ICU care.[61,62] Family presence on ICU rounds and open visiting hours are associated with improved satisfaction and communication.[64,65]

caretakers both medically and emotionally for hospital discharge, and determining the most appropriate discharge location. Patients frequently experience muscle wasting, weakness, and dysphagia after critical illness.[26] Evaluation by physical therapists and occupational therapist can be helpful to determine whether patients require additional inpatient rehabilitation or home therapy, and evaluation by speech language pathologists is important to determine whether patients require dietary modification (eg, pureed foods, thickened liquids) or nil per os precautions.

At present, issues of survivorship are rarely discussed during hospitalization.[27] Many patients are unaware of their sepsis diagnosis,[28] and even fewer are aware of the potential long-term sequelae. Ideally, this education regarding survivorship concerns should begin in the hospital and continue in the postdischarge setting. Fortunately, there are now many online resources whereby patients and families can learn about sequelae of sepsis and critical illnesses (**Box 2**).

After Discharge

Management of sepsis survivors in the early posthospital period should focus on ongoing rehabilitation, adaptation to functional impairments, emotional support for patients and caretakers, and active surveillance and prevention of further medical deterioration. Given the high rate of death,[5] disability,[4] and health care utilization[13] in sepsis survivors, it is also important to discuss overall goals of care. Patients with presepsis disability and further decline following sepsis hospitalization may be interested in transitioning to a palliative focus. But, despite reduced quality of life (QOL) relative to age-matched population norms,[29,30] long-term sepsis survivors are often satisfied with their QOL and would undergo ICU treatment again,[31] so patient-specific conversation is needed.

Box 2 Selected online resources for sepsis survivorship	
Web site	Selected information available at the site
www.sepsisalliance.org	• Signs/symptoms of sepsis • Description of common sequelae • More than 400 "Faces of Sepsis": written tributes to lost loved ones and stories of survivors
www.myicucare.org/thrive	• Several white-board videos for patients and families, including videos on preparing for hospital discharge after critical illness, post–intensive care syndrome, and wellness after critical illness • Information on virtual and in-person peer support groups for critical illness survivors
www.icusteps.org	• Information on in-person support groups in the United Kingdom • Informational pamphlets for patients and families, including a guide to the intensive care unit (ICU)
www.healthtalk.org	• Video interviews describing patient and family experiences of the ICU
www.icudelirium.org/patients	• Information about common sequelae of critical illness, including patient testimonials • Information about the Vanderbilt ICU recovery center

PHARMACOLOGIC STRATEGIES
Treatment of Sepsis

We recommend rapid treatment with broad-spectrum antibiotics, fluid resuscitation, source control, and vasopressors, in accordance with the Surviving Sepsis Campaign[32] guidelines. We support shorter antibiotic courses for patients with rapid clinical resolution and/or improved procalcitonin level to minimize microbiome disruption, which in turn increases patients' risk for recurrent sepsis.[33] Using procalcitonin to tailor antibiotic duration results in less antibiotic exposure, without increased short-term mortality. In observational studies, increased antibiotic exposure (both the duration of treatment and the number of drug classes) is independently associated with increased risk of recurrent sepsis.[34] So, shortened antibiotic courses may also decrease patients' risk for recurrent sepsis, which is the most common reason for hospital readmission in this population. Because exposure to an increased number of drug classes is also associated with increased risk for subsequent sepsis, it is worthwhile to consider (and attempt to avoid) exposure to additional drug classes during the process of antibiotic deescalation.

Stress Ulcer Prophylaxis

Stress ulcer prophylaxis is widespread in the ICU, but risk of bleeding is low, and concentrated among patients with coagulopathy or respiratory failure.[35] Thus, we do not recommend stress ulcer prophylaxis in patients without either of these risk factors, as maintaining acidic gastric acid is a protective factor against infection. Indeed, stress ulcer prophylaxis, in particular proton pump therapy, has been associated with increased risk for *Clostridium difficile* infection and pneumonia.[36] When stress ulcer prophylaxis is indicated (for respiratory failure or coagulopathy), we recommend H2 receptor agonists over proton pump inhibitors to minimize risk for subsequent infection.

Pharmacologic Management of Pain and Agitation

Patients frequently experience pain and discomfort during the ICU. Patients were traditionally treated with deep sedation while mechanically ventilated, but this practice has been associated with longer duration of mechanical ventilation, higher rates of delirium, poor long-term cognitive function, and higher long-term mortality.[37,38] Thus, the current standard as described in the Pain, Agitation, and Delirium guidelines (and supported by the Surviving Sepsis Campaign Guidelines[32]) is to use "lighter" sedation.[39] This can be achieved by a variety of strategies, including treating pain first in conjunction with routine pain assessments using a validated pain assessment scale (and thereby limiting need for sedation); using intermittent rather than continuous sedation medications; using a sedation scale (eg, Richmond Agitation Sedation Scale) to target light levels of continuous sedation; and performing daily awakening trials during which continuous sedative medications are turned off and restarted only if needed.[39]

Beyond treating pain and targeting light sedation, the choice of sedative agent is also important. Benzodiazepines have been associated with increased risk for delirium, which is in turn associated with worse long-term outcomes. Propofol and dexmedetomidine are short-acting continuous sedative medications that are preferred over benzodiazepines for patients requiring continuous sedation.

Medications Associated with Intensive Care Unit–Acquired Weakness

Observational studies suggest that several medications (eg, corticosteroids, aminoglycosides, and in particular neuromuscular blocking agents [NMBs]) may exacerbate

ICU-acquired weakness through direct toxicity to nerves, muscles, or both. However, the quality of these data is low due to confounding by indication and other methodological limitations.[40] At present, the Surviving Sepsis Campaign guidelines have weak recommendations for using 48 hours of NMBs in patients with sepsis-induced acute respiratory distress syndrome (ARDS) and Pao_2/Fio_2 less than 150 based on a 340-person, multicenter randomized controlled trial (RCT) showing a mortality benefit.[32,41] In this study, there was no increase in ICU-acquired weakness in the NMB arm, but all patients were deeply sedated, half of the control arm received at least 1 dose of NMB, and there was no long-term follow-up of weakness. Thus, considerable equipoise remains, and uptake of NMBs has been low.[42] While we await further RCT data on the safety and efficacy of NMB from the ongoing Reevaluation of Systemic Early Neuromuscular Blockade Trial (ROSE),[43] we prefer to reserve NMB for only the sickest patients with sepsis-related ARDS (eg, those with Pao_2/Fio_2 <75).

Medication Reconciliation and Titration

Medication reconciliation at the time of hospital discharge is particularly important for patients with sepsis, who are likely to have had multiple medication adjustments during their hospitalization.[44] Chronic medications are frequently held and forgotten, whereas medications to treat acute symptoms may be continued inadvertently.[45–47] In a recent prospective study, 24% of patients who were prescribed an atypical antipsychotic for acute delirium during critical illness had the medication continued at discharge, despite a black-box warning for long-term use and scant evidence that atypical antipsychotics are helpful for acute symptoms.[48] Beyond getting the medication list correct, it is important to consider that the dosages of chronic medications may need to be adjusted as a result of physiologic changes during sepsis hospitalization (eg, reduced muscle mass or decline in glomerular filtration rate).

NONPHARMACOLOGIC STRATEGIES
Intensive Care Unit Diaries

ICU diaries are written accounts of a patient's hospitalization, typically created by bedside nurses and family members. They describe the hospital course in lay terms and often include drawings or photographs, helping patients to understand what transpired while they were sedated. Providing a diary at 1 month is associated with lower rates of posttraumatic stress disorder (PTSD) in patients and relatives at 3 months.[49,50] Although diaries are provided by many hospitals in Scandinavia and western Europe,[51] they are rarely used in the United States. Describing the hospital course in simple terms may provide similar benefit, and is commonly included in many ICU follow-up clinics.[52]

Early Activity and Mobility

Early mobility, including progressively increasing a patient's activity level to the goal of ambulation during invasive mechanical ventilation, has been shown to be safe and effective at reducing short-term physical disability associated with critical illness, as well as at reducing delirium.[53,54] Patients randomized to early mobility interventions have better physical function at ICU and hospital discharge. They also are more likely to be discharged directly home (43% vs 24% discharged to home, $P = .06$).[53] Although early mobility interventions have not been shown to improve long-term physical function, skeletal muscle weakness has been associated with both early and late mortality after critical illness.[55] Thus, it is reasonable to suspect that the improvements in functional status at discharge do indeed translate to better long-term outcomes.

It is important to note that the main benefit of mobility interventions seems to be the prevention of acute muscle loss. Skeletal muscle wasting begins within 24 hours of critical illness,[56] so mobility interventions must occur as soon as possible. Interventions that begin later in the ICU stay,[57] after ICU discharge[58] or after hospital discharge,[59] have generally not been successful.

Cognitive Therapy

In a single-center pilot feasibility study, ICU survivors randomized to cognitive and physical rehabilitation showed improved executive functioning by 3 months.[60] However, another single-center pilot study testing a multifaceted intervention, including early cognitive therapy delivered twice a day during the ICU, found no difference in cognitive function at 3 months.[61] Larger studies are needed to assess early and later cognitive therapy.

Family Engagement

Family engagement has been recognized as an increasingly important goal in ICU care for several reasons. First, family members often serve as surrogate decision-makers when patients are unable to voice their own wishes. Second, families provide invaluable support during a patient's recovery. With increasing fragmentation of health care delivery, family members may be the only people capable of placing the sepsis hospitalization within the broader context of a patient's overall recovery. Third, critical illness has a profound effect on families, many of whom experience stress and depression as a result of the their caregiving or surrogate decision-maker role.[28,62] Effective family engagement includes showing respect for the family's values and goals, sharing information on a patient's status in a timely fashion, and actively partnering with families to develop treatment plans.[63] Family presence on ICU rounds and open visiting hours are increasingly accepted ways to incorporate families into ICU care.[64,65]

Intensive Care Unit Follow-up Clinics

Specialized post-ICU clinics have been proposed as a strategy for improving long-term outcomes after critical illness.[52] These clinics are common in the United Kingdom, where approximately one-third of ICUs run a follow-up clinic.[66] Over the past few years, there has also been growing interest in ICU follow-up clinics within the United States. The first centers were the Critical Care Recovery Center at Indiana University and the Vanderbilt ICU Recovery Center,[67] and several additional centers are now building similar clinics. The exact organization of these clinics varies across centers, and no optimal model has been identified.[66]

The evidence in support of ICU follow-up clinics is limited. The largest study to date evaluated the impact of a self-directed physical therapy program and visits to a nurse-led follow-up clinic at 3 and 9 months.[52] During the clinic visit, patients had a medication review, discussion of their ICU course, physiologic screen, evaluation for specialty referral, a visit to their ICU, and a formal letter to their primary care physician. There was no improvement in QOL, PTSD, depression, costs, or mortality among patients randomized to the intervention.[52] There are several possible explanations for this negative trial. The trial enrolled unselected ICU survivors, did not formally integrate families into the intervention, and did not see patients in clinic until 3 months after ICU discharge. Furthermore, the medical complexity of ICU survivors may require an interdisciplinary approach, as is used in many ICU follow-up clinics.[67]

SELF-MANAGEMENT STRATEGIES
Symptom Management

Patients often experience anxiety, fear, and agitation during ICU stays, but sedative medications commonly used to treat these symptoms are associated with worse long-term outcomes, particularly when given in high doses. There is a growing body of literature supporting patient-controlled symptom management as an adjunct or replacement to nurse-administered sedation. For example, in a 373-person RCT, patient-directed music therapy resulted in reduced anxiety and reduced sedative dosing compared with usual care or noise-cancelling headphones.[68] A current RCT is testing whether patient-controlled sedative therapy with dexmedetomidine is safe and effective compared with nurse-administered sedation.[69]

Exercise and Rehabilitation

Evidence for self-directed rehabilitation is mixed. In a study of 126 ICU patients, randomization to receiving a 6-week rehabilitation manual was associated with improved physical function at 8 weeks and 6 months.[70] However, in a study of 286 ICU patients randomized to a 3-month rehabilitation manual coupled with referral to a nurse-run ICU follow-up clinic showed no improvement in physical function at 6 months or 1 year. It is possible that the benefit of self-directed rehabilitation does not persist more than a few months. In older patients recently discharged from the hospital, self-directed exercise programs have been associated with greater mobility, but also with an increased number of falls, suggesting that self-directed rehabilitation programs are not without risk.

Peer-to-Peer Support

There is a long tradition of peer support groups for chronic conditions, such as cancer, diabetes, and mental health and substance disorders. Recently, peer support groups have also been formed for critical illness survivors and families, such as ICUSteps[71] in the United Kingdom and Society for Critical Care Medicine's Thrive Network[72] in the United States. In these support groups, critical illness survivors share their experiences, provide empathy, and give and receive practical advice on navigating life with new disabilities.[73] Patients and caretakers benefit from giving and receiving support.[73] These groups may also serve as a venue to discuss the role of religion and spirituality in recovery, which are often neglected by clinicians.[73] Although the peer-support model is appealing, the optimal structure and process of these groups has yet to be determined.

EVALUATION, ADJUSTMENT, RECURRENCE
Evaluation

Sepsis survivors are at high risk for further medical deterioration in the weeks to months following hospital discharge. By 3 months, more than 40% of older survivors are readmitted to the hospital at least once.[14,74] Many of these readmissions are for potentially preventable causes, most commonly infection, heart failure exacerbation, acute renal failure, chronic obstructive pulmonary disease exacerbation, and aspiration pneumonia.[14] Thus, in addition to addressing new disabilities, early outpatient care should focus on active screening for and mitigating risk of these common problems.

Adjustment

As a result of impaired mobility, many patients are unable to continue previous activities and hobbies. Patients may be newly dependent on spouses and family members to complete activities of daily living, such as bathing and dressing. Because of this loss of independence, patients may feel helpless, embarrassed, or angry.[28] Family members also experience significant life changes following a loved one's sepsis hospitalization. Family members have new or growing responsibilities as a caretaker, and completing domestic chores that the patient can no longer complete.[28] These new responsibilities coupled with the stress of the patient's illness may lead family members to feel frustration, guilt, anxiety, stress, and depression.[28,62] Beyond recognizing and validating patients' and families' experiences and emotion, clinicians should refer interested patients and families to peer-to-peer support groups and online resources (**Box 2**) where they can learn more about survivorship issues.

Recurrence

The most common cause of hospital readmission in sepsis survivors is infection. A full 6% of older Americans who survive a sepsis hospitalization return to the hospital within 3 months for another bout of sepsis, whereas nearly a quarter return for some sort of infection.[14] However, on closer review of these readmissions (not merely examining the principal diagnosis codes), as many as one-half to two-thirds of all readmissions appear to be infection-related.[15,75–77] There is an even split between new infections and relapsed/recurrent infections,[75] suggesting that these readmissions are not merely treatment failures.

There are many reasons for which sepsis survivors are at high risk for subsequent infection. First, the demographic and health factors that placed patients at risk for their first episode of sepsis are often still present. Second, sepsis is often followed by a period of relative immune suppression, during which time patients are at heightened risk for subsequent infections.[78,79] Third, as a result of both infection and its treatment, patients experience microbiome disruption, which may further increase risk for subsequent sepsis.[33,80]

Beyond standard infection-prevention measures (hand-washing, avoidance of sick contacts, keeping vaccines up to date), there are no specific therapies to boost patients' immune system after sepsis. In the future, immune-therapy may be used to restore immune function, and diet and probiotics may be used to restore the gut microbiome.[77]

SUMMARY

Although acute survival from sepsis has improved dramatically in recent years, a large fraction of sepsis survivors experience poor long-term outcomes. In particular, sepsis survivors have high rates of weakness, cognitive impairment, hospital readmission, and late death. To improve long-term outcomes, in-hospital care should focus on early, effective treatment of sepsis; minimization of delirium, distress, and immobility; and preparing patients for hospital discharge. In the posthospital setting, medical care should focus on addressing new disability and preventing medical deterioration, providing a sustained period out of the hospital to allow for recovery.

REFERENCES

1. Kaukonen KM, Bailey M, Suzuki S, et al. Mortality related to severe sepsis and septic shock among critically ill patients in Australia and New Zealand, 2000-2012. JAMA 2014;311:1308–16.
2. Prescott HC, Kepreos KM, Wiitala WL, et al. Temporal changes in the influence of hospitals and regional healthcare networks on severe sepsis mortality. Crit Care Med 2015;43:1368–74.

3. Iwashyna TJ, Speelmon EC. Advancing a third revolution in critical care. Am J Respir Crit Care Med 2016;194:782–3.
4. Iwashyna TJ, Ely EW, Smith DM, et al. Long-term cognitive impairment and functional disability among survivors of severe sepsis. JAMA 2010;304:1787–94.
5. Prescott HC, Osterholzer JJ, Langa KM, et al. Late mortality after sepsis: propensity matched cohort study. BMJ 2016;353:i2375.
6. Needham DM, Davidson J, Cohen H, et al. Improving long-term outcomes after discharge from intensive care unit: report from a stakeholders' conference. Crit Care Med 2012;40:502–9.
7. Pandharipande PP, Girard TD, Ely EW. Long-term cognitive impairment after critical illness. N Engl J Med 2013;369:1306–16.
8. Parker AM, Sricharoenchai T, Raparla S, et al. Posttraumatic stress disorder in critical illness survivors: a metaanalysis. Crit Care Med 2015;43:1121–9.
9. Davydow DS, Gifford JM, Desai SV, et al. Depression in general intensive care unit survivors: a systematic review. Intensive Care Med 2009;35:796–809.
10. Nikayin S, Rabiee A, Hashem MD, et al. Anxiety symptoms in survivors of critical illness: a systematic review and meta-analysis. Gen Hosp Psychiatry 2016;43: 23–9.
11. Angus DC. The lingering consequences of sepsis: a hidden public health disaster? JAMA 2010;304:1833–4.
12. Iwashyna TJ, Cooke CR, Wunsch H, et al. Population burden of long-term survivorship after severe sepsis in older Americans. J Am Geriatr Soc 2012;60: 1070–7.
13. Prescott HC, Langa KM, Liu V, et al. Increased 1-year healthcare use in survivors of severe sepsis. Am J Respir Crit Care Med 2014;190:62–9.
14. Prescott HC, Langa KM, Iwashyna TJ. Readmission diagnoses after hospitalization for severe sepsis and other acute medical conditions. JAMA 2015;313: 1055–7.
15. Prescott HC. Variation in postsepsis readmission patterns: a cohort study of veterans affairs beneficiaries. Ann Am Thorac Soc 2017;14:230–7.
16. Woon FL, Dunn CB, Hopkins RO. Predicting cognitive sequelae in survivors of critical illness with cognitive screening tests. Am J Respir Crit Care Med 2012; 186:333–40.
17. Iwashyna TJ. Trajectories of recovery and dysfunction after acute illness, with implications for clinical trial design. Am J Respir Crit Care Med 2012;186:302–4.
18. Girard TD, Jackson JC, Pandharipande PP, et al. Delirium as a predictor of long-term cognitive impairment in survivors of critical illness. Crit Care Med 2010;38:1513–20.
19. Davydow DS, Zatzick D, Hough CL, et al. In-hospital acute stress symptoms are associated with impairment in cognition 1 year after intensive care unit admission. Ann Am Thorac Soc 2013;10:450–7.
20. Morandi A, Brummel NE, Ely EW. Sedation, delirium and mechanical ventilation: the 'ABCDE' approach. Curr Opin Crit Care 2011;17:43–9.
21. Brummel NE, Balas MC, Morandi A, et al. Understanding and reducing disability in older adults following critical illness. Crit Care Med 2015;43:1265–75.
22. Marra A, Ely EW, Pandharipande PP, et al. The ABCDEF bundle in critical care. Crit Care Clin 2017;33:225–43.
23. Girard TD, Kress JP, Fuchs BD, et al. Efficacy and safety of a paired sedation and ventilator weaning protocol for mechanically ventilated patients in intensive care (Awakening and Breathing Controlled trial): a randomised controlled trial. Lancet 2008;371:126–34.

24. Balas MC, Vasilevskis EE, Olsen KM, et al. Effectiveness and safety of the awakening and breathing coordination, delirium monitoring/management, and early exercise/mobility bundle. Crit Care Med 2014;42:1024–36.

25. Barnes-Daly MA, Phillips G, Ely EW. Improving hospital survival and reducing brain dysfunction at seven California community hospitals: implementing PAD guidelines via the ABCDEF bundle in 6,064 patients. Crit Care Med 2017;45:171–8.

26. Zielske J, Bohne S, Brunkhorst FM, et al. Acute and long-term dysphagia in critically ill patients with severe sepsis: results of a prospective controlled observational study. Eur Arch Otorhinolaryngol 2014. http://dx.doi.org/10.1007/s00405-014-3148-6.

27. Govindan S, Iwashyna TJ, Watson SR, et al. Issues of survivorship are rarely addressed during intensive care unit stays. Baseline results from a statewide quality improvement collaborative. Ann Am Thorac Soc 2014;11:587–91.

28. Gallop KH, Kerr CE, Nixon A, et al. A qualitative investigation of patients' and caregivers' experiences of severe sepsis. Crit Care Med 2015;43:296–307.

29. Winters BD, Eberlein M, Leung J, et al. Long-term mortality and quality of life in sepsis: a systematic review. Crit Care Med 2010;38:1276–83.

30. Yende S, Austin S, Rhodes A, et al. Long-term quality of life among survivors of severe sepsis. Crit Care Med 2016;44:1461–7.

31. Cuthbertson BH, Elders A, Hall S, et al. Mortality and quality of life in the five years after severe sepsis. Crit Care 2013;17:R70.

32. Rhodes A, Evans LE, Alhazzani W, et al. Surviving sepsis campaign: international guidelines for management of sepsis and septic shock: 2016. Intensive Care Med 2017. http://dx.doi.org/10.1007/s00134-017-4683-6.

33. Prescott HC, Dickson RP, Rogers MA, et al. Hospitalization type and subsequent severe sepsis. Am J Respir Crit Care Med 2015;192:581–8.

34. Baggs J, Jernigan J, McCormick K, et al. Increased Risk of Sepsis during Hospital Readmission following exposure to certain antibiotics during hospitalization. IDSA conference abstract, 2016. Available at: https://idsa.confex.com/idsa/2016/webprogram/Paper58587.html. Accessed September 8, 2017.

35. Cook DJ, Fuller HD, Guyatt GH, et al. Risk factors for gastrointestinal bleeding in critically ill patients. Canadian Critical Care Trials Group. N Engl J Med 1994;330:377–81.

36. Krag M, Perner A, Møller MH. Stress ulcer prophylaxis in the intensive care unit. Curr Opin Crit Care 2016;22:186–90.

37. Kress JP, Gehlbach B, Lacy M, et al. The long-term psychological effects of daily sedative interruption on critically ill patients. Am J Respir Crit Care Med 2003;168:1457–61.

38. Shehabi Y, Bellomo R, Reade MC, et al. Early intensive care sedation predicts long-term mortality in ventilated critically ill patients. Am J Respir Crit Care Med 2012;186:724–31.

39. Barr J, Fraser GL, Puntillo K, et al. Clinical practice guidelines for the management of pain, agitation, and delirium in adult patients in the intensive care unit. Crit Care Med 2013;41:263–306.

40. Puthucheary Z, Rawal J, Ratnayake G, et al. Neuromuscular blockade and skeletal muscle weakness in critically ill patients: time to rethink the evidence? Am J Respir Crit Care Med 2012;185:911–7.

41. Papazian L, Forel JM, Gacouin A, et al. Neuromuscular blockers in early acute respiratory distress syndrome. N Engl J Med 2010;363:1107–16.

42. Bellani G, Laffey JG, Pham T, et al. Epidemiology, patterns of care, and mortality for patients with acute respiratory distress syndrome in intensive care units in 50 countries. JAMA 2016;315:788–800.

43. Huang DT, Angus DC, Moss M, et al. Design and rationale of the reevaluation of systemic early neuromuscular blockade trial for acute respiratory distress syndrome. Ann Am Thorac Soc 2017;14:124–33.

44. Stollings JL, Bloom SL, Huggins EL, et al. Medication management to ameliorate post-intensive care syndrome. AACN Adv Crit Care 2016;27:133–40.

45. Bell CM, Brener SS, Gunraj N, et al. Association of ICU or hospital admission with unintentional discontinuation of medications for chronic diseases. JAMA 2011; 306:840–7.

46. Morandi A, Vasilevskis EE, Pandharipande PP, et al. Inappropriate medication prescriptions in elderly adults surviving an intensive care unit hospitalization. J Am Geriatr Soc 2013;61:1128–34.

47. Scales DC, Fischer HD, Li P, et al. Unintentional continuation of medications intended for acute illness after hospital discharge: a population-based cohort study. J Gen Intern Med 2016;31:196–202.

48. Tomichek JE, Stollings JL, Pandharipande PP, et al. Antipsychotic prescribing patterns during and after critical illness: a prospective cohort study. Crit Care 2016;20:378.

49. Jones C, Bäckman C, Capuzzo M, et al. Intensive care diaries reduce new onset post traumatic stress disorder following critical illness: a randomised, controlled trial. Crit Care 2010;14:R168.

50. Jones C, Bäckman C, Griffiths RD. Intensive care diaries and relatives' symptoms of posttraumatic stress disorder after critical illness: a pilot study. Am J Crit Care 2012;21:172–6.

51. ICU-diary.org. Available at: http://www.icu-diary.org/diary/start.html. Accessed April 12, 2017

52. Cuthbertson BH, Rattray J, Campbell MK, et al. The practical study of nurse led, intensive care follow-up programmes for improving long term outcomes from critical illness: a pragmatic randomised controlled trial. BMJ 2009;339:b3723.

53. Schweickert WD, Pohlman MC, Pohlman AS, et al. Early physical and occupational therapy in mechanically ventilated, critically ill patients: a randomised controlled trial. Lancet 2009;373:1874–82.

54. Schaller SJ, Anstey M, Blobner M, et al. Early, goal-directed mobilisation in the surgical intensive care unit: a randomised controlled trial. Lancet 2016;388: 1377–88.

55. Puthucheary Z, Prescott H. Skeletal muscle weakness is associated with both early and late mortality after acute respiratory distress syndrome. Crit Care Med 2017;45:563–5.

56. Puthucheary ZA, Rawal J, McPhail M, et al. Acute skeletal muscle wasting in critical illness. JAMA 2013;310:1591.

57. Moss M, Nordon-Craft A, Malone D, et al. A randomized trial of an intensive physical therapy program for patients with acute respiratory failure. Am J Respir Crit Care Med 2016;193:1101–10.

58. Walsh TS, Salisbury LG, Merriweather JL, et al. Increased hospital-based physical rehabilitation and information provision after intensive care unit discharge: the recover randomized clinical trial. JAMA Intern Med 2015;175:901–10.

59. Connolly B, Salisbury L, O'Neill B, et al. Exercise rehabilitation following intensive care unit discharge for recovery from critical illness. Cochrane Database Syst Rev 2015;(6):CD008632. (ed. Connolly B). (John Wiley & Sons, Ltd).

60. Jackson JC, Ely EW, Morey MC, et al. Cognitive and physical rehabilitation of intensive care unit survivors. Crit Care Med 2012;40:1088–97.

61. Brummel NE, Girard TD, Ely EW, et al. Feasibility and safety of early combined cognitive and physical therapy for critically ill medical and surgical patients: the activity and cognitive therapy in ICU (ACT-ICU) trial. Intensive Care Med 2014;40:370–9.

62. Cameron JI, Chu LM, Matte A, et al. One-year outcomes in caregivers of critically ill patients. N Engl J Med 2016;374:1831–41.

63. Brown SM, Rozenblum R, Aboumatar H, et al. Defining patient and family engagement in the intensive care unit. Am J Respir Crit Care Med 2015;191: 358–60.

64. Davidson JE. Family presence on rounds in neonatal, pediatric, and adult intensive care units. Ann Am Thorac Soc 2013;10:152–6.

65. Chapman DK, Collingridge DS, Mitchell LA, et al. Satisfaction with elimination of all visitation restrictions in a mixed-profile intensive care unit. Am J Crit Care 2016; 25:46–50.

66. Griffiths JA, Barber VS, Cuthbertson BH, et al. A national survey of intensive care follow-up clinics. Anaesthesia 2006;61:950–5.

67. Huggins EL, Bloom SL, Stollings JL, et al. A clinic model: post-intensive care syndrome and post-intensive care syndrome-family. AACN Adv Crit Care 2016;27: 204–11.

68. Chlan LL, Weinert CR, Heiderscheit A, et al. Effects of patient-directed music intervention on anxiety and sedative exposure in critically ill patients receiving mechanical ventilatory support: a randomized clinical trial. JAMA 2013;309: 2335–44.

69. Project Information - NIH Reporter. Efficacy of self-management of sedative therapy by ventilated ICU patients. Available at: https://projectreporter.nih. gov/project_info_description.cfm?aid=9263829&icde=33867669&ddparam=& ddvalue=&ddsub=&cr=1&csb=default&cs=ASC&pball=. Accessed April 13, 2017

70. Jones C, Skirrow P, Griffiths RD, et al. Rehabilitation after critical illness: a randomized, controlled trial. Crit Care Med 2003;31:2456–61.

71. Welcome - ICUsteps. Available at: http://www.icusteps.org/. Accessed April 13, 2017

72. Patients and Families | SCCM | Connect With Patients and Families. Available at: http://www.myicucare.org/Thrive/Pages/Find-In-Person-Support-Groups.aspx. Accessed April 11, 2017

73. Mikkelsen ME, Jackson JC, Hopkins RO, et al. Peer support as a novel strategy to mitigate post-intensive care syndrome. AACN Adv Crit Care 2016;27:221–9.

74. Liu V, Lei X, Prescott CH, et al. Hospital readmission and healthcare utilization following sepsis in community settings. J Hosp Med 2014;9:502–7.

75. Sun A, Netzer G, Small DS, et al. Association between index hospitalization and hospital readmission in sepsis survivors. Crit Care Med 2016;44(3):478–87.

76. Donnelly JP, Hohmann SF, Wang HE. Unplanned readmissions after hospitalization for severe sepsis at academic medical center-affiliated hospitals. Crit Care Med 2015. http://dx.doi.org/10.1097/CCM.0000000000001147.

77. Prescott HC. Toward a nuanced understanding of the role of infection in readmissions after sepsis. Crit Care Med 2016;44:634–5.

78. Boomer JS, To K, Chang KC, et al. Immunosuppression in patients who die of sepsis and multiple organ failure. JAMA 2011;306:2594–605.

79. Hotchkiss RS, Monneret G, Payen D. Immunosuppression in sepsis: a novel understanding of the disorder and a new therapeutic approach. Lancet Infect Dis 2013;13:260–8.
80. Zaborin A, Smith D, Garfield K, et al. Membership and behavior of ultra-low-diversity pathogen communities present in the gut of humans during prolonged critical illness. mBio 2014;5:e01361–414.
81. Heyland DK, Stelfox HT, Garland A, et al. Predicting performance status 1 year after critical illness in patients 80 years or older. Crit Care Med 2016;44:1718–26.
82. Brummel NE, Jackson JC, Pandharipande PP, et al. Delirium in the ICU and subsequent long-term disability among survivors of mechanical ventilation*. Crit Care Med 2014;42:369–77.
83. Ferrante LE, Pisani MA, Murphy TE, et al. Factors associated with functional recovery among older intensive care unit survivors. Am J Respir Crit Care Med 2016;194:299–307.
84. Brummel NE, Bell SP, Girard TD, et al. Frailty and subsequent disability and mortality among patients with critical illness. Am J Respir Crit Care Med 2016. http://dx.doi.org/10.1164/rccm.201605-0939OC.
85. Ferrante LE, Pisani MA, Murphy TE, et al. Functional trajectories among older persons before and after critical illness. JAMA Intern Med 2015;175:523–9.
86. Stein-Parbury J, McKinley S. Patients' experiences of being in an intensive care unit: a select literature review. Am J Crit Care 2000;9:20–7.
87. Strom T, Martinussen T, Toft P. A protocol of no sedation for critically ill patients receiving mechanical ventilation: a randomised trial. Lancet 2010;375:475–80.
88. Riker RR, Shehabi Y, Bokesch PM, et al. Dexmedetomidine vs midazolam for sedation of critically ill patients: a randomized trial. JAMA 2009;301:489–99.
89. Reade MC, Finfer S. Sedation and delirium in the intensive care unit. N Engl J Med 2014;370:444–54.
90. Ely EW, Shintani A, Truman B, et al. Delirium as a predictor of mortality in mechanically ventilated patients in the intensive care unit. JAMA 2004;291:1753.
91. van Eijk MMJ, van Marum RJ, Klijn IA, et al. Comparison of delirium assessment tools in a mixed intensive care unit. Crit Care Med 2009;37:1881–5.

Moving?

Make sure your subscription moves with you!

To notify us of your new address, find your **Clinics Account Number** (located on your mailing label above your name), and contact customer service at:

Email: journalscustomerservice-usa@elsevier.com

800-654-2452 (subscribers in the U.S. & Canada)
314-447-8871 (subscribers outside of the U.S. & Canada)

Fax number: 314-447-8029

Elsevier Health Sciences Division
Subscription Customer Service
3251 Riverport Lane
Maryland Heights, MO 63043

*To ensure uninterrupted delivery of your subscription, please notify us at least 4 weeks in advance of move.